D0141763

NOT TO LEAVE
ROESCH LIBRARY
UNIVERSITY OF DAYTON

KIRBY'S GUIDE TO FITNESS AND MOTOR PERFORMANCE TESTS

NOT TO LEAVE
ROESCH LIBRARY
UNIVERSITY OF DAYTON

UNIVERSITY
UNIVERSITY OF BATH

KIRBY'S GUIDE TO FITNESS AND
MOTOR PERFORMANCE TESTS

Edited by

Ronald F. Kirby, Ed.D.
Southeast Missouri State University

NOT TO LEAVE
ROESCH LIBRARY
UNIVERSITY OF DAYTON

DISCARDED
FROM
UNIVERSITY OF DAYTON
ROESCH LIBRARY

BenOak Publishing Company
Cape Girardeau, Missouri 63702-0474
1991

BenOak Publishing Company
P.O. Box 474
Cape Girardeau, MO 63702-0474
United States of America
(314) 334-8789

ISBN 0-962-90983-1

Library of Congress Catalog Card Number: 91-70120

Production supervisor and design:
Priscilla Michaels

Illustrations by:
Frank Ozaki

Copyright © 1991 by BenOak Publishing Company. All rights reserved. No part of this book may be reproduced in any manner or by any means without permission in writing from the Publisher.

Printed in the United States of America.

REFERENCE

QP
201
55
1991

94 09284

To my parents

Alvena and Darrell Kirby

94 09284

PREFACE

The purpose of this measurement book is to provide students, teachers and researchers with a reference tool they may use to enhance their productivity. Secondarily, it is hoped that the publication of this book will stimulate the development of better fitness and motor performance tests as well as encourage future test constructors to provide more detailed information about the tests which they develop.

The book is unique in that it fills a void in exercise science, kinesiology, physical education and sport science for a reference tool which gives comprehensive information regarding the tests of components of fitness and motor performance. The eleven fitness and motor performance components given coverage are: agility, balance, cardiorespiratory endurance, coordination, flexibility, kinesthesis, muscular endurance, power, reaction time, speed and strength. This book presents both a description of 193 tests and a review of each test written by 124 different measurement experts from Canada and the United States. Included in the description of each test are the following topics: reference(s), additional sources, purpose, objectivity, reliability, validity, age and sex, equipment, space requirements and design, directions, scoring and norms.

This book not only addresses the problem of helping students and professionals locate the available tests for measuring a specific component, but most importantly, the specially prepared reviews provide an authoritative means to help them select the mostappropriate test for their specific situation. The reviewers address both the scientific and practical aspects of the tests. In addition, the reviewers present the strengths and weaknesses of the tests, suggestions on how they can be best administered and safety precautions which one should be aware of before administering such tests.

It is my pleasure to extend thanks to the 124 reviewers who contributed so significantly to the production of this book. Without their contributions, it would not have become a reality. Special thanks is also extended to Michele Sweitzer, who typed the manuscript and handled the tremendous volume of correspondence associated with this project.

Ronald F. Kirby

CONTENTS

Chapter 1

INTRODUCTION

PURPOSE AND SCOPE OF THE BOOK

The purpose of this measurement book is to provide a reference tool which students, teachers and researchers may use to enhance their productivity. This reference is designed to be comprehensive by providing descriptions and reviews of 193 fitness and motor performance tests. Single item fitness and motor performance tests, as differentiated from test batteries, are included. Tests which require equipment, with the exception of weight training machines, costing more than approximately $1000 are not included. Since this reference is unique to the disciplines of exercise science, kinesiology, physical education, and sport science, the editor included as many tests as possible. In the attempt to be comprehensive and because most fitness and motor performance tests had never been reviewed, some dated and weaker tests have been included. A number of tests which obviously no longer applied to the modern day situation were, however, omitted.

Finally, although every effort was made to be comprehensive, the editor presumes that some tests were simply overlooked. It is hoped that the tests which were inadvertently omitted will be brought to the editor's attention so they may be included in future editions of this reference. Test constructors are encouraged to submit their tests to the editor to ensure their inclusion in future editions.

REVIEWERS OF THE TESTS

The reviewers of the tests were volunteers recruited with a letter of solicitation mailed to Measurement Council members of the American Alliance for Health, Physical Education, Recreation and Dance. The 124 reviewers who participated in this project are listed below. The test(s) that each reviewer evaluated is listed after the reviewer's name and address.

MATT ADAMS
Undergraduate Student
Department of Physical Education
Frostburg State University
Frostburg, MD 21532
BASKETBALL FOUL SHOT TEST

THOMAS M. ADAMS, II, Ed.D.
Professor of Physical Education
Arkansas State University
Jonesboro, AR 72401
FLEISHMAN SHUTTLE RUN TEST
JUMP WITH WEIGHTS TEST

BARBARA E. AINSWORTH, Ph.D.
Assistant Professor of Physical Education, Exercise and Sport Science
University of North Carolina
Chapel Hill, NC 27599-8700
REPEATED 220 YARD SPRINT TEST
SHARKEY STEP TEST

STEVEN J. ALBRECHTSEN, Ph.D.
Director, Human Performance Laboratory
University of Wisconsin-Whitewater
Whitewater, WI 53190
PULL UP TEST
YMCA PHYSICAL WORKING CAPACITY TEST

SYNE ALTENA, Ed.D.
Professor of Physical Education
Dordt College
Sioux Center, IA 51250
OHIO STATE UNIVERSITY STEP TEST (CALLAN MODIFICATION)
SQUAT JUMPS TEST

EUGENE R. ANDERSON, Ph.D.
Associate Professor of Health, Physical Education and Recreation
University of Mississippi
University, MS 38677
ONE FOOT BALANCE TEST
300 YARD SHUTTLE RUN TEST

PAUL A. ANDERSON, Ph.D.
Assistant Professor of Physical Therapy
University of Maryland
Baltimore, MD 21201
ANKLE EXTENSION TEST
SIDEWARD LEAP TEST

CHARLES J. ANSORGE, Ph.D.
Professor of Physical Education
University of Nebraska - Lincoln
Lincoln, NE 68588-0229
CLARKE CABLE TENSION
STRENGTH TESTS

CHARLES W. ASH, Ph.D.
Associate Professor of Physical Education
State University of New York at Cortland
Cortland, NY 13045
MONTANA BICYCLE TEST
SIT UP TEST

THOMAS E. BALL, Ph.D.
Assistant Professor of Physical Education
Northern Illinois University
DeKalb, IL 60115
BENCH PRESS TEST
MEDICINE BALL PUT (SITTING
ON FLOOR) TEST

DEBRA A. BALLINGER, Ph.D.
Assistant Professor of Health, Physical
Education and Recreation
Old Dominion University
Norfolk, VA 23529-0196
STATIC PUSH UP (HOLD HALF
PUSH UP) TEST
WRIST FLEXIBILITY TEST

LINDA R. BARLEY, Ed.D.
Professor of Health and Physical Education
York College - CUNY
Jamaica, NY 11451
ALTERNATE HAND WALL TOSS TEST
ARM RAISING SIDEWARD 90
DEGREES TEST

HARRY BEAMON, Ed.D.
Professor of Health, Physical Education, and
Recreation
Tennessee State University
Nashville, TN 27209-1561
TIMED BENCH PRESS TEST

BARRY BEEDLE, Ed.D.
Associate Professor of Health, Physical
Education and Leisure
Elon College
Elon College, NC 27244-2177
PULL UP WITH WEIGHTS TEST
SPIDER SPRINT TEST

DAVID E. BELKA, Ph.D.
Associate Professor of Physical Education
Miami University
Oxford, OH 45056
BALL THROW TEST
FOOTBALL 20 YARD SHUTTLE TEST

PHILLIP BISHOP, Ed.D.
Associate Professor of Health and Physical
Education
University of Alabama
Tuscaloosa, AL 35487
BENCH JUMPS TEST
LEIGHTON FLEXOMETER TEST

CYNTHIA B. BOOK, Ph.D.
Field Research Manager
American Guidance Service
Circle Pines, MN 55014-1796
BRIDGE UP TEST

LOUIS BOWERS, Ph.D.
Professor of Physical Education
University of South Florida
Tampa, FL 33620
LEG RAISING TEST

JANELLE BRAATZ, M.S.
Assistant Professor of Physical Education
Black Hills State University
Spearfish, SD 57999
FRONT TO REAR SPLITS TEST

ELAINE BUDDE, Ph.D.
Professor of Physical Education
Roanoke College
Salem, VA 24153
GRASS DRILL TEST
PRONATION AND SUPINATION TEST

E. R. BUSKIRK, Ph.D.
Professor of Applied Physiology
The Pennsylvania State University
University Park, PA 16802
MODIFIED PUSH UP TEST
NARSS MODIFIED HARVARD STEP TEST

KIM CARTER
Undergraduate Student
Department of Physical Education
Frostburg State University
Frostburg, MD 21532
BASKETBALL FOUL SHOT TEST

DONALD R. CASADY, Ph.D.
Professor of Exercise Science
University of Iowa
Iowa City, IA 52241
CALF RAISE TEST
STANDING VERTICAL ARM PRESS TEST

SAMUEL CASE, Ph.D.
Professor of Physical Education
Western Maryland College
Westminster, MD 21157
KASCH PULSE RECOVERY TEST
MEDICINE BALL PUT (SITTING IN CHAIR) TEST

CRAIG J. CISAR, Ph.D.
Associate Professor of Human Performance
San Jose State University
San Jose, CA 95192-0054
OHIO STATE UNIVERSITY STEP TEST
VERTICAL ARM PULL TEST (DISTANCE)

WILLIAM F. CLIPSON, Ed.D.
Emeritus Professor of Physical Education
University of Alabama
Tuscaloosa, AL 35486
FORWARD BEND OF TRUNK TEST
MEDICINE BALL PUT (STANDING) TEST

DOYICE J. COTTEN, Ed.D.
Professor of Physical Education
Georgia Southern University
Statesboro, GA 30460
SQUAT THRUST OR BURPEE TEST
VERTICAL POWER JUMP (WORK) TEST

N. KAY COVINGTON, Ph.D.
Assistant Professor of Health, Recreation and Physical Education
Southern Illinois University at Edwardsville
Edwardsville, IL 62026-1126
SIT UP WITH WEIGHTS TEST

PHYLLIS T. CROISANT, Ph.D.
Associate Professor of Physical Education
Eastern Illinois University
Charleston, IL 61920
CARLSON FATIGUE CURVE TEST
SHOULDER AND WRIST ELEVATION TEST

DAVID E. CUNDIFF, Ph.D.
Professor of Health and Physical Education
Campbellsville College
Campbellsville, KY 42718
SUBMAXIMAL WALK TEST

JOHN DAGGER, Ph.D.
Assistant Professor of Physical Education
University of Illinois
Chicago, IL 60680
ALTERNATE LEG JUMP FOR DISTANCE TEST
HEXAGON RAIL WALKING (FLEISHMAN'S) TEST

JACQUELINE A. DAILEY, Ed.D.
Health, Physical Education and Recreation
Program Coordinator
University of Wisconsin-Whitewater
Whitewater, WI 53190
KNEE FLEXION TEST
STORK STAND TEST

MARY L. DAWSON, Ph.D.
Associate Professor of Health, Physical Education and Recreation
Western Michigan University
Kalamazoo, MI 49008
MODIFIED BASS DYNAMIC BALANCE TEST

JAMES DECKER, Ph.D.
Assistant Professor of Health, Physical Education, Recreation and Safety
East Carolina University
Greenville, NC 27858-4353
CORBIN BALL HANDLING TEST
EUROFIT BICYCLE ERGOMETER TEST (PWC170)

J. JESSE DEMELLO, Ed.D.
Associate Professor of Health and Physical
Education
Louisiana State University in Shreveport
Shreveport, LA 71115
DISTANCE RUN/WALK TESTS
PHOSPHATE RECOVERY TEST

DALE E. DEVOE, Ph.D.
Associate Professor of Exercise and
Sport Science
Colorado State University
Fort Collins, CO 80523
PROGRESSIVE INVERTED
BALANCE TEST
SHOULDER ROTATION TEST

LINUS J. DOWELL, Ed.D.
Chair, Graduate Programs
Department of Health and Physical Education
Texas A & M University
College Station, TX 77843
AUTO TIRE TEST
MARGARIA ANAEROBIC POWER TEST

MICHAEL J. DURNIN, M.A.
Instructor of Physical Education
University of Puget Sound
Tacoma, WA 94816
FOOTBALL 60 YARD SHUTTLE TEST

BLANCHE W. EVANS, Ed.D.
Exercise Physiologist
Indiana State University
Terre Haute, IN 47809
MODIFIED PULL UP (NCYFSII) TEST
SICONOFI STEP TEST

HAROLD B. FALLS, Ph.D.
Professor of Biomedical Sciences
Southwest Missouri State University
Springfield, MO 65804
UNIVERSITY OF MONTREAL TRACK
TEST (UM-TT)

R. A. FAULKNER, Ph.D.
Associate Professor of Physical Education
University of Saskatchewan
Saskatoon, Canada S7N 0W0
TRUNK AND NECK EXTENSION TEST

CONNIE FOX, Ed.D.
Assistant Professor of Physical Education
Northern Illinois University
DeKalb, IL 60115
AAHPER SHUTTLE RUN (POTATO
RACE) TEST
SHOULDER FLEXIBILITY TEST

B. DON FRANKS, Ph.D.
Professor of Kinesiology
Louisiana State University
Baton Rouge, LA 70803
KRAUS WEBER FLOOR TOUCH TEST
PWC170 PHYSICAL WORKING
CAPACITY TEST

SCOTT E. FRAZIER, P.E.D.
Assistant Professor of Physical Education
University of Wisconsin-Stevens Point
Stevens Point, WI 54481
12 MINUTE CYCLING TEST

BARRY A. FRISHBERG, Ph.D.
Associate Professor of Health and Physical
Education
South Carolina State University
Orangeburg, SC 29117
GONIOMETER TEST

JAMES B. GALE, Ph.D.
Professor of Physical Education and Health
Sciences
Sonoma State University
Rohnert Park, CA 94928
LSU STEP TEST
ONE REPETITION MAXIMUM (1-RM)
LEG STRENGTH TESTS

DOUGLAS J. GOAR, Ph.D.
Chair and Associate Professor of Health,
Physical Education and Recreation
Kentucky State University
Frankfort, KY 40601
DIPS TEST
ILLINOIS AGILITY RUN TEST

SCOTT GOING, Ph.D.
Assistant Research Scientist,
Exercise and Sport Sciences
University of Arizona
Tucson, AZ 85721
PRESS TEST

M. GOLDMAN, Ph.D.
Professor of Physical Education
University of Massachusetts-Boston Harbor Campus
Boston, MA 02125
DISTANCE PERCEPTION JUMP TEST
SCOTT OBSTACLE RACE TEST

JOYCE GRAENING, D.A.
Assistant Professor of Physical Education
University of Arkansas
Fayetteville, AR 72701
LATHAM YARDSTICK REACTION TIME TEST
MODIFIED SIT AND REACH TEST

JOHN B. GRATTON, Ed.D.
Chair, Division of Kinesiology and Health Science
Bee County College
Beeville, TX 78102
ISOMETRIC LEG SQUAT (WALL SIT) TEST

JAMES E. GRAVES, Ph.D.
Assistant Research Scientist, College of Medicine
University of Florida
Gainesville, FL 32610
BENCH SQUAT TEST
20M SHUTTLE RUN TEST

JOSEPH J. GRUBER, Ph.D.
Professor of Physical Education
University of Kentucky
Lexington, KY 40506-0219
MARGARIA-KALAMEN ANAEROBIC POWER TEST
QUEENS COLLEGE STEP TEST

DON HARDIN, Ph.D.
Professor of Kinesiology
University of Texas at El Paso
El Paso, TX 79968
BACK LIFT OR WING LIFT TEST
SPEED HOP TEST

JOHN L. HAUBENSTRICKER, Ph.D.
Professor of Physical Education
Michigan State University
East Lansing, MI 48824
EDGREN AND MODIFIED SIDE STEP TESTS

JOY L. HENDRICK, Ph.D.
Assistant Professor of Physical Education
State University College at Cortland
Cortland, NY 13045
TWO WAY ALTERNATE RESPONSE TEST

RONALD K. HETZLER, Ph.D.
Assistant Professor of Health, Physical Education and Recreation
University of Hawaii at Manoa
Honolulu, HI 96822
DASH FOR A SPECIFIED DISTANCE TEST
HIP FLEXOR TEST

DAVID R. HOPKINS, P.E.D.
Associate Professor of Physical Education
Indiana State University
Terre Haute, IN 47809
FLEISHMAN DYNAMIC FLEXIBILITY TEST

LARRY D. ISAACS, Ph.D.
Professor of Health, Physical Education and Recreation
Human Performance Laboratory
College of Education and Human Services
Wright State University
Dayton, OH 45435
CARDIOVASCULAR EFFICIENCY FOR GIRLS AND WOMEN (SKUBIC & HODGKINS) TEST
GRIP TO DESIGNATED AMOUNT TEST

JIMMY H. ISHEE, Ph.D.
Associate Professor of Physical Education
University of Central Arkansas
Conway, AR 72032
BALANCE STABILIZATION TEST
SHOULDER FLEXIBILITY FACTOR TEST

LEIGH F. KIEFFER, Ph.D.
Professor of Physical Therapy and Exercise Science
S.U.N.Y. at Buffalo
Buffalo, NY 14214
STANDING LONG (BROAD) JUMP TEST

THOMAS J. KILROY, M.Ed.
Assistant Professor of Physical Education
Paul Smiths College
Paul Smiths, NY 12970
DIP STRENGTH TEST

JAMES KLINZING, Ph.D.
Associate Professor of Health, Physical
Education and Recreation
Cleveland State University
Cleveland, OH 44115
CANADIAN HOME FITNESS TEST
SPEED CURVE TEST

ROBERT KOSLOW, P.E.D.
Chair and Professor of Physical Education and
Sport
James Madison University
Harrisonburg, VA 22807
SIT AND REACH TEST

BILL KOZAR, Ph.D.
Associate Professor of Physical Education
Boise State University
Boise, ID 83725
PUSH-PULL TO DESIGNATED
AMOUNT TEST
SHUTTLE RUN TEST

LARRY M. LANDIS, Ph.D.
Professor of Social Science
Black Hills State University
Spearfish, SD 57999
FRONT TO REAR SPLITS TEST
KINESTHETIC OBSTACLE TEST

CHARLES M. LAY, Ph.D.
Associate Professor of Physical Education
Mississippi State University
Mississippi State, MS 39762
DODGING RUN TEST

BRENDA LICHTMAN, Ph.D.
Associate Professor of Health and Kinesiology
Sam Houston State University
Huntsville, TX 77341
REACTIVE AGILITY TEST
SHOULDER FLEXIBILITY-HORIZON-
TAL ABDUCTION TEST

RICHARD LITWHILER, Ed.D.
Associate Professor of Physical Education
Georgia Southwestern College
Americus, GA 31709
COZENS' DODGING RUN TEST
MARGARIA-CHALOUPKA ANAEROBIC
POWER TEST

BEN R. LONDEREE, Ed.D.
Associate Professor of Health and Physical
Education
University of Missouri-Columbia
Columbia, MO 65211
COTTEN GROUP CARDIOVASCULAR
STEP TEST (MODIFIED OHIO STATE
STEP TEST)
ONE REPETITION MAXIMUM (1-RM)
UPPER BODY STRENGTH TESTS

RUSSELL H. LORD, Ed.D.
Professor and Chair, Educational Foundations
and Counseling
Eastern Montana College
Billings, MT 59101-0298
THE SPEED TEST
3 MILE WALKING TEST (NO RUNNING)

HERBERTA M. LUNDEGREN, Ph.D.
Professor of Physical Education and Leisure
Studies
The Pennsylvania State University
University Park, PA 16802
BASS STICK TESTS

PRISCILLA MACRAE, Ph.D.
Associate Professor of Sports Medicine
Pepperdine University
Malibu, CA 90263
NELSON FOOT REACTION TEST

MATTHEW T. MAHAR, Ed.D.
Assistant Professor of Physical Education
Springfield College
Springfield, MA 01109
ENDURANCE SHUTTLE RUN TEST

MICHAEL MANGUM, Ph.D.
Assistant Professor of Physical Education and
Leisure Management
Columbus College
Columbus, GA 31993
HANGING HALF-LEVER TEST
12 MINUTE SWIMMING TEST

JAMES M. MANNING, Ph.D.
Associate Professor of Movement Science and
Leisure Studies
The William Paterson College at New Jersey
Wayne, NJ 07470
WINGATE ANAEROBIC TEST
YMCA LEG EXTENSION
STRENGTH TEST

SHERRY L. FOLSOM-MEEK, Ph.D.
Assistant Professor of Physical Education
University of Missouri
Columbia, MO 65211
FLAMINGO BALANCE TEST
SHUFFLEBOARD DISTANCE
PERCEPTION TEST

MARK J. MEKA, M.S.
Assistant Professor of Health and Physical
Education
Lake Tahoe Community College
South Lake Tahoe, CA 95702
ARM HANG OR FLEXED ARM
HANG TEST
BALANCE BEAM WALK TEST

KATHLEEN MILLER, Ph.D.
Professor of Health and Physical Education
Associate Dean, School of Education
University of Montana
Missoula, MT 59812
FLEISHMAN EXTENT FLEXIBILITY TEST
YMCA BENCH PRESS TEST

PERRY F. MILLER, Ed.D.
Professor of Health and Physical Education
Southwest Missouri State University
Springfield, MO 65804
LOOP-THE-LOOP RUN TEST
NELSON BALANCE TEST

DUANE MILLSLAGLE, Ed.D.
Associate Professor of Physical Education
Northern State University
Aberdeen, SD 57401
DASH FOR A SPECIFIED TIME TEST

SUSAN M. MOEN, Ph.D.
Assistant Professor of Physical Education
Dallas Baptist University
Dallas, TX 75211
FAIRBANKS SUBMAXIMAL TEST

JAMES R. MORROW, JR., Ph.D.
Professor of Health and Human Performance
University of Houston
Houston, TX 77204-5331
HARVARD STEP TEST
MARGARIA-DEVRIES ANAEROBIC
POWER TEST

RICHARD MUNROE, Ed.D.
Associate Professor of Exercise and Sport
Sciences
University of Arizona
Tucson, AZ 85721
ARM PULL (HORIZONTAL) TEST
VERTICAL JUMP TEST

CHERYL NORTON, Ed.D.
Associate Professor of Human Performance
Metropolitan State College
Denver, CO 80204
ANKLE FLEXION (STANDING) TEST
GALLAGHER & BROUHA TEST FOR
HIGH SCHOOL GIRLS (MODIFICATION
OF HARVARD STEP TEST)

REGINALD T-A. OCANSEY, Ph.D.
Assistant Professor of Physical Education
State University of New York,
College at Brockport
Brockport, NY 14420
LINE WALK TEST
30 SECONDS ROPE JUMPING TEST

LYNN B. PANTON, M.S.
Department of Exercise and Sport Sciences
University of Florida
Gainesville, FL 32610
20M SHUTTLE RUN TEST

DALE G. PEASE, Ph.D.
Associate Professor and Chair, Health and
Human Performance
University of Houston
Houston, TX 77204-5331
NELSON CHOICE RESPONSE
MOVEMENT TEST

MARY L. PUTMAN, Ph.D.
Assistant Professor of Health and Physical
Education
Glassboro State College
Glassboro, NJ 08028
DYNAMIC POSITIONAL BALANCE TEST
RIGHT BOOMERANG RUN TEST

LORRAINE REDDERSON, Ed.D.
Professor of Physical Education
Lander College
Greenwood, SC 29646
LSU AGILITY OBSTACLE COURSE TEST
SIDE SPLITS TEST

T. GILMOUR REEVE, Ph.D.
Professor of Health and Human Performance
Auburn University
Auburn, AL 36849-5323
FOUR-WAY ALTERNATE
RESPONSE TEST
WALKING A STRAIGHT LINE WITH
TURNS TEST

RAY R. REIDER, M.Ed.
Assistant Professor of Health and Physical
Education
Gettysburg College
Gettysburg, PA 17325
CABLE JUMP TEST

JAMES A. RICHARDSON, Ed.D.
Assistant Professor of Exercise Science and
Wellness
The University of South Dakota
Vermillion, SD 57069
F-EMU STEP TEST (MODIFIED OHIO
STATE STEP TEST)
MODIFIED PULL UP TEST

JOANNE ROWE, Ph.D.
Assistant Professor of Physical Education
University of Louisville
Louisville, KY 40292
ANKLE FLEXION AND EXTENSION TEST
SQUAT STAND (TIP UP) TEST

JEFFREY C. RUPP, Ph.D.
Associate Professor of Health, Physical
Education, Recreation and Dance
Georgia State University
Atlanta, GA 30303
PUSH UP TEST

MARGARET J. SAFRIT, Ph.D.
Henry-Bascom Professor
University of Wisconsin-Madison
Madison, WI 53706
THREE MINUTE HEIGHT-ADJUSTED
STEP TEST

MYRNA M. SCHILD, Ed.S.
Assistant Professor of Physical Education
Southern Illinois University
Edwardsville, IL 62026
PARTIAL CURL UP TEST

ELIZABETH J. SCHUMAKER, D.P.E.
Associate Professor of Physical Education
Stetson University
DeLand, FL 32720
CANADIAN AEROBIC FITNESS TEST
QUADRANT JUMP TEST

JANET A. SEAMAN, P.E.D.
Professor of Physical Education
California State University
Los Angeles, CA 90032
BARROW (TEXAS) ZIGZAG RUN TEST
STICK BALANCE TEST

TERESA SHARP, M.Ed.
Research Assistant in Clinical Nutrition
Vanderbilt University Medical Center
Nashville, TN 37232-8285
MODIFIED PULL UP TEST
(BAUMGARTNER)
ROCKPORT WALK TEST

SHARON SHIELDS, Ph.D.
Associate Professor of Teaching and Learning
Peabody College of Vanderbilt University
Nashville, TN 37232-8285
MODIFIED PULL UP TEST
(BAUMGARTNER)
ROCKPORT WALK TEST

EDGAR W. SHIELDS, JR., Ph.D.
Associate Professor of Physical Education,
Exercise and Sport Science
University of North Carolina
Chapel Hill, NC 27599-8605
PUSH AND PULL STRENGTH TESTS
UNDERHAND, BACKWARD SHOT
THROW TEST

BETHANY SHIFFLETT, Ph.D.
Associate Professor of Human Performance
San Jose State University
San Jose, CA 95192-0054
TWO-HAND PUSH TEST

FRANK SMITH, Ph.D.
Dean, School of Education
St. Edward's University
Austin, TX 78704
HIP ADDUCTOR FLEXIBILITY TEST
STATIC VISUALIZATION TEST

WILLIE S. SMITH, Ed.D.
Associate Professor of Physical Education
North Carolina Central University
Durham, NC 27707
BOARD BALANCE TEST
TEXAS SHUTTLE RUN FOR
DISTANCE TEST

WILLIAM R. SPIETH, Ph.D.
Professor of Physical Education
Georgia Southern College
Statesboro, GA 30460
NELSON HAND REACTION TEST

ROBERT E. STADULIS, Ed.D.
Associate Professor of Physical Education
Kent State University
Kent, OH 44242
NELSON SPEED OF MOVEMENT TEST

JIM L. STILLWELL, P.E.D.
Chair, Human Performance Studies
The University of Alabama
Tuscaloosa, AL 35487
SUICIDE DRILL TEST
TRUNK PULL TEST

NANCY STUBBS, Ed.D.
Assistant Professor of Physical Education
Wichita State University
Wichita, KS 67208
CHIN UP (SUPINATED GRIP) TEST

FREDERICK C. SURGENT, Ed.D.
Professor of Physical Education
Frostburg State University
Frostburg, MD 21532
BASKETBALL FOUL SHOT TEST

JOSEY H. TEMPLETON, Ph.D.
Assistant Professor of Health and
Physical Education
The Citadel
Charleston, SC 29409
LEG LIFTS TEST
SEMO AGILITY TEST

DONNA J. TERBIZAN, Ph.D.
Assistant Professor of Health, Physical
Education and Recreation
North Dakota State University
Fargo, ND 58105
KENT STATE UNIVERSITY STEP TEST
THOMSON ANAEROBIC CAPACITY TEST

NOLAN A. THAXTON, D.P.E.
Professor of Physical Education
Medgar Evers College of
The City University of New York
Brooklyn, NY 11225
LEWIS NOMOGRAM TEST

WALTER R. THOMPSON, Ph.D.
Director, Laboratory of Applied Physiology
School of Human Performance and Recreation
The University of Southern Mississippi
Hattiesburg, MS 39406-5142
MANAHAN-GUTIN ONE-MINUTE
STEP TEST
STATIC GRIP ENDURANCE TEST

LARRY W. TITLOW, Ph.D.
Professor of Physical Education
University of Central Arkansas
Conway, AR 72032
ABSOLUTE ENDURANCE OF UPPER
BODY TEST
ASTRAND-RYHMING TEST

RICHARD TRIMMER, Ph.D.
Professor of Physical Education
Chico State University
Chico, CA 95929
HEXAGON OBSTACLE TEST

KATHLEEN TRITSCHLER, Ed.D.
Assistant Professor of Sport Studies
Guilford College
Greensboro, NC 27410
HAND GRIP STRENGTH TEST
HIP ADDUCTOR STRETCH TEST

MARY LOU VEAL, Ed.D.
Assistant Professor of Exercise and
Sport Science
University of North Carolina
Greensboro, NC 27412-5001
AGILITY-COORDINATION (AGCO) TEST
HAWAII BALANCE ON ONE FOOT TEST

FRANK M. VERDUCCI, Ed.D.
Professor of Physical Education
San Francisco State University
San Francisco, CA 94132
BOSCO'S MECHANICAL POWER
JUMP TEST

PAUL G. VOGEL, Ph.D.
Associate Professor of Physical Education
Michigan State University
East Lansing, MI 48824
GALLAGHER & BROUHA TEST FOR
HIGH SCHOOL BOYS (MODIFICATION
OF HARVARD STEP TEST)

DOUGLAS L. WEEKS, Ph.D.
Assistant Professor of Exercise Science
Ball State University
Muncie, IN 47306
SHOT PUT TEST

JEANNE WENOS, P.E.D.
Assistant Professor of Physical Education
Western Washington University
Bellingham, WA 98225
BASS DYNAMIC BALANCE TEST

SUE W. WHITE, M.Ed.
Assistant Professor of Physical Education
Black Hills State University
Spearfish, SD 57999
FRONT TO REAR SPLITS TEST
KINESTHETIC OBSTACLE TEST

DARLENE YEE, Ed.D.
Associate Professor of Health Education
San Francisco State University
San Francisco, CA 94132
YMCA 3 MINUTE STEP TEST

THE REVIEW PROCESS

The reviews were written and submitted over a one year period initiated in October, 1989. The reviews were written according to the following guidelines.

General Suggestions for Reviews

*Adapted from *The Ninth Mental Measurements Yearbook* (1985). Mitchell, J. V. (ed.). University of Nebraska-Lincoln, Lincoln, NE: Buros Institute of Mental Measurements, pp xvi-xvii.

1. The reviews were to be written with the following major objectives in mind:

A. To provide test users with carefully prepared evaluations of motor performance tests for their guidance in selecting and using the tests.

B. To stimulate progress toward better constructed tests by commending good work, by censuring poor work and by suggesting improvements.

C. To encourage test constructors to present more detailed information on the construction, objectivity, reliability, validity and potential applications and misapplications of their tests.

2. Each review was to begin on a new piece of paper with the name of the test typed in **bold** or CAPITAL LETTERS as a center heading at the top of the page. Just below the name of the test, reviewers were to type their name, degree, title, position, and address (e.g., Joe E. Exercise, Ph.D., Professor of Physical Education, Southeast Missouri State University, Cape Girardeau, Missouri 63701).

3. The reviews were to be openly critical and written in a scholarly and unbiased manner. Consideration was to be given to each question listed below under the heading "Specific Aspects of Physical Tests for Reviews."

4. The reviews were to be written in concise paragraph form. Each review was to be concluded with a summary containing lists of the strengths and weaknesses of the test and a general recommendation of the test.

5. The reviews were to be clearly written with both students and professionals in mind.

6. The reviews were to present a clear idea of the test's relative importance and value compared to similar tests.

7. Information presented in the description of the test was not to be repeated in the review. The description of the test sent to the reviewer was the same description which appears in this book just above each review. Reviewers were requested to pencil in changes they felt were needed in the test descriptions.

8. The reviews were to be typed double space. The maximum length of the review was not to exceed three pages.

9. Three copies of the final review were to be prepared with two copies to be submitted to the editor and one copy to be retained by the reviewer.

10. The reviews were to be edited, but no major changes were to be made without the consent of the reviewer.

11. The editor reserved the right to reject any review which did not meet the above standards.

Specific Aspects Of Physical Tests For Reviews

1. Scientific Aspects

A. Did the test measure the physical component as commonly defined in the literature (i.e., was the test valid)?

B. Did the test measure the physical component consistently (i.e., was the test reliable)?

C. Did the test measure consistently when given by different testers (i.e., was the test objective)?

D. Did the test require the active participation of another person who could have affected the performance of the examinee?

2. Practical Aspects

A. Were the facility and/or space requirements likely to cause a problem(s)?

B. Was the equipment requirement likely to cause a problem(s)?

C. Was the test easy to administer or were the leadership and expertise requirements too great? The reviewer was also to consider the number of people required to administer the test.

D. Did the test require an excessive amount of time to administer?

E. Were an adequate number of trials recommended?

F. Was the test suitable to be used as a drill to promote learning and/or conditioning?

G. Was the test suitable for the intended age and/or ability level(s)? Did the test discriminate among its intended users?

H. Did the test have any dangerous aspects to it? If yes, what were they?

I. Was the scoring objective? For example, could people have easily scored themselves and used the test for self evaluation?

J. Was the test of suitable precision for research purposes?

K. Were norms available for the test? Age groups? Sex? Up to date?

3. Summary

A. Major strengths of the test were to be listed in brief statements and numbered 1, 2, 3, etc.

B. Major weaknesses of the test were to be listed in brief statements and numbered 1, 2, 3, etc.

C. Overall recommendation was to be written in paragraph form:

1. Excellent test - was completely acceptable for research and/or teaching for the following reasons.

2. Acceptable test - was adequate for research and/or teaching with the following cautions and/or qualifications.

3. Unacceptable test - was inadequate for research and/or teaching for the following reasons.

THE TEST DESCRIPTIONS

The test descriptions were prepared by the editor. Although it was the editor's objective to be as comprehensive as possible in terms of the number of tests included, in some cases it was deemed unnecessary to reproduce the tests in their entirety. This approach was followed primarily because complete descriptions are provided in the original sources and secondarily because of space limitations imposed on this work. The reader is encouraged to locate and use the original references of the tests he/she has selected for potential use.

In preparation of the tests' descriptions, the editor attempted to present information on each of the following major topics: reference(s), other sources, purpose, objectivity, reliability, validity, age and sex, equipment, space requirements and design, directions, scoring, and norms. A brief explanation of why these major topics were included for every test is provided immediately after each major topic heading presented below.

Reference(s):

To provide the primary source for the test which was used extensively in the preparation of the test's description. It is intended that the reader will use these references after he/she has narrowed the choice of tests for possible employment.

Other Sources:

To provide a listing of the last name of the author(s) of measurement and evaluation books published since 1980 which contain information about the test. It is intended that these listings will increase efficiency in locating additional information about each test. The complete bibliographical information of the textbooks included under this topic are listed in *Appendix A: Measurement and Evaluation Books in Exercise Science, Physical Education and Sport Science Published Since 1980.*

Purpose:

To provide the purpose of the test as presented by the test constructors. In situations where the test constructors did not report the purpose of their test, it was written by the editor.

Objectivity:

To provide information with which the reader may judge if the test measures consistently when given by two different testers.

Reliability:

To provide information with which the reader may judge if the test measures consistently when given by the same tester two or more times.

Validity:

To provide information with which the reader may judge if the test measures the physical component as commonly defined in the literature.

Age and Sex:

To provide information about the group for which the test is intended. In cases where the test constructors did not report this information, the editor made an arbitrary decision about the suitability of the test for various age groups and gender.

Equipment:

To provide information about the equipment needed to administer the test properly.

Space Requirements and Design:

To provide information about the type and the amount of space needed to administer the test. The design is intended to describe how the test should be constructed within the suggested area.

Directions:

To provide information about how the test is administered.

Scoring:

To provide information on how the test is scored.

Norms:

To provide sources, if available, of norms to use in the interpretation of the test's results. The complete bibliographical information for these listed references may be found at the back of this book in *Appendix B: References.*

Chapter 2

AGILITY

RUNNING TYPE AGILITY TESTS

AAHPER SHUTTLE RUN (POTATO RACE) TEST

References.

AAHPER (1965) *Youth fitness test manual.* Washington, DC: American Association for Health, Physical Education and Recreation, pp 19, 28, 36, 45, 50, 55, 59-60.

Metheny, E. et al. (1945). Physical performance levels for high school girls. *Journal of Health and Physical Education,* 16:308-311, 354-357.

Additional Sources.

Barrow et al. (1989, p. 117); Baumgartner & Jackson (1982, pp. 218-220); Baumgartner & Jackson (1987, pp. 281-282);

Baumgartner & Jackson (1991, p. 264); Clarke & Clarke (1987, pp. 159-160, 166-167, 215-216); Hastad & Lacy (1989, pp. 257-259, 286-287); Jensen & Hirst (1980, p. 148);

Johnson & Nelson (1986, pp. 227-228, 374); Kirkendall et al. (1987, pp. 152-153); Kirkendall et al. (1980, pp. 271-272);

Miller (1988, p. 127); Safrit (1981, p. 241); Safrit (1986, pp. 277-279); Safrit (1990, pp. 409-411).

Purpose.

To measure the ability of an examinee to change directions quickly and abruptly while running.

Objectivity.

Not reported.

Reliability.

Not reported.

Validity.

Not reported.

Age and Sex.

Females and males, age 9 - college.

Equipment.

Marking tape, two wooden blocks 5cm x 5cm x 10cm (2" x 2" x 4"), and a stopwatch.

Space Requirements and Design.

A clear, level area approximately 3m x 15m (10' x 45') with two parallel lines approximately 2m (6') in length marked 9.15m (30') apart in the center of the area. One of the lines is considered the starting line and the two wooden blocks are placed on the other line about 1m (3') apart.

Directions.

The examinee takes a standing position behind the starting line and upon the signal, "Ready, Go," runs to the other line (9.15m, 30' away), bends over, picks up one block and returns to the starting line where he/she places the block beyond the line. The examinee then returns to the other line and picks up the second block, turns around and runs across the starting line carrying the block in her/his hand. The first block must be placed on the floor - it cannot be thrown. Two trials are given.

Scoring.

The score is the best time, measured to the nearest tenth of a second, in which the course is run.

Norms.

American Alliance (1975, pp. 28, 36, 45, 50, 55, 59, 60) boys, girls, men and women; American Alliance (1990, p. 47) boys and girls; Alabama (1988, pp. 13-15, 24-25) boys and girls;

Barrow et al. (1989, p. 121) boys and girls; Baumgartner & Jackson (1982, p. 219) boys and girls; Baumgartner & Jackson (1987, pp. 282, 286) boys and girls; Baumgartner & Jackson (1991, pp. 262, 267) boys and girls;

Canadian Association (1980, pp. 37-60) boys and girls (3 blocks); Chrysler/AAU (1990, p. 6) boys and girls (3 blocks); Clarke & Clarke (1987, p. 162) boys and girls;

Evans (1973, p. 386) rugby players (60' apart); Fleishman (1964A, p. 49) boys and girls (60' apart); Hastad & Lacy (1989, p. 258) boys and girls; Hawaii (1989, pp. 19-20) boys and girls; Johnson & Nelson (1986, pp. 229, 373-376, 382) boys and girls;

Kirkendall et al. (1987, p. 158) boys and girls; Kirkendall et al. (1980, pp. 277, 285-286, 332-333) boys and girls; McCaughan (1975, p. 14) boys (60' apart); Metheny et al. (1945, p. 309) girls;

Miller (1988, pp. 127, 234) boys and girls; National Marine (no date, p. 12) boys and girls (180' apart); Ostyn et al. (1980, pp. 107, 127-140) boys (5m apart); President's Council (1987, p. 1) USSR boys and girls;

President's Council (1989, p. 8) boys and girls; Rhode Island (1989, pp. 23-26) boys and girls; Safrit (1986, p. 279) boys and girls; Simons et al. (1990, p. 102, 97) girls (50m, 480m); Virginia (1988, pp. 36-37) boys and girls.

REVIEW

CONNIE FOX, Ed.D.

Assistant Professor
Physical Education
Northern Illinois University
DeKalb, IL 60115

The test is described as measuring the ability to change directions quickly and accurately while running. This objective speaks to the motor fitness area of agility. Typically, agility is defined as the ability to change directions quickly and accurately. This test is a valid measure of agility, but not a particularly useful one. Sports and most activities do not require a direction reversal, but a change from forward to lateral or similar change.

The test is a reliable measure, particularly if testers are given the opportunity to practice. However, the score is the best time of two trials. This procedure lowers reliability because it does not measure typical performance but measures the best performance, which may include luck. Another problem with the test's reliability lies in the use of 2" x 2" x 4" wood blocks. This is approximately the size of a blackboard eraser and not similar to any common physical education equipment. Testers are likely to use erasers, and

chalk dust on the floor results. This can cause a slippery surface after several examinees have run, thus raising the times for the second trial.

The test is as objective as is possible with a stopwatch. Inconsistency in the use of the watch would account for the error. No other individual will affect the performance of the examinee.

The test is highly applicable from a practical standpoint. There are no problems with facilities or space. The space required includes floor markings 30' apart, which are fairly standard on most gym floors. No equipment is needed - save the blocks required. These blocks are inexpensive and can be bought from lumber stores. The test is not difficult or time consuming to set up. It may require considerable time to administer because examinees are tested one at a time for two trials. This can be reduced by running two watches on two examinees simultaneously.

The Shuttle Run Test is not suitable for a drill to teach or condition for agility. If the test were extended over several lengths, it might be more valuable. It is suitable for all age ranges listed and does discriminate well. It is not suitable for self testing unless a large clock were available for examinees to time themselves. The test is suitable for research purposes and is appropriately normed. Due to the age of norms, it may be necessary to re-norm.

SUMMARY

Major Strengths:

1. Quick to set up and explain.

2. Quick to administer.

3. Valid, objective measure of direction reversal agility.

Major Weaknesses:

1. Time consuming because not applicable for group testing.

2. The inappropriate use of blackboard erasers for equipment could deposit chalk dust and endanger safety.

Overall, the Shuttle Run is acceptable and useful if given with the above reservations considered. It is an excellent test for research due to its objectivity and validity. It is not a good conditioning test due to its brevity.

AGILITY-COORDINATION (AGCO) TEST

Reference.
O'Dwyer, S. (1987). AGCO: The construction of an agility-coordination test. Paper presented at First World Congress of Science and Football, Liverpool.

Additional Sources.
None.

Purpose.
To measure the agility and coordination of an examinee.

Objectivity.
r = 1.00 was obtained between O'Dwyer and another tester.

Reliability.
r = .87 for test-retest separated by thirteen days.

Validity.
r = .74 between the Agility-Coordination Test and the Shuttle Run Test. r = .48 between the Agility-Coordination Test and the Lateral Moving Test.

Age and Sex.
Not reported.

Equipment.
One mat 2m x 1.2m (6' x 4') that has a parallel mark 30cm (12") from one long edge, 3 chairs, 2 foam rubber plates 20cm x 20cm x 5cm (8" x 8" x 2"), marking tape, and stopwatch.

Space Requirements and Design.
A clear, level area approximately 15m (50') square. Inside this area, the test pattern is laid out in a rectangle (Figure 2-1). The starting line with the mat is off of one corner. Eight meters ahead in the next corner is square one (30cm or 12") and 7 meters to the left in the third corner is square two (30cm or 12"). The finish line is at the fourth corner. Sufficient distance should be between the finish line and any obstacles so the examinee can safely stop. Three meters from the inside edge of square one and four meters from square two, the two form plates are placed one on each side of the straight line connecting the two squares. The three chairs are arranged two meters apart in a zigzag pattern between the starting line and square one. The first and third

chairs are positioned two meters to the left of a straight line connecting the corner at the starting line and the corner of square one. Chair two is placed on this straight line with its back facing away from the rectangle. The backs of chairs one and three face the inside of the rectangle.

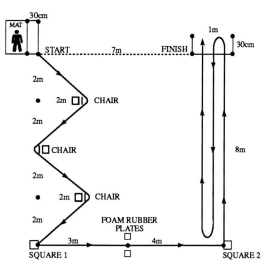

Figure 2-1. AGCO Agility - Coordination Test.

Directions.

The examinee assumes a supine position on the starting mat outside the 30cm mark. On command, "Ready, Go," the examinee gets to her/his feet, runs to the left of the first chair and continues to run to the right and left of the next two chairs. After placing one foot in square one, the examinee changes direction and runs toward square two. While running toward square two, the examinee picks up both foam rubber plates, one in each hand, and then places one on top of the other in square two. The examinee makes a 90 degree turn toward the finish line. One foot must be placed past the finish line as the examinee reverses direction and returns to square two to pick up the foam rubber plates. The examinee runs across the finish line with a foam rubber plate in each hand. One practice trial and two legal trials are given. A retrial is given to anyone who becomes confused running the circuit.

Scoring.

The score is the average time of the two trials. The time for each trial is recorded to the nearest tenth of a second. The examinee is given a tenth of a second penalty for each of the following:

1. When the examinee touches the chairs.

2. When the examinee does not place a foot in square one.

3. When the examinee does not place the foam rubber plates in square two.

4. When the examinee does not cross the finish line with the foot when returning to square two.

Norms.

Not reported.

REVIEW
MARY LOU VEAL, Ed.D.
Assistant Professor
Exercise and Sport Science
University of North Carolina
Greensboro, NC 27412-5001

The Agility-Coordination (AGCO) Test is reported to have extremely high objectivity between the test constructor and one other tester and relatively high reliability of .87. However, the test does not fare well in validity. Comparisons are made with the Shuttle Run Test and the Lateral Moving Test, both of which are well known and accepted agility measures, but validity scores are low, especially compared to the latter test. There is no effort made to demonstrate validity of the AGCO with any known measure of coordination. The test is designed to be administered to one examinee at a time.

While the space requirement of 50' x 50' is large, it is a reasonable requirement for school gymnasiums. However, the test constructor does not make clear the space requirement outside of the actual test area, especially at the finish line.

Administration of the test appears to be relatively easy since only a stopwatch and a single tester are required. The time required to administer the test is not reported, and since norms are not provided, the time requirements for two trials per examinee are completely unknown. It does appear that the test could be set up for practice drills, but since the space requirement is relatively large, it appears that only two practice areas could be set up in a typical gymnasium. It would be difficult to arrange for practice in a physical education class of 30 or more students.

While the test directions tell us that 50 examinees were tested, there is no mention of the age or gender of those examinees. It is impossible to guess the intended examinees, but this reviewer would rule out the test for elementary or junior high students, given the somewhat complicated test pattern and instructions. The absence of norms means that the prospective test user does not know if the test discriminates among its intended users.

Scoring appears to be a simple matter of using the stopwatch correctly. The test constructor has given specific instructions for a penalty of a tenth of a second each for four different infractions of test rules.

SUMMARY

Major Strengths:

1. High reliability and objectivity.

2. Good validity when correlated with the Shuttle Run Test.

3. Easy and precise to administer.

Major Weaknesses:

1. Absence of norms.

2. No indication of intended age or gender.

3. Unsuitable for use in physical education classes due to the large area needed to test one examinee and complicated test pattern.

4. Questionable validity as a test of agility and coordination.

The AGCO is unacceptable for school use as an agility measure since the Shuttle Run Test is available and more suitable for that audience. The AGCO test may be more suitable for research purposes, although the reviewer is not convinced that the test has been shown to be anything other than a weak agility measure. It appears to measure something other than agility, since the validity score is so low, but the evidence that it measures coordination is not presented in these instructions.

AUTO TIRE TEST

Reference.
McCloy, C. H., & Young, N. D. (1954). *Tests and measurements in health and physical education.* New York, Appleton-Century-Crofts, pp 81-82.

Additional Sources.
Kirkendall et al. (1980, p. 246); Kirkendall et al. (1987, p. 123).

Purpose.
To measure the ability of an examinee to place her/his feet accurately while running.

Objectivity.
Not reported.

Reliability.
r = .97.

Validity.
r = .69.

Age and Sex.
Suitable for females and males, high school through college.

Equipment.
Marking tape, tape measure, 10 auto tires, and a stopwatch.

Space Requirements and Design.
A clear, level area approximately 3m x 15m (10' x 45') with the 10 automobile tires, their centers 1.83m (6') apart, arranged in two columns of five tires each. The two columns are 1.22m (4') apart. The center of the first tire in the right column is .91m (3') from the starting line while the first tire in the left column is 1.83m (6') from the starting line (Figure 2-2).

Directions.
The examinee takes a standing position behind the starting line and upon the signal, "Ready, Go," places the right foot into the center of the first tire in the right column and then the left foot into the center of the first tire in the left column. The examinee repeats this pattern until all tires have been stepped into. The examinee then turns to the left and returns to the finish line by following the same stepping pattern.

Scoring.
The score is the time (the editor assumes it is

Figure 2-2. Auto Tire Test.

measured to the nearest tenth of a second) to complete the round trip.

Norms.
Not reported.

REVIEW

LINUS J. DOWELL, Ed.D.
Chair, Graduate Programs
Health and Physical Education
Texas A & M University
College Station, TX 77843

The Auto Tire Test as it is described in the literature is not a valid test since there is not a decrement in scoring for stepping on the tires or missing the target area. Without this as a part of the test scoring, the test does not measure the ability to accurately place the feet. A reported

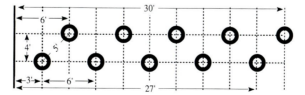

Figure 2-2. Auto Tire Test.

validity coefficient of .69 appears high if the purpose is to measure the ability to place the feet accurately while running.

The test, however, is very reliable as a reported reliability of .97 would indicate. There is no reason to believe that one would not get the same results each time the test was given. In like manner, the test is objective since the measurement taken is time on the stopwatch. The test does not require the assistance of another individual.

Facilities and space requirements are not a problem. However, the accumulation of water in the tires can cause problems if the tires are left outside in the rain. Administration of the test is very simple and requires almost no expertise. Time constraints are minimal for the test, although two trials might yield a more accurate assessment of agility than a single trial. This test has been used for years as a drill to promote learning and conditioning in football, though today most football teams use a series of suspended ropes instead of tires for the same drill or test.

The only discrimination that may occur is to examinees of very short stature where the distance between the tires may prove too great for them to traverse. The test can be dangerous if an examinee hangs a foot in a tire and falls face first into another tire, although this rarely happens.

Falls during this test normally lead only to abrasions of arms and legs which come into contact with the ground.

Scoring is objective and examinees may test themselves with a stopwatch while running the tires. Without penalty assessment for missed foot placement, the validity of this test is not high enough to be considered for research purposes. Norms for the Auto Tire Test were not found.

SUMMARY

Major Strengths:

1. Ease in preparing for the test.

2. Low cost.

3. Ability to test large groups in a short period of time.

4. Easy administration.

Major Weaknesses:

1. Lack of penalty for stepping on or missing tires.

2. The distance between tires for examinees of shorter stature.

This is an acceptable test for teaching and drill purposes. This test does not meet the criteria, that is, to place the feet accurately, without some means of penalizing faulty foot placement. The Auto Tire Test, designed by McCloy, should be used only as a drill, or for achievement testing and not for research.

BARROW (TEXAS) ZIGZAG RUN TEST

References.
Barrow, H. M. (1953). A test of motor ability for college men. Unpublished doctoral dissertation, Indiana University.

Barrow, H. M., & McGee, R. (1979). *A practical approach to measurement in physical education.* Philadelphia: Lea & Febiger, pp 141-143.

(Texas) Governor's Commission on Physical Fitness (no date). *Texas physical fitness - Motor ability test.* Austin, TX, pp 11-13.

Additional Sources.
Baumgartner & Jackson (1982, p. 217-218); Baumgartner & Jackson (1987, p. 204); Baumgartner & Jackson (1991, p. 224-225); Hastad & Lacy (1989, pp. 282, 295-296);

Johnson & Nelson (1986, p. 362-365); Miller (1988, pp. 127-128; Mood (1980, p. 237); Safrit (1986, p. 354); Safrit (1990, pp. 523-526).

Purpose.
To measure the ability of an examinee to run a specified course.

Objectivity.
r = .99.

Reliability.
r = .80.

Validity.
Construct validity was established (Texas, no date).

Age and Sex.
Females and males, age 8 - college.

Equipment.
Five high jump type standards (plastic cones or similar obstacles may be used), marking tape, stopwatch, and a tape measure.

Space Requirements and Design.
A clear, level area approximately 5m x 8m (15' x 24') with a rectangle of 3.05m x 4.88m (10' x 16') marked off in the center of the area. A standard is placed in each corner and one in the center of the marked off rectangle (Figure 2-3).

Directions.
The examinee takes a standing position behind the starting line, which is an extension of the 3.05m line, to the right of the bottom right corner standard. Upon the signal, "Ready, Go," the ex- aminee runs a figure eight pattern by going to the: (1) left of the center standard, (2) right of the top right corner standard, (3) right of the top left corner standard, (4) left of the center standard, (5) right of the bottom left corner standard, and (6) right of the bottom right corner standard. It marks the end of one lap when the examinee crosses the starting line . Three such figure eight laps are required for each trial with the stopwatch being stopped when the examinee crosses the finish line, an extension of the 4.88m line at the bottom right standard. In the Barrow Test, if the examinee hits or grasps a standard or fails to follow the prescribed pattern, no score is recorded for that trial and a retrial is given. In the Texas test, one practice trial and two legal trials are given.

Scoring.
In the Barrow Test, the score is the time measured to the nearest tenth of a second required to run the three laps. In the Texas Test, the score is the sum time of the two trials measured to the nearest tenth of a second.

Norms.
Barrow & McGee (1979, p. 143) men; Baumgartner & Jackson (1982, p. 218) boys and girls; Baumgartner & Jackson (1987, p. 205) boys and girls; Baumgartner & Jackson (1991, p. 245) boys and girls;

Hastad & Lacy (1989, 296-297) boys and girls; Johnson & Nelson (1986, pp. 280, 363-364) boys and men; Miller (1988, p. 128) boys; Mood (1980, pp. 238-239) boys and men; Safrit (1986, pp. 356-357) boys and men; Safrit (1990, 524-525) girls and women; Texas (special pamphlet with no copyright date or page numbers) boys and girls.

NOTE: The U.S. Nordic Ski Team Agility Run is nearly identical to the above tests - see Arnot and Gaines (1986, p. 228).

REVIEW

JANET A. SEAMAN, P.E.D.

Professor of Physical Education
California State University
Los Angeles, CA 90032

This test has the potential to measure agility and maneuverability. Performance on the test should correlate favorably with athletic ability and sport performance, attesting to its construct validity. The surface on which the performance is run, however, could adversely affect validity. Scoring is objective. Both versions use time measured in tenths of a second.

The reliability of scores is contingent upon the examinee's understanding of the instructions and whether or not subsequent administrations are performed on the same surface. It appears to be a quick and easy test to administer, once the area is marked off and the standards (obstacles) set in place. It requires equipment that is common to nearly any context and only one tester is needed to administer it accurately.

Understanding the instructions could be troublesome for some examinees. One trial does not assure that all examinees understand what they are to do. This test could be administered to an entire class in one day, but in so doing, for some examinees, it would probably adversely affect reliability and validity.

This test would be suitable as a drill for any age level and would be appropriate for use in classifying examinees for ability groupings, grading, or program evaluation. It should be used with caution with groups of language disabled, learning disabled, or mentally retarded unless sufficient trials are allowed to insure that the examinees understand the task. In its present form, it does not appear to be useful for research purposes for the reasons cited above. The currency of the norms is unknown since the Texas version published norms in an undated manuscript and the Barrow version, although published in a 1979 textbook, may or may not reflect a renorming since its original version appeared in 1953.

SUMMARY

Major Strengths:
1. The Zigzag Run Test is easy to administer in a short amount of time with commonly available equipment.
2. It has the potential to discriminate among a wide range of examinees.
3. It can be used as a drill or training device to give examinees the opportunity to practice maneuvering their bodies around obstacles in a safe and nonthreatening context.

Major Weaknesses:
1. There are not enough practice trials allowed for the naive examinees who have difficulty grasping the concepts of the task.
2. The physical design of the test area is unclear, leaving room for variability from test site to test site as well as among intraadministrations at the same site, thereby adversely affecting validity and reliability.

The Zigzag Run can serve as an useful tool in classifying examinees for ability groupings across a wide age and ability range. It also appears to have a useful purpose in identifying athletic ability for sports requiring maneuverability.

The Zigzag Run could be used as a pretest and posttest to measure the effectiveness of agility enhancing programs and could be used satisfactorily for this purpose with examinees with special needs to measure changes on this parameter. It is suggested that the tester further standardize the physical set up to assure that the test conditions are the same in each administration.

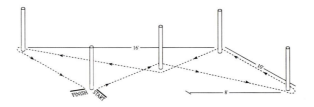

Figure 2-3. Barrow (Texas) Zigzag Run.

COZENS' DODGING RUN TEST

References.

Cozens, F. W. et al. (1937). *Achievement scales in physical education activities for secondary school girls and college women*. New York: A. S. Barnes, pp 33-34.

Johnson, B. L., & Nelson, J. K. (1986). *Practical measurements for evaluation in physical education*. Edina, MN: Burgess Publishing, p 233.

Additional Source.

Jensen & Hirst (1980 pp. 146-148).

Purpose.

To measure the ability of an examinee to change directions laterally while running forward.

Objectivity.

Not reported.

Reliability.

Not reported.

Validity.

Not reported.

Age and Sex.

High school and college females.

Equipment.

Five hurdles from track and field, marking tape, and a stopwatch.

Space Requirements and Design.

A clear, level rectangular area approximately 6m x 15m (20' x 45') with one hurdle (A) placed in the lower left hand corner. A short starting line (approximately .60m or 2' in length) is marked off with tape to the right of the hurdle. The other four hurdles are placed parallel to this original hurdle at distances of: 4.57m (15') = B, 8.23m (27') = D, 6.40m (21') = C, and 10.06m (33') = E. In addition, these four hurdles are positioned in four 91cm (3') lanes to the right of the original hurdle so that the left edge of the next hurdle falls on a straight line even with the right edge of the previous hurdle (Figure 2-4).

Directions.

The examinee takes a standing position behind the starting line and upon the signal, "Ready, Go," runs to the left and around the first hurdle (B), around the right end of the next hurdle (C), around the left end of the next hurdle (D) and completely around the last hurdle (E). The ex-aminee then runs the course back to and around the first hurdle (A) and repeats the same course. The test is completed when the examinee crosses the finish line after completing two laps. Two trials are given.

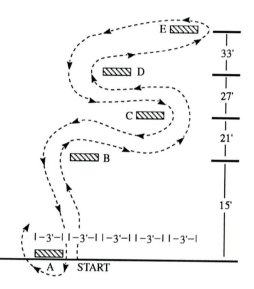

Figure 2-4. Cozens' Dodging Run.

Scoring.

The score is the best time measured to the nearest tenth of a second required to complete the two laps of the course.

Norms.

Cozens et al. (1937, pp. 90-91) girls and women; Johnson & Nelson (1986, p. 233) men and women.

REVIEW

RICHARD LITWHILER, Ed.D.

Associate Professor
Physical Education
Georgia Southwestern College
Americus, GA 31709

This test of agility is similar in many respects to a number of basic tests of running forward and changing directions right and left. The generally accepted definition of "agility" appears to be the ability to change the whole body and body segment direction quickly and accurately in a coordinated manner. While this test does have similar attributes to many shuttle runs, zigzag runs, chair runs, boomerang and figure eight runs, it lacks a component which measures change of direction of the body up and down, twisting, turning and other similar locomotor functions. With respect to the many other agility tests, one may suggest that this test is valid if the required component tested is restricted to running forward and switching directions quickly and accurately to the right and left.

Very little information has been reported specifically on the reliability of this test, probably because it has not been accepted as a standard since it was developed in 1937. Comparing the results of similar tests, one should be able to attain a reliability correlation of .90 to .95 or higher.

Likewise, very little information can be found on the objectivity of the test, but based on other such tests, an objectivity correlation of above .95 should be attained.

This test does not require another active participant; therefore, the performance is dependent on the examinee. However, a more accurate measure of agility might be achieved if the tester starts the watch on the first movement of the examinee rather than on the signal, "Ready, Go," as suggested in the directions. This procedure would eliminate the factor of reaction time which could prejudice the test in favor of those with good anticipatory ability.

The space requirement is well within the means of most programs and, in most situations, several stations could be set up. One might question the use of track hurdles in the test. They may not be readily available in many situations; and they also may cause a safety problem in that they are designed to tip over in only one direction if hit, and the counter balance feet may be stepped on if an examinee cuts too close to the hurdle. Properly spaced chairs might do just as well.

This test does not require an excessive amount of time to administer and can be supervised by one tester per test station. The two trials suggested in the directions should be sufficient unless an examinee violates a direction or runs into a hurdle, in which case another trial should be given. Although the test was originally designed for girls and college women, it has been adapted for college men by Johnson and Nelson (1986). Unfortunately, very few norms are available for this test.

SUMMARY

Major Strengths:

1. Easy to set up, administer and score.

2. Should be highly objective and reliable.

3. Does not take a great deal of time to administer and is easy for the examinee to understand.

4. Could be used for both sexes and all ages from middle school through college and could possibly be adapted for elementary school children.

Major Weaknesses:

1. Not generally in use, therefore no norms.

2. Possible safety hazard with track hurdles as noted in the discussion.

3. Limited practicality in that it measures only forward running with change of direction right and left.

4. Shortness of the test reduces the range of the scores, thus causing difficulty in distinguishing good from poor performance.

5. Does not measure agility other than that initiated by the legs.

The weaknesses of this test far outweigh the strengths, thus it is an unacceptable test. Any test of such a general nature should have a large volume of literature to support its continued use. The fact that a test is not well received does not necessarily make it a bad test, but, in this case, there are too many other agility tests which have norms for various age groups and both sexes. It may well be that the best agility test has not yet been developed. Until it is, one should choose a test which most closely meets the specific skill desired. At this time, this test is inadequate for use in research and teaching.

DODGING RUN TEST

Reference.
McCloy, C. H., & Young, N. D. (1954). *Tests and measurements in health and physical education.* New York: Appleton-Century-Crofts, p. 80.

Additional Sources.
Kirkendall et al. (1980, p. 246); Kirkendall et al. (1987, p. 123); Verducci (1980, pp. 258-259).

Purpose.
To measure the ability of an examinee to change directions laterally while running forward.

Objectivity.
Not reported.

Reliability.
r = .93.

Validity.
r = .82.

Sex and Age.
Suitable for females and males, age 10 through college.

Equipment.
Four hurdles from track and field, marking tape, and a stopwatch.

Space Requirements and Design.
A clear, level area approximately 3m x 15m (10' x 45') with a starting line 1.83m (6') in length. Four hurdles positioned parallel to the starting line: 3.66m (12'), 5.49m (18'), 7.31m (24'), and 9.14m (30') from the starting line. The hurdles are positioned along a straight line which is perpendicular to the starting line (Figure 2-5).

Directions.
The examinee takes a standing position to the right of the starting line and upon the signal, "Ready, Go," runs to the left of the first hurdle. The examinee continues weaving between and around the remaining hurdles down and back. The examinee completes the test by running to the right of and behind the 1.83m (6') starting line, then crossing the line where he/she started.

Scoring.
The score is the time (the editor assumes it is measured to the nearest tenth of a second) required to complete the lap.

Norms.
McCloy & Young (1954, p. 80) median time for junior high students.

REVIEW

CHARLES M. LAY, Ph.D.

Associate Professor
Physical Education
Mississippi State University
Mississippi State, MS 39762

The Dodging Run measures the physical component of agility as described in the purpose. Therefore, the test is valid. A reliability coefficient (N = 10) was computed by utilizing the test-retest method and yielded a r = .647, P.05. The reported reliability of the test is .93. The directions and scoring of the test are clearly stated; therefore, objectivity was found to be good.

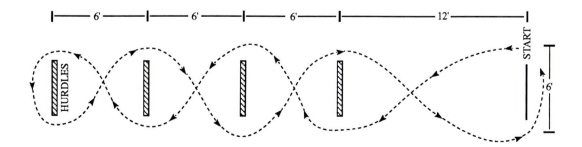

Figure 2-5. Dodging Run.

Regarding the practical aspects of the test, the facility and space requirements do not cause a problem. However, the use of chairs in place of hurdles did present a problem and is considered potentially dangerous. The examinees tend to bump the chairs and place their hands on them causing the chair(s) to fall. This could be dangerous as the examinee may have to run past the chair again. The test requires little time to administer. Administrative expertise requirements are minimal. Examinees could score themselves. The test could also be used for agility conditioning.

SUMMARY

Major Strengths:

1. Minimal equipment.

2. Space requirements no burden.

3. Scoring and directions are easy to understand.

Major Weaknesses:

1. Need for at least 15 feet behind the starting line should be stated in directions.

2. Chairs will fall and present a safety problem - hurdles or perhaps cones, should be used.

3. When chairs are used, two assistants are needed to pick up and reset those that fall.

4. Must wear proper shoes.

The Dodging Run is acceptable for teaching or individual self evaluation. There will be too much inter and intra variability for use in quality research.

FLEISHMAN SHUTTLE RUN TEST

Reference.

Fleishman, E. A. (1964B). *The structure and measurement of physical fitness.* Englewood Cliffs: Prentice Hall, pp 93, 112, 128, 163-164.

Additional Sources.

None.

Purpose.

To measure the ability of an examinee to change directions quickly and abruptly while running.

Objectivity.

Not reported.

Reliability.

r = .85 by test-retest method.

Validity.

Not reported.

Age and Sex.

Suitable for females and males, age 10 - college.

Equipment Requirements.

A stopwatch and marking tape.

Space Requirements and Design.

A clear, level area approximately 3m x 30m (10' x 90') with two parallel lines (one the starting line and the other the finish line) approximately 2m (6') in length and 18.29m (60') apart marked off in the center of the area.

Directions.

The examinee takes a standing position behind the starting line and upon the command, "Ready, Go," runs and places one foot in the area beyond the finish line. The examinee then returns and places one foot beyond the starting line completing one round trip. The examinee quickly repeats another round trip and then completes the test by running straight through the finish line. In other words, the examinee runs two and one-half round trips covering a total distance of 91.44m or 300 feet. The tester should observe the examinee turn at each line and encourage a tight turn. The examinee may touch the area beyond the lines with either foot.

Scoring.

The score is the time required to complete the two and one-half round trips measured to the nearest tenth of a second.

Norms.

Fleishman (1964B, pp. 93, 112) men, boys and girls.

NOTE: Fleishman (1964B, p. 83) also presents a shuttle run in which two parallel lines are marked 4.57m (15') apart. The score is the time required to complete five round trips between the two lines.

REVIEW

THOMAS M. ADAMS, II, Ed.D.
Professor of Physical Education
Arkansas State University
Jonesboro, AR 72401

Fleishman (1964B) offers a shuttle run designed to measure an examinee's ability to change directions quickly when running. Tests of this nature are frequently used as field tests to obtain a broad determination of an examinee's speed and agility and, to a lesser extent, explosive strength.

No coefficient of validity was reported, suggesting a certain amount of face validity was accepted. In defense however, the test design is consistent with other similar shuttle run field tests and within these limitations, can be considered valid.

The reported test-retest reliability coefficient was .85. This value is generally, yet somewhat arbitrarily considered acceptable. Users should feel comfortable that the results of the Fleishman Shuttle Run Test are dependable.

No measure of objectivity was provided. Given the numerical, nonsubjective method of scoring, the preciseness of the timing equipment (i.e., a stopwatch), and the simplicity of the test, the test should allow for meaningful measurement information. The most prominent factor influencing the test's objectivity is the exactness or accuracy of measurement recorded by the tester serving as the timer.

From a practical standpoint the test does require a reasonably large amount of floor space. Because of the abrupt changes in direction required of examinees during the test, a non skid, smooth, flat surface is advised. If floor space is available, the test could be effectively administered indoors.

The test can be administered in just a few minutes. Testers in environments such as the classroom, where time restrictions exist, should find the time requirements of the test within acceptable limits.

The test can be easily and safely administered by two testers. The first serves as a starter, timer, and observer. The second serves only as an observer, and simply notes whether the examinee has stepped over the second line before turning. Both testers should encourage examinees to touch over the respective lines, to take a small turning radius, and to run as quickly as possible. As a result of the technical error associated with "hand timing," a third tester serving as a second timer is strongly encouraged.

An examinee's score is the time, recorded to the nearest tenth of a second, it takes to complete one run. If two timers have been used, the average of the two watches should serve as the score. Only one trial is indicated. Since some

examinees learning effect may occur, the best time recorded over several trials would seem more appropriate.

Norms are available for females and males between the ages of 12 and 18. Given that the data was developed in the mid 1960's, studies identifying their current applicability seem warranted.

SUMMARY
Major Strengths:
1. The test requires limited, inexpensive, and readily available equipment.

2. The test can be administered safely and easily.

Major Weaknesses:
1. The means and standard deviation norms provided may be dated and are limited to examinees between the ages of 12 and 18.

2. Scoring is influenced by the ability of the tester to measure running time accurately.

3. Only one trial is required.

In summary, the Fleishman Shuttle Run may be considered an acceptable, practical, field test that provides a meaningful measure of an examinee's ability to quickly change directions while running. For research purposes, more accurate measurements of running time could be obtained using an automated digital timer.

FOOTBALL 20 YARD SHUTTLE TEST

Reference.
Redding, D. (1989). Head strength and conditioning coach, Kansas City Chiefs. Personal Correspondence, December 6.

Additional Sources.
None.

Purpose.
To measure the ability of an examinee to change directions quickly and accurately while running.

Objectivity.
Not reported.

Reliability.
Not reported.

Validity.

Not reported.

Age and Sex.
Not reported, but suitable for females and males, age 6 - adult.

Equipment.
A stopwatch.

Space Requirements and Design.
A 9.15m (10 yd) area on a football field with three parallel lines marked 4.57m (5 yds) apart.

Directions.
The examinee takes a three point stance with the down hand on and the feet straddling the middle line. When ready, the examinee moves laterally to touch an outside line; reverses direction and runs past the middle to touch the other outside line; and reverses direction and runs past the middle line. The examinee may initially move right or left, but during the second trial, he/she must initially move in the opposite direction taken in the first trial. The tester should start the stopwatch on the initial movement of the down hand and stop the stopwatch when the examinee crosses the middle line the second time after having run 20 yards.

Scoring.
The score is the best time, measured to the nearest tenth of a second, of the two trials.

Norms.
Not reported.

REVIEW

DAVID E. BELKA, Ph.D.

Associate Professor
Physical Education
Miami University
Oxford, OH 45056

The purpose of the evaluation device is explained clearly, but no information is available about validity, reliability or objectivity.

The Football 20 Yard Shuttle is easy to administer and the directions are very clear. While no reliability data is available, it appears that both reliability and objectivity could be very high. The evaluation takes very little time for administration and the use of a stopwatch provides a score which is often motivational for many examinees. Results can be recorded quickly. Very little site preparation is needed and very little training is necessary to learn to administer the task. The task requires three changes of direction within 20 yards and requires examinees to begin in a football stance.

Lack of validity, reliability, and applicability data are major problems. Increasing the number of trials and averaging the trial scores might result in an acceptable reliability. Another weakness is the lack of specific directions about exactly how to move: Is sidewards shuffling allowed or recommended? Is a pulling motion recommended or expected? The manner of touching the line (i.e., with hand or foot) was not specified. Failure to provide norms or acceptable performance criteria limits the meaningfulness of the task.

SUMMARY
Major Strengths:

1. Administration simplicity, including time.

2. Directions are clear.

3. Results are clear.

4. Examinees can use results as motivation for subsequent trials.

Major Weaknesses:

1. Lack of specificity in performance procedures.

2. No norms are available.

3. Only face validity supports this test.

4. No reliability or objectivity data are available.

This is not a test, but a task. It may be an acceptable task, but it is an unacceptable test.

FOOTBALL 60 YARD SHUTTLE TEST

Reference.
Redding, D. (1989). Head strength and conditioning coach, Kansas City Chiefs. Personal Correspondence, December 6.

Additional Sources.
None.

Purpose.
To measure the ability of an examinee to change directions quickly and accurately while running.

Objectivity.
Not reported.

Reliability.
Not reported.

Validity.
Not reported.

Age and Sex.
Not reported, but suitable for females and males, age 10 - adult.

Equipment.
A stopwatch.

Space Requirements and Design.
A 13.72m (15 yd) area on a football field with four parallel lines marked 4.57m (5 yds) apart. The first line is labeled the starting line, the second line the 5 yard line, the third line the 10 yard line and the fourth line the 15 yard line.

Directions.
The examinee takes a three point stance just behind the starting line facing the other three lines. When ready, the examinee runs forward to touch the 5 yard line and returns to touch the starting line, reverses direction and runs to touch the ten yard line and returns to touch the starting line, reverses direction and runs to touch the 15 yard line, and returns by sprinting past the starting line. The tester starts the stopwatch on the initial movement of the down hand and stops the stopwatch when the examinee crosses the starting line at the end of the third round trip after completing a total of 60 yards of running. Two trials are given.

Scoring.
The score is the best time, measured to the nearest tenth of a second, of the two trials.

Norms.
Not reported.

REVIEW

MICHAEL J. DURNIN, M.A.

Instructor of Physical Education
University of Puget Sound
Tacoma, WA 94816

The analysis of the measurement instrument outlined above has led to various questions and concerns. The basic question of validity, reliability, and objectivity are of greatest concern. There are also questions relating to the procedures applied to this instrument.

In regard to validity, it is the opinion of this reviewer that the test was designed with logical validity in mind. Upon review of the test's purpose and the test's procedures, it is apparent the test also measures the variables of conditioning (especially if used with ages 10 to adult) and acceleration, due to the numerous changes of direction.

The reliability should be easily computed based upon the multiple times the testing instrument has been used.

The objectivity for this testing instrument leads to many questions relating to the procedures or directions of the test write up. While a football field is required; are we distinguishing between artificial turf or grass? What type of footwear is required? Is the examinee being tested required to touch the line with a hand or a foot? With a more specific statement of requirements, this test would have a greater degree of objectivity.

In regard to the administration of the instrument, the test appears to be easy to set up. Problems with time constraints could occur with only one testing station and a multiple number of examinees. This would be even more apparent if two trials were desired.

There is a high degree of skill involved with the implementation of the change of direction. With this in mind, the test should be used in a drill situation prior to actual testing.

SUMMARY

Major Strengths:

1. Simplicity in administration.
2. Good test of agility skill in running, which is involved in many activities.
3. Good potential to measure improvement over various time periods.

Major Weaknesses:

1. Time factor with only one test station.

2. Continuity in testing on same surface (especially if testing on grass).

3. Conditioning factor with younger examinees.

Overall, this is an acceptable test if the same procedures are used every time. The test should state standard requirements in regard to the type of surface to be run on and the type of shoes to be worn. Also, a standard should be incorporated with respect to what happens when an examinee slips while performing this test.

If the above concerns are met, this could be an excellent test of agility while running.

ILLINOIS AGILITY RUN TEST

References.
O'Connor, M. E., & Cureton, T. K. (1945). *Motor fitness tests for high school girls*. *Research Quarterly*, 16(4):302-314.

Hastad, D. N., & Lacy, A. C. (1989). *Measurement and evaluation in contemporary physical education* . Scottsdale, AZ: Gorsuch Scarisbrick Publishers, pp 252-253.

Additional Source.
Bosco & Gustafson (1983, pp. 112-114).

Purpose.
To measure the ability of an examinee to change positions of the whole body and then run a weaving pattern.

Objectivity.
Not reported.

Reliability.
r = .92 test-retest of high school females.

Validity.
r = .46 with composite score of 18 other tests measuring six different motor fitness components.

Age and Sex.
Suitable for females and males, age 10 - college.

Equipment.
Eight chairs (plastic cones could be substituted), marking tape, and a stopwatch.

Space Requirements and Design.
A clear, level area approximately 5m x 15m (15' x 45') with a chair placed in each corner of a rectangle 3.66m x 9.14m (12' x 30') and a column of four chairs placed down the center of the 3.66m width with a distance of 3.05m (10') between them. At one end of the 9.14m length, a starting line is drawn next to one chair while a finishing line is drawn next to the other chair 9.14m (12') away. These lines should be approximately 2m (6') in length and laid out perpendicular to the 9.14m sides of the rectangle (Figure 2-6).

Directions.
The examinee assumes a prone position behind the starting line. Upon the signal, "Ready, Go," the examinee gets to her/his feet and runs straight ahead to the left of and around the chair.

The examinee then runs to the last chair of the middle row and begins running a weaving pattern down and back. Upon the completion of the round trip, the examinee runs to the left of and around the last chair of the right row of chairs. From there the examinee runs straight ahead to cross the finish line. The examinee is timed from the signal, "Go" until he/she crosses the finish line.

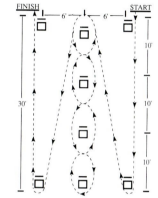

Figure 2-6. Illinois Agility Run.

Scoring.
The score is a "pass" or "fail" depending on whether the examinee was successful or not in running the test course in less than 24 seconds. An optional method of scoring is to measure the time, to the nearest tenth of a second, required to run the test course. The best score of three trials is recorded.

Norms.
Cureton (1951, p. 68) men; McCristal & Adams (1965, p. 131) men; O'Connor & Cureton (1945, p. 314) girls; Getchell (1983, p. 66) men and women; Greenberg & Pargman (1989, p. 314) (age and sex not specified).

REVIEW

DOUGLAS J. GOAR, Ph.D.

Associate Professor and Chair
Division of Health, Physical
Education and Recreation
Kentucky State University
Frankfort, KY 40601

The Illinois Agility Run first appeared in the "Motor Fitness Tests for High School Girls" published by O'Connor and Cureton (1945). It is only one of many dodge and run agility tests which have appeared individually or as components of motor ability or motor fitness test batteries over the past half century.

Agility is generally defined as the ability to change body movement position and/or direction rapidly, accurately, and under control. Research has shown that agility, regardless of how it is defined or measured, is highly related to and may be dependent upon other factors such as height, weight, balance, strength, power, reaction time, response time, movement time, coordination, and flexibility. Because of these relationships, a high probability for a learning factor may exist between repeated trials for all dodge and run agility tests as a group. It should also be noted that some authors qualify the definition of agility so that it is movement in response to unanticipated stimuli. The dodge and run type agility tests, as a group, do not include unanticipated stimuli as a test parameter but rather require movement on predetermined paths using predictable movement patterns. Further research focused specifically on agility and its dependencies upon other psychomotor factors would seem warranted to define more clearly the validity of the dodge and run family of tests, including the Illinois Agility Run, as assessment instruments.

Reliability, or the consistency with which the Illinois Agility Run test measures agility, has little, if any, value until the validity of what is being measured can be more precisely defined. However, reliability has been reported at $r = .77$ for young boys ages 7-13 and $r = .92$ for young men ages 17-26 and for high school girls. Objectivity, or the consistency of measurement when administered by different examiners has not been reported.

In quick review of the professional literature and measurement textbooks in physical education or exercise science, only one current textbook reference to the Illinois Agility Run could be found. The time needed to administer the test when the 24 second pass fail criterion is considered as a planning guide is excessive. When coupled with the three trials recommended for each examinee, it would not be unreasonable to need one minute for each trial by each examinee to administer this test. For a class of 30, that would consume two class periods. The nature of the course layout is also far more extensive than some other tests in the dodge run family. Further, the perceived requirement to monitor administration of the test closely would probably dedicate a teacher to this task, requiring an additional teacher to keep other class members gainfully occupied during the testing period. Normative data is out of date and incomplete, and there is little, if any, evidence to suggest that this test is widely used. The questionable validity of the Illinois Agility Run renders it inappropriate for most research purposes.

SUMMARY

In summary, it appears that, due to lack of a definitive definition of agility, the Illinois Agility Run would lack the validity necessary for use as a research instrument. However, the very nature of this problem may mean that it would be a very viable area for research itself. As a teaching tool, it does provide some indications for individual improvement in the before and after evaluation, however, the tester would have to be well organized and provide other activity to make worthy use of class time. The limited inclusion of this test in current measurement and evaluation publications, coupled with the lack of professional interest in developing and maintaining current normative date, would seem to indicate a professional lack of interest in this test.

LOOP-THE-LOOP RUN TEST

References.
Gates, D. D., & Sheffield R.P. (1940). Tests of change of direction as measurements of different kinds of motor ability in boys of the seventh, eighth, and ninth grades. *Research Quarterly*, 11:136-147.

McCloy, C. H., & Young, N. D. (1954). *Tests and measurements in health and physical education*, New York: Appleton Century-Crofts, pp 78-79.

Additional Sources.
None.

Purpose.
To measure the ability of an examinee to change directions while running.

Objectivity.
Not reported.

Reliability.
r = .97 when first trial was correlated against second trial (Gates and Sheffield, 1940, pp. 138 - 139).

Validity.
r = .77 for males and r = .71 for females but method is not stated (McCloy & Young, 1954, pp. 78).

Age and Sex.
Junior high males.

Equipment.
Six Indian Clubs (plastic cones may be substituted), marking tape, and a stopwatch.

Space Requirements and Design.
A clear, level area approximately 13m (40') square with a starting line approximately 2m (6') laid off near the lower left hand corner (Figure 2-7). The Indian clubs are arranged in a staircase design 2.74m (9') apart and with the top of the stairs to the right of the starting line. The first club is located directly forward of the starting line. The second club is located to the right of the first club on a line parallel with the starting line. The third club is located a perpendicular distance of 5.49m (18') from the starting line directly forward of the second club. The fourth club is located to the right of the third club on a line parallel with the starting line. The fifth club is located directly forward of the fourth at a per-pendicular distance of 8.23m (27') from the starting line. The sixth club is located to the right of the fifth club on a line parallel to the starting line.

Directions.
The examinee takes a standing position behind the starting line and upon the signal, "Ready, Go," runs to the right and counterclockwise around the first Indian club. The examinee runs to the left and clockwise around the second Indian club and continues on in the same pattern of alternately running to the right of one club and then to the left of the next until he/she has run around each club during one complete round trip. The stopwatch is started on the signal, "Go," and stopped when the examinee crosses the starting/finishing line.

Scoring.
The score is the time (the editor assumes it is measured to the nearest tenth of a second) to run one complete trip.

Norms.
McCloy & Young (1954, p. 79) junior high school boys.

REVIEW

PERRY F. MILLER, Ed.D.
Professor
Health and Physical Education
Southwest Missouri State University
Springfield, MO 65804

The Loop-the-Loop Run is designed to measure the ability to change directions while running. The physical performance component of agility is defined as "the ability of the body to change directions rapidly and accurately." That being the case, then it can be said that this test would be a valid measure of agility. Since the cones are spaced only 9' apart, change of direction ability should be of more importance than speed.

The stated reliability coefficient is .97 on a test-retest. Reliable results should be obtained as long as there is not confusion on the examinee's part as to the pattern to follow. Placing directional arrows on the floor showing the path around the cones might be helpful. Since the measurement is strictly a timing chore, achieving objectivity should not be difficult. As long as adequate instructions are given to the examinee as to the movement pattern through the cones, objectivity should not be a problem.

The most obvious problem in the use of the test would be in getting the course set accurately. It may require use of trigonometry to get the correct distances and the exact 90 degree angles to achieve the perpendicular and parallel relationships required. Once the set up is completed, testing should go quickly. Although there is no mention of multiple trials, it would not be difficult, or terribly time consuming, to give more than one trial. Becoming familiar with the movement pattern should improve performance scores.

This test does not have any hazardous aspects to it as long as rubber or plastic cones are used and there are no hazards close to the course. Use of the same or similar movement pattern could certainly be used as a drill for purposes of improving agility or rapid directional change.

Limited norms are available for certain populations. Constructing new local norms should not be a problem. While the original test was directed toward junior high males, there seems to be no reason why it would not be applicable to most any population group. It would appear to be an enjoyable and challenging test.

SUMMARY

Major Strengths:

1. The ease of administering the test once it has been set up.

2. The objectivity.

3. The reliability.

Major Weaknesses:

1. The difficulty in getting the course set up exactly as specified.

2. The possibility of confusion on the examinee's part in following the prescribed pattern.

3. The availability of existing norms for population groups other than junior high males.

Overall, this test is an acceptable test, one that could be used for evaluation and research. The major concern lies in the subjectivity of the performance component agility.

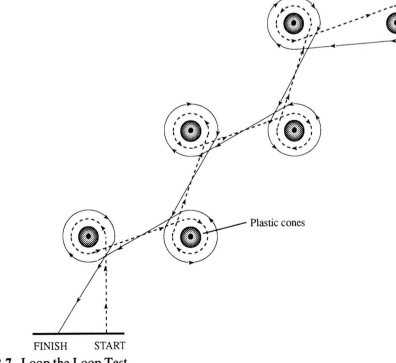

Plastic cones

FINISH   START

Figure 2-7. Loop the Loop Test.

LSU AGILITY OBSTACLE COURSE TEST

Reference.
Johnson, B. L., & Nelson, J. K. (1986). *Practical measurements for evaluation in physical education.* Edina, MN: Burgess Publishing, pp 231-233.

Additional Sources.
None.

Purpose.
To measure the ability of an examinee to run a zigzag pattern, to change directions 180 degrees quickly and accurately while running and to change position of the whole body rapidly.

Objectivity.
r = .98 between two testers of college females and males.

Reliability.
r = .91 between two trials.

Validity.
Face validity and construct validity were assumed.

Age and Sex.
Females and males, age 10 - college.

Equipment.
Seven plastic cones and a stopwatch.

Space Requirements and Design.
A badminton court without a net (an area approximately 108m x 15m or 30' x 50') (Figure 2-8). The starting line is on the side of the court between the back service line for doubles play and the back boundary line. Plastic cones are placed: (1) straight ahead from the starting line in the corner of the court bounded by the doubles sideline and the back boundary line; (2) in the corner of the alley bounded by the short service line and the sideline on the same side of the court as the starting line; (3) in the middle of the court; (4), (5), and (6) are placed in the alley on the side of the court opposite the starting line with (4) in the corner bounded by the short service line and the sideline, (5) even with the net, and (6) in the corner bounded by the short service line and the sideline and; (7) in the corner bounded by the short service line and the sideline on the same side as the starting line. Cones 2 and 6 are near the short service line on the same side of the net that the starting line is located while cones 4 and

7 are on the opposite side of the net. All four cones are placed in the corners nearest to where the net would be.

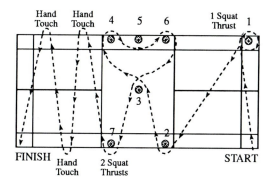

Figure 2-8. LSU Agility Abstacle Course.

Directions.
The examinee lies in a supine position with her/his feet behind the starting line. When ready and without any signal being given, the examinee stands upright and runs to the left and around the cone 1 directly ahead. The examinee executes one squat thrust and then runs to the left and around cone 2, to the right of cone 3, to the left of cone 4, right of cone 5, left of cone 6, right of cone 3 and left of cone 7. Once past cone 7, the examinee executes two squat thrusts and then runs quickly to the opposite sideline. The examinee touches the floor beyond the sideline and runs for the other sideline, touches the floor, and runs back to the other sideline. After touching the floor beyond the sideline, the examinee runs across the other sideline at which time the stopwatch is stopped. The finish line is located in the other corner on the same side of the court the starting line is located, but on the opposite side of the net. The examinee should finish by running across the sideline between the back service line for doubles and the back boundary line. The stopwatch is started when the examinee starts the initial movement to get to her/his feet.

Scoring.

The score is the time, measured to the nearest tenth of a second, needed to complete the course. A .5 second penalty is added each time the squat thrust is not executed in the correct four count sequence.

Norms.

Johnson & Nelson (1986, p. 233) men and women.

REVIEW

LORRAINE REDDERSON, Ed.D.

Professor of Physical Education
Lander College
Greenwood, SC 29646

The LSU Agility Test was administered to 15 physical education major students in a tests and measurements class laboratory. Results of the test were correlated with results of the Right Boomerang (r = .48), Loop-the-Loop (r = .48), Zigzag (r = .48), 40 Yard Maze Run (r = .85), and the Illinois Agility (r = .88). Presuming the criteria tests are valid, it can be said that the LSU Agility Obstacle Course is valid.

The 15 students took the test twice. The correlation coefficient for test-retest was .89. It can therefore be pronounced reliable. Only the course instructor administered the test.

The space requirements for this test are excellent because of the use of badminton courts. Administering tests are always easier if lines are already present on the floor rather than having to measure and record new marked areas. The equipment needed is minimal and the alternatives for the necessary equipment are good. One tester is enough and the time consumed in administration is efficient. The test should have two trials because of the learning factor. The test is suitable for college students and does discriminate among examinees due to body structure and the ability to do squat thrusts. The test is not dangerous and examinees can score themselves providing timing devices are available. The test is not recommended for research purposes.

SUMMARY

Major Strengths:

1. The use of a badminton court.

2. The combination of squat thrusts and speed in changing directions.

Major Weaknesses:

1. The difficulty of judging the execution of the squat thrusts.

2. The number of trials.

The test is unacceptable in its present form due to the way in which the directions are written. Even though the test appears to be valid and reliable, the simplicity elements are poor. Since there are so many other good agility tests available, any other choice would be more desirable.

RIGHT BOOMERANG RUN TEST

References.

Gates, D. D., & Sheffield R. P. (1940). Tests of change of direction as measurements of different kinds of motor ability in boys of the seventh, eighth, and ninth grades. *Research Quarterly*, 11:136-147.

McCloy, C. H., & Young, N. D. (1954). *Tests and measurements in physical education*. New York: Appleton Century-Crofts, pp 78-79.

Additional Sources.

Bosco & Gustafson (1983, pp. 115-116); Hastad & Lacy (1989, pp. 259-260); Jensen & Hirst (1980, p. 148);

Johnson & Nelson (1986, pp. 230-231); Kirkendall et al. (1980, pp. 245-246); Kirkendall et al. (1987, pp. 122-123); Miller (1988, pp. 122-123).

Purpose.

To measure the ability of an examinee to change directions to the right while running.

Objectivity.

Not reported.

Reliability.

r = .92 when first trial was correlated against second trial (Gates & Sheffield, 1940, pp. 138 - 139).

Validity.

r = .82 for males and r = .72 for females but method is not stated (McCloy & Young, 1954, p. 78).

Age and Sex.

Suitable for females and males, age 10 - college.

Equipment.

Three Indian clubs (plastic cones), one high jump standard, marking tape, and a stopwatch.

Space Requirements and Design.

A clear, level area approximately 12m (36') square with the high jump standard in the center. A 2m starting line 4.57 (15') in front of the high jump standard. Indian clubs are placed 4.57m (15') from the high jump standard in each of the other three directions (Figure 2-9).

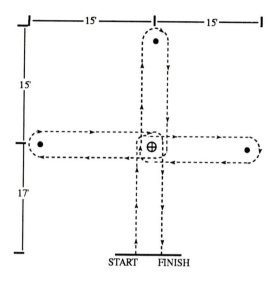

Figure 2-9. Right Boomerang Run.

Directions.

The examinee takes a standing position behind the starting line and upon the signal, "Ready, Go," runs to the left of the high jump standard. After passing the jump standard, the examinee turns right and runs to the left of the Indian club, turns right and once past the club, runs back to the left of the jump standard. The examinee once again turns right around the jump standard and runs to the left of the club opposite the starting line, turns right and runs back to the jump standard. Once past the standard, the examinee turns right and runs to the left of the third Indian club, turns right and heads back to the jump standard. Once past the standard, the examinee turns right and runs across the finish line. In other words, the examinee executes quarter right turns at the high jump standard and half right turns at the Indian clubs.

Scoring.

The score is the time (the editor assumes it is measured to the nearest tenth of a second) required to run the complete course.

Norms.

McCloy & Young (1954, p. 79) boys and girls; Johnson & Nelson (1986, pp. 231-232) boys, men and women.

REVIEW

MARY L. PUTMAN, Ph.D.

Assistant Professor
Health and Physical Education
Glassboro State College
Glassboro, NJ 08028

The Right Boomerang Run measures the ability to change directions to the right while running and typifies similar tests of agility. Agility is defined as the ability to change direction of movement rapidly and is most frequently measured with running tests. Consequently, speed is often related to agility. Acceptable validity coefficients for both female (r = .72) and male (r = .82) performers are reported.

This test requires the examinee to change directions only to the right. Athletic and physical education activities more often involve bilateral body movement. In addition, left handed examinees could be at a slight disadvantage. This is one of the oldest tests of running agility. There are more current tests which incorporate bilateral body movement.

The reliability coefficient (r = .92) is very high which is indicative of the use of an internal consistency method for determining reliability. The minimum number of two trials was used to calculate this reliability coefficient. A stability reliability is considered to be a better indicator of consistency of measurement for psychomotor tests. The test constructors do not report objectivity coefficients. The test can be adequately and accurately administered by one tester provided the interpretation of the directions is correct and the tester has experience in the use of a stopwatch.

The decisions and procedures involved in the test administration can be easily satisfied and do not require any specialized training on the part of a qualified tester. The equipment and facilities needed are available in most school based and nonschool based settings. The test must be performed on a surface which provides proper traction, and examinees must wear appropriate footwear.

The testing station must be accurately prepared. The testing procedures provide for one tester which is adequate. It is strongly recommended that there be a second test course provided or, a time prior to the test day be arranged for practice. Research has shown that the scores on measures of agility increase with practice and produce the best result with four or five trials. The examinees may perform initial pretest practice trials to reduce the time needed for the actual testing and provide the most valid and reliable results. The number of trials is not indicated. Most agility measures require a minimum of two trials. The test constructors have indicated that mean scores and ranges are available for boys and girls. Local norms and/or criterion scores would need to be developed for other age and gender groups.

The development and use of tests for motor ability, of which agility measures are a component, has declined in the last two decades. The increase in technology and expertise in the area of measurement and evaluation have made measurement specialists, researchers, and practitioners question the validity of tests designed to measure constructs or traits. General motor ability tests do not correlate highly with sport skill tests, are not appropriate to use for ability grouping, and have limited use in research.

SUMMARY

Major Strengths:

1. The test requires a minimal amount of equipment and space which makes it adaptable to school based and nonschool based settings.

2. An individual with training in measurement and evaluation at the undergraduate level would have the expertise necessary to administer this test.

3. Examinees generally enjoy the challenge involved with agility testing.

Major Weaknesses:

1. The test constructors do not provide gender and age specific norms and/or criterion scores for all age groups. Local norms would have to be developed by professionals interested in using this measure.

2. This test measures the unilateral ability to change directions to the right which is less common than bilateral movements and introduces a bias toward left handers.

3. Tests of motor ability have limited value for prediction, grouping, or research.

This is an acceptable test of running agility. There are several more recent and better tests of this motor ability. The use of results for prediction or grouping must be done cautiously. Task specific tests are more valid and reliable in the evaluation of performance.

SCOTT OBSTACLE RACE TEST

References.
Scott, M. G. (1939). The assessment of motor ability of college women through objective tests. *Research Quarterly,* 10:63-83, October.

Scott, M. G. (1943). Motor ability tests for college women. *Research Quarterly,* 14(4):402-405.

Additional Sources.
Hastad & Lacy (1989, pp. 278-279); Johnson & Nelson (1986, pp. 368-369); Safrit (1986, pp. 349-351; Safrit (1990, pp. 520-523).

Purpose.
To measure the ability of an examinee to execute various changes of body position while running.

Objectivity.
Not reported.

Reliability.
r = .91 test-retest method.

Validity.
r = .65 correlated with McCloy general motor ability test scores and r = .58 when correlated with composite criterion of total points, expert ratings and other sports items.

Age and Sex.
Females, high school and college.

Equipment.
Three high jump standards, a light weight crossbar at least 2m (6') in length, marking tape, and a stopwatch.

Space Requirements and Design.
A clear, level area approximately 5m x 17m (15' x 55') with the obstacle course laid out in the center (Figure 2-10).

Directions.
The examinee takes a supine position at A with the heels of the feet at the starting line. Upon the signal, "Ready, Go," the examinee gets to her feet and runs straight ahead making sure both feet are placed inside each of the three rectangles. The examinee continues on and passes to the right of the lone high jump standard (E) and circles it in a counterclockwise direction. After one and one-half revolutions, the examinee runs

to the crossbar and proceeds to go under it. The examinee quickly gets to her feet and runs to the last line (H), then back to the other line (G), back to the last line (H), and back to the other line (G). The examinee completes the course by running across the last line (H). In other words, the examinee shuttles back and forth between the two lines until she reaches the finish line (H) a third time. The examinee must touch the lines with her hand each time except when she runs across the line the last time. The test procedure should be demonstrated and ample practice should be allowed before testing is begun.

Scoring.
The score is the time, measured to the nearest tenth of a second, required to complete the course.

Norms.
Hastad & Lacy (1989, p. 277) women; Johnson & Nelson (1986, pp. 370-371) girls and women; Safrit (1986, pp. 352-353) girls and women; Scott (1939, p. 82) women; Scott (1943, pp. 404-405) women.

REVIEW

M. GOLDMAN, Ph.D.
Professor of Physical Education
University of Massachusetts-Boston
Harbor Campus
Boston, MA 02125

The Scott Obstacle Race, which is sometimes used as a test of agility, is in reality a segment of the Scott Motor Ability test first published in 1939. This test was originally normed on high school girls and college aged women, and agility was not specifically mentioned as a test parameter. If this test is to be used as a test of agility - or for anything else - its validity must be questioned. The Scott test has apparently never been validated against tests that measure the same kinds of agility as the Obstacle Race appears to assess.

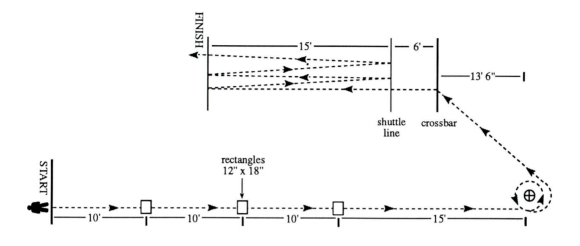

Figure 2-10. Scott Obstacle Race.

The Scott test presents a multitude of problems for the user. The objectivity of the test is probably quite low even though the reliability cited is certainly respectable. The standard diagram that accompanies the Scott test is open to interpretation and the written materials do not help to resolve discrepancies. For example, a line is shown on the diagram that is even with the single jump standard and parallel to the crossbar placement. This "line" is to be used solely as a reference point for the correct placement of the crossbar and the shuttle run lines and is not a part of the test. Yet this phantom line commonly appears as a bold line on almost all diagrams of the Scott layout. Coming off the counterclockwise run around the jump standard, the examinee should cut diagonally to the crossbar in order to get the best time possible. Even though the path of the run is shown as a diagonal on published diagrams, some testers who give this test require examinees to first cross the reference line before proceeding to the crossbar. The confusion is understandable - the use of the line is not specified anywhere in the test directions.

Further, while familiarity with motor performance tests would lead one to assume that the jump boxes at the start of the test are to be 18" long and 12" wide to accommodate the length of the foot, the directions do not specify which is the length and which is the width. This is a small but necessary detail. Likewise, there is no requirement for locking down any of the high jump standards. An examinee circling the lone standard could very easily cause the standard to fall and roll into the testing path. An examinee diving under the crossbar may dislodge the bar along with the standards. These are serious safety hazards that the Scott test does not address. Also, nowhere in the instructions do we receive any clue as to the height of the crossbar from the floor. Without this information, there certainly cannot be objectivity claimed for the test. While the directions do state that a light weight crossbar be used, no safety precautions are given in spite of the obvious, and multiple, hazards of this portion of the test.

For all practical purposes an area at least the length of a basketball court and almost half the width of one should be reserved for the test if safety factors in regard to space are to be observed. Because this test requires precise measurements, it is time consuming to set up.

The Scott test is not difficult to administer and each examinee can be tested efficiently since there is but a single trial. However, it may take some time for examinees to learn the pattern of the run. Along with the primary tester, there should be several trained assistants posted at each of the jump standards for the sake of safety. The Scott test contains the suggestion that a second examinee begin the test before the preceding examinee has completed it. This could present serious problems with safety.

Separate T-scales are available for high school girls and college women. They are undated and no assumptions may be made concerning them or the examinees involved in deriving them.

SUMMARY

The Scott test is unacceptable because it is, among other failings, invalid. While it may in fact measure some aspects of agility, many changes must be made in the Scott test before it can be used with confidence. It is not worth the effort.

As an alternative, the LSU Agility Obstacle Course should be seriously considered.

The LSU test does require that badminton court markings be available, and the pattern that the examinee must follow to complete the LSU test does seem to satisfactorily overcome many of the objections to the Scott test. The LSU test is widely published and has relatively recent norms for both females and males.

SEMO AGILITY TEST

References.
Kirby, R. F. (1971). A simple measure of agility. *Coach and Athlete,* 32(11):30-31.

Johnson, B. L., & Nelson, J. K. (1986). *Practical measurements for evaluation in physical education.* Edina, MN: Burgess, p 230.

Additional Source.
Miller (1988, p. 126).

Purpose.
To measure the ability of an examinee to change directions and move sideways, backward, and forward.

Reliability.
r = .88 between trials one and two.

Objectivity.
r = .97 between two test administrators.

Validity.
r = .72 between the test and the dodging run, r = .63 between the test and the AAHPER shuttle run and r = -.61 between the test and the sidestep test.

Age and Sex.
Females and males, high school and college.

Equipment.
Four plastic cones and a stopwatch.

Space Requirements and Design.
The free throw lane of a basketball court or a rectangle 3.66m x 5.79m (12' x 19') with a cone placed in each corner (Figure 2-11).

Directions.
The examinee takes a standing position outside the free throw lane under the basket with her/his back to the free throw line. Upon the signal, "Ready, Go," the examinee sidesteps to the right across the free throw lane passing to the outside of the cone. The examinee then backpedals diagonally across the free throw lane passing to the inside of the cone. The examinee then sprints forward parallel to the side of the free throw lane passing to the outside of the cone where the examinee started the test. From there, the examinee backpedals diagonally across the free throw lane passing to the inside of the cone and then sprints forward parallel to the side of the free throw lane. Once past the cone, the examinee sidesteps to the left across the free throw lane to finish the test. A cross over step cannot be used while sidestepping and the examinee's back must remain perpendicular to an imaginary line connecting the corner cones while backpedaling. The tester should stop an examinee who disregards the correct procedures and count it as a trial. Several practice trials should be given followed by two legal trials.

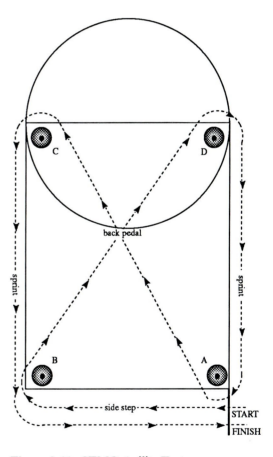

Figure 2-11. SEMO Agility Test.

Scoring.
The score is the best time of two trials measured to the nearest tenth of a second.

Norms.
Johnson & Nelson (1986, p. 230) men and women.

REVIEW

JOSEY H. TEMPLETON, Ph.D.

Assistant Professor
Health and Physical Education
The Citadel
Charleston, SC 29409

The SEMO Agility Test measures accuracy and speed of changing direction while moving as well as an aspect of agility not found in many agility tests - backpedaling diagonally. Although a greater correlation between the SEMO Test and other tests of agility would be desirable, agility performance is believed to be specific to the task and such correlations are generally low. The addition of backpedaling to the SEMO Test could greatly influence its correlation to other agility tests, but it is still a very valid measure. It should prove excellent for measuring agility for sports requiring lateral, forward, and backward changes of direction. The results of the test for reliability and objectivity indicate very good correlations. Since there is not involvement other than the examinee and the tester, there should be no external adverse influences on the examinee's performance.

The equipment and the facility required for the SEMO Agility Test are readily available, and the leadership and expertise required to administer this test are easily within the capabilities of any physical educator. The test is easily administered by a single tester, however, the instructions are unclear.

Questions concerning performance are: (1) Does the examinee begin the test standing "directly" under the basket or "with her/his back" to the cone to the left of the basket? (2) After the first and second "backpedaling," is the "inside of the cone" between the two cones on the corners of the free throw line or between the two cones on the lane line? How close must the examinee be to the "inside" of the cone before sprinting? (3) On the last "side step" is the examinee actually outside the free throw lane (out of bounds) under the basket? (4) Does the watch start on the word "go" or when the examinee begins to move? (5) Exactly where should the examinee be when the watch is stopped? These directions could be

clarified with a diagram and/or numbering of the cones with the number references included in the diagram. A clarification of the body position during the "backpedaling" and a limitation of the number of practice trials should be set. Side stepping and backpedaling skills should be practiced separately rather than in an actual test trial. The length of the rest between the trials should be designated.

The amount of time required to administer this test to one examinee at a time would be excessive and it is likely that a test which could be administered to several examinees at a time would be selected.

Two trials for this test seem to be adequate if the examinees had previous opportunities to practice the side stepping and backpedaling skills and understood the floor pattern of the test.

The test could serve as a learning or conditioning drill for several sports, but it should be done starting from the left of the basket as well as from the right of the basket.

The test would be suitable for high school and college examinees if the directions were more precise. It might be worthwhile to consider going around the cones each time to avoid an examinee's possible tendency to "cut the corners." The test possibly discriminates against examinees who have average or low athletic ability and have a preferred starting movement to the right rather than to the left.

The test might also discriminate against lesser skilled examinees who are not proficient in backpedaling skills. The recent *JOPERD* article (January, 1990, pp. 33-35) by Barrett and Gaskin raises the question of the safety of a similar activity for average or low skilled students. "As a planned activity in a physical education class, running backwards in a relay race (running swiftly rather than safely) is questionable at best." Although the case discussed in the article referred to an injured female in a sixth grade class, a high school or college physical education teacher should also consider the ability and safety of her/his students when performing similar skills for time and score.

The scoring is completely objective and could be done by partners if the directions were more specific. Using partners would require more space and equipment but the entire class could be tested in less time. Examinees could score themselves, but it might be difficult. They would have to concentrate on the starting and stopping of the watch as well as the performance of the test. The test could be used to evaluate the improvement of agility.

No norms appear to be available for this test.

SUMMARY

Major Strengths:

1. It encompasses all aspects of agility - moving forward, sideways, and backward.

2. It can be administered with readily available equipment.

3. It is easy to score.

Major Weaknesses:

1. The directions are not specific.

2. Only one examinee can be tested at a time.

3. It might be dangerous for poorly skilled examinees.

The SEMO Agility Test would be an acceptable test for research and teaching if it included more specific directions. To test agility, the examinees should already be proficient in sprinting forward, backpedaling, and sidestepping in both directions. The test would also be more acceptable if more than one examinee could be tested at a time (perhaps have one on each of several "drawn" free throw lanes) with partners listening for the time which was being called by the tester. The test could be excellent for use as a training drill for the movement patterns of several sports.

SHUTTLE RUN TEST

Reference.
Committee of Experts on Sports Research (1988). *Eurofit: Handbook for the eurofit tests of physical fitness,* Rome, Italy, pp 16, 56-57.

Additional Sources.
None.

Purpose.
To measure the ability of an examinee to change directions quickly and abruptly 180 degrees while running.

Objectivity.
Had to be high to meet their criteria, but an exact figure is not reported (Committee, 1988, p. 16).

Reliability.
Had to be high to meet their criteria, but an exact figure is not reported (Committee, 1988, p. 16).

Validity.
Had to be high to meet their criteria, but an exact figure is not reported (Committee, 1988, p. 16).

Age and Sex.
Females and males, age 6 - 18.

Equipment.
Marking tape, four plastic cones, a tape measure, and a stopwatch.

Space Requirements and Design.
A clear, level, slip proof surface approximately 3m x 10m (10' x 30') with two parallel lines, each 1.20m (3.9') long, marked off 5m (16.4') apart in the center of the 10m length. A plastic cone is placed on each end of the two lines in order to set the lines off.

Directions.
The examinee stands behind one line and upon the command, "Ready, Go," runs as fast as possible to the other line, reverses direction and returns to the starting line. This counts as one cycle and a total of five are required. The examinee must touch both feet beyond the line and between the two cones each time except at the end of the fifth cycle when he/she should run past the finish line without slowing. One trial is given.

Scoring.
The score is the time, measured to the nearest tenth of a second, needed to complete the five cycles.

Norms.
Not reported.

REVIEW

BILL KOZAR, Ph.D.
Associate Professor
Physical Education
Boise State University
Boise, ID 83725

A shuttle run is frequently used as a test of agility since on the surface at least, it appears to meet the criteria established by the definition of agility and thus achieve face validity. The Eurofit Shuttle Run is similar to several others (AAHPERD, 1976; McCloy & Young, 1954). The major differences involve a shorter running distance, more changes in direction, and the omission of the blocks of wood called for in the AAHPERD test. The reduction in running distance, and the use of five rather than two or three cycles of the course, places a greater emphasis on changes in direction and less reliance on running speed. This results in the test being more in line with the generally accepted definition of agility.

No validity, reliability or objectivity figures are reported. However, according to the guidelines published in the Eurofit Handbook, the tests selected for inclusion had to be high in all three to meet their criteria. McCloy and Young (1954) presented validity and reliability measures of .829 and .932 respectively for a similar shuttle run test.

This test is valid only in terms of the limited type of agility it measures (i.e., a total body agility which emphasizes the use of the legs in a closed environment). Its validity would be considerably lower as a measure of the type of agility a gymnast needs on the uneven bars, or that of a basketball player trying to anticipate and react rapidly and precisely to several unpredictable stimuli occurring in an open, dynamic environment.

Comparing the similarity of this test to other shuttle run tests which have reported acceptable reliability coefficients, this test should prove quite reliable. Also, assuming good testing procedure, a competent timer, and an accurate timing device, this test should have adequate objectivity.

The simplicity of the test adds greatly to its use with large numbers in a variety of testing situations. The space requirements are considerably less than other shuttle run tests, allowing for both indoor and outdoor use as well as the possibility of multiple stations.

The materials section calls for a "slip proof" floor; a slip resistant floor would be a more realistic requirement. Of equal importance from a physics standpoint is the type of footwear worn by examinees. A surface which is near slip proof for a basketball type shoe may not be for a soccer type shoe. Instructions to the tester should recommend that footwear be standardized as much as possible. Instructions also state that the examinee should not slip or slide during the test. What the tester is to do if the examinee does slip and/or slide is not addressed.

The turn lines are only 1.2 meters long with traffic cones set up as boundaries. The implication is that the examinee must remain within the boundaries set up by the 1.2 meter lines. This narrow turning diameter may place an inordinate emphasis on precision at the expense of rapidity in turning for adults.

Most fitness items exhibit a learning effect over trials. Therefore, it would seem appropriate to have at least one practice trial, or several trials with the best one recorded, instead of allowing only one trial.

Since motivation is such an important performance variable, some standard instructions beyond running as fast as possible should be provided. One tester may allow class/club mates to exhort the examinee on to optimal performance while another tester may not allow this type of extrinsic reinforcement.

SUMMARY

Major Strengths:

1. Test simplicity should result in high reliability and objectivity measures.

2. Limited space requirements facilitate its use in most test situations.

3. Only one individual is needed to administer the test.

4. Safety - assuming normal screening is followed.

5. Objective scoring.

Major Weaknesses:

1. Specific agility measured by the test does not correlate highly with other measures of agility.

2. Some attempt to standardize footwear as well as the running surface is needed.

3. More than one trial would be desirable.

4. Instructions to the tester should be more specific regarding what constitutes an invalid trial and control of outside motivators.

5. Absence of norms.

The Eurofit Shuttle Run does adequately measure the specific agility needed in making rapid and precise changes in running direction. It is acceptable as one of several items measuring physical fitness.

SPIDER SPRINT TEST

Reference.
Groppel, J. L. (1989). How fit are you? Take this fitness test. *Tennis,* 24(12):97-100.

Additional Sources.
None.

Purpose.
To measure an examinee's running agility and speed.

Objectivity.
Not reported.

Reliability.
Not reported.

Validity.
Not reported.

Age and Sex.
Tennis players, boys and girls through adults.

Equipment.
A stopwatch, five tennis balls, and a towel.

Space Requirements and Design.
One-half of a singles tennis court with a towel placed on the center mark at the baseline. Two balls are placed on the corners of the singles court at the baseline and the other three balls are placed at the junctions where the sidelines meet the service line and where the two service lines meet (Figure 1-12).

Directions.
The examinee stands behind the towel facing the net and upon the command, "Ready, Go," runs to deuce court corner, picks up the ball and returns it to the towel in such a way that it does not roll away. The examinee retrieves the remaining four balls, one at a time, and returns them to the towel in the same manner following a counterclockwise progression. The tester should remove each ball after it has been placed on the towel in order to reduce the possibility of the examinee stepping on a ball.

Scoring.
The score is the time, measured to the nearest tenth of a second, it takes from the signal, "Go," until the fifth ball is placed on the towel.

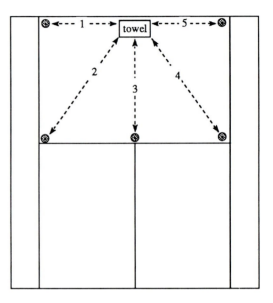

Figure 2-12. Spider Sprint Test.

Norms.
Groppel (1989, p. 99) boys, girls, men and women (tennis players).

REVIEW

BARRY BEEDLE, Ed.D.
Associate Professor
Health, Physical Education,
and Leisure/Sports Management
Elon College
Elon College, NC 27244-2177

It is difficult to determine if the test has any validity, reliability, or objectivity because they are not reported. Although agility is not a difficult fitness component to measure, it is probably specific to the sport; therefore, the test constructor should incorporate movements which simulate the game of tennis. The test does not require the active participation of another individual which makes the scoring more objective.

The test is very practical and can be used as a conditioning drill during or at the end of practice. It does not require much space or time, is easy to administer, does not require expensive equipment, and should be relatively easy to score.

Because the test is a maximal one apparently designed to assess some aspect of fitness, probably anaerobic fitness, the test constructor should have developed this test for specific age levels. The test may not be appropriate for very young tennis players. The test probably discriminates between those who have good anaerobic fitness from those who do not, but it does not discriminate between good and bad tennis players. Norms were not reported; since validity, reliability, and objectivity were not reported, this test would not be appropriate for either research purposes or grading purposes.

SUMMARY

Major Strengths:

1. For the most part, the test is very practical. It requires very little equipment and very little space.

2. It is easy to administer.

3. It is not time consuming.

4. It can be used as a drill or for self evaluation.

5. The test is scored very easily.

Major Weaknesses:

1. Validity, reliability, objectivity, and norms were not reported.

2. This agility test is not specific to the game of tennis.

3. Because this test is strenuous, it is not appropriate for very young or older tennis players unless they have had some previous conditioning.

This test is acceptable for use as a drill. It is not acceptable for research or for grading purposes and may not be acceptable as an agility test in tennis because it is not specific enough to the game of tennis. In order for a test to be considered useful for research or for teaching, it should be valid and reliable. The test constructor does not report either.

TEXAS SHUTTLE RUN FOR DISTANCE TEST

Reference.
(Texas) Governor's Commission on Physical Fitness (no date). *Texas physical fitness - motor ability test.* Austin, TX, pp 10-12.

Additional Sources.
None.

Purpose.
To measure the ability of an examinee to change directions quickly and abruptly 180 degrees while running.

Objectivity.
Not reported.

Reliability.
Not reported.

Validity.
Not reported.

Age and Sex.
Females and males, age 8 - 18.

Equipment.
Marking tape and a stopwatch.

Space Requirements and Design.
A clear, level area approximately 3m x 21m (10' x 70'). Five parallel lines of any length are marked 4.57m (15') apart in the middle of the area. The first line of the five is considered the starting line.

Directions.
The examinee takes a standing position behind the starting line. Upon the signal, "Ready, Go," the examinee runs and touches or crosses the fifth line, 18.29m (60') away, with one foot. The examinee reverses direction and runs back to the starting line and touches or crosses it with one foot. During one such round trip, the examinee crosses eight lines. The examinee repeats the pattern as many times as possible in 15 seconds. At the end of the 15 seconds, a whistle is blown and the spot where the examinee was located when the whistle sounded is noted. One practice trial and two legal trials are given.

Scoring.
The score is the total number of lines crossed during the two trials. Eight points are awarded for a round trip, four down and four back.

Norms.
Texas (no date, no page numbers) boys and girls.

REVIEW

WILLIE S. SMITH, Ed.D.
Associate Professor
Physical Education
North Carolina Central University
Durham, NC 27707

The validity of this test is acceptable at face value as it represents an adequate measure of agility as defined in the literature. While construct validity is evidenced, technical materials on objectivity, reliability and validity are not furnished. The test requires the active participation of a tester who starts, times, and then spots the finish of the examinee's performance. As a result, the examinee's performance outcome could be significantly affected as it is largely dependent upon the tester's precision in managing the scoring process.

Facility, space, and equipment requirements are well defined and are unlikely to pose a problem administratively. While the test poses no difficulty in this regard and can be administered by a single tester, precision in using the stopwatch, and spot locating the examinee's end performance is necessary. The test is not time consuming, and the number of trials recommended is appropriate thus making it quite suitable for use as a motivational tool and conditioning drill among the groups and age levels for which it was designed. While the test is safe and free of any difficult task assignments, scoring objectivity is largely dependent upon the accuracy and precision of the tester. Although examinees could conceivably self score the test for evaluative purposes, it is not viewed to be of suitable precision for research purposes. Norms are furnished for intended age groups and sexes.

SUMMARY

Major Strengths:

1. It is safe, easy to administer, and quite suitable for both females and males of the age levels intended.

2. It is both a good motivational tool and conditioning drill.

3. Large numbers of examinees can be tested during a single class period.

Major Weaknesses:

1. Technical materials on validity, reliability, and objectivity are not furnished.

2. Examinee starting position could be more clearly defined (i.e., feet parallel or staggered; arms hanging or hands on hips).

3. Examinees are permitted a choice of manuevers to reverse directions (i.e., foot may either touch or cross the line). Examinees should be directed to employ one technique only when performing the task.

4. While space requirements and design are clearly indicated, some mention should be made of indoor and outdoor surface differences as well as recommended footwear for examinees.

The absence of correlation coefficients on validity, reliability, and objectivity makes this test unacceptable for research or for teaching purposes. This information should be provided for the sex and age levels intended. Also, examinees should be provided a task demonstration prior to trials. Although space requirements and design are clearly indicated, differences between indoor and outdoor surfaces could affect performance outcome and should be addressed. Overall, the test could prove valuable as a motivational tool or conditioning drill.

NON-RUNNING TYPE AGILITY TYPE TESTS

GRASS DRILL TEST

Reference.
Fleishman, E. A. (1964B). *The structure and measurement of physical fitness.* Englewood Cliffs: Prentice Hall, p 85.

Additional Sources.
None.

Purpose.
To measure the ability of an examinee to change directions continuously while moving on both hands and feet.

Objectivity.
Not reported.

Reliability.
Not reported.

Validity.
Not reported.

Age and Sex.
Not reported, but suitable for females and males, age 10 - college.

Equipment.
Two folding chairs, marking tape, and a stopwatch.

Space Requirements and Design.
A clear, level area approximately 2m x 4m (6' x 12') with the front edges of two folding chairs facing each other and positioned 2.13m (7') apart. A starting line (approximately 2m long) is drawn even with the back edge of one chair and perpendicular to an imaginary line connecting the two chairs (Figure 2-13).

Directions.
The examinee takes a position behind the starting line with her/his body weight on both hands and feet. Upon the signal, "Ready, Go," the examinee crawls around the first chair next to the starting line, between the two chairs, around the second chair, back between the two chairs, and over the starting line. This figure eight pattern is repeated until four laps are completed.

Scoring.
The score is the time (the editor assumes it is measured to the nearest tenth of a second) required to complete the four laps.

Norms.
Fleishman (1964B, p. 93) men.

REVIEW

ELAINE BUDDE, Ph.D.
**Professor of Physical Education
Roanoke College
Salem, VA 24153**

The test is basically an agility test (agility defined as the ability to maneuver the body or the ability to make successive movements in different directions efficiently and rapidly). Agility is highly task specific, thus there is no valid measure of overall agility. However, attempts have been made to validate statistically stated test objectives on other available agility tests. No information is provided on the validity of this test. The test information fails to indicate any study of reliability and objectivity.

Space requirements should not cause any administrative problems, but the design specifications are not clear as to the surfaces that might be appropriate. A question should also be raised regarding footwear requirements.

The equipment needed should be easy to obtain and handle. Directions for the test are quite simple and the test should be easy to administer. A timer to score the test is the only individual required for the procedure. A student can perform this task. Only one trial is recommended for the test and there is no evidence that there is any statistical rationale for this decision. Test users should assess test reliability (not reported) and make decisions on an appropriate number of trials based on the statistical information obtained. In all probability, more than one trial should be used.

One would not expect that individuals would perform equally well on different types of agility tests. Therefore, this test would be most suitable for use as a learning and/or diagnostic tool for assessment of performance on this specific agility task. The test lacks statistical evaluation necessary to be used for research and using performance on this attribute as part of grading procedures is highly questionable.

The test appears to be suitable for the stated age groups. Consideration should be given to the fact that examinees may inadvertently bump the chairs that serve as obstacles. The very limited normative data presented is outdated and should not be used.

SUMMARY

Major Strengths:

1. The test presents an interesting approach to measuring a specific agility movement.

2. The test is easy to administer, practical, and requires little space and equipment.

3. The test seems appropriate for diagnostic purposes and for learning to change directions continuously while moving on both hands and feet.

Major Weaknesses:

1. The test fails to address the question of validity.

2. The test has not been assessed to determine reliability and objectivity.

3. The scoring procedure (i.e., number of trials) is questionable.

4. Elements such as practice, footwear, repeating the trial, and use of the test have not been addressed.

5. Normative data is inadequate and outdated.

The test is so old that appropriate data is not provided. The test is unacceptable for research or teaching due to the lack of vital basic statistical information.

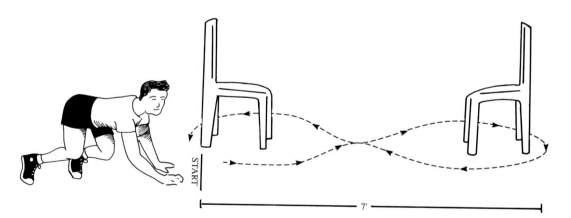

Figure 2-13. Grass Drill.

EDGREN AND MODIFIED SIDE STEP TESTS

References.
Edgren, H. D. (1932). An experiment in the testing of ability and progress in basketball. *Research Quarterly,* 3(1):159-171.

McCloy, C. H., & Young, N.D. (1954). *Tests and measurements in health and physical education.* New York: Appleton-Century-Crofts, pp 80-81.

State Education Department (1977). *The New York State physical fitness screening test: For boys and girls grades 4-12,* Albany, NY: State Education Department, pp 8-9, 32-42.

State Education Department of Public Instruction (1977). *North Carolina motor fitness battery.* Raleigh, NC: State Education Department of Public Instruction. In Barrow, H. M., & McGee, R. (1979). *A practical approach to measurement in physical education.* Philadelphia: Lea and Febiger, pp 201-203, 207.

Additional Sources.
Clark & Clarke (1987, p. 163); Hastad & Lacy (1989, pp. 254-255, 293); Jensen & Hirst (1980, pp. 148-149); Kirkendall et al. (1980, p. 244); Kirkendall et al. (1987, p. 122).

Purpose.
To measure the ability of an examinee to change directions quickly and abruptly while moving laterally.

Objectivity.
Not reported.

Reliability.
$r = .98$ (McCloy & Young, 1954, p. 80 - method is not reported).

Validity.
$r = .70$ (McCloy & Young - method is not reported).

Age and Sex.
Not reported, but suitable for children through adults.

Equipment.
Marking tape and a stopwatch.

Space Requirements and Design.
A clear, level area approximately 2m x 6m (6' x 25') with three lines approximately 2m (6') in length marked parallel to each other. In the McCloy and Young and New York versions, the lines are 1.22m (4') apart and in the North Carolina version, the lines are 3.66m (12') apart. In the original Edgren test, there were just two lines marked 2.44m (8') apart, representing the width of the free throw lane at that time.

Directions.
The examinee takes a standing position straddling the center line. Upon the signal, "Ready, Go," the examinee sidesteps to the right until the right foot crosses the right line. The examinee then reverses direction and sidesteps to the left until the left foot crosses the left line. The examinee continues the sidestepping pattern for 10 seconds (McCloy & Young; New York versions) or for 30 seconds (North Carolina version). The examinee must face the same direction throughout the test and he/she cannot cross the feet. In the original Edgren test, the examinee completed five round trips (i.e., moving five times to the right and five times to the left).

Scoring.
In McCloy and Young version, the score is the number of times the examinee crosses the center line in 10 seconds. In the New York version, the score is the number of lines crossed in 10 seconds. In the North Carolina version, the score is the number of lines crossed or touched in 30 seconds. In the original Edgren test, the score is time needed to complete the five round trips between the two lines.

Norms.
Barrow & McGee (1979, p. 207) boys and girls; Corbin & Lindsey (1983, p. 126) men and women; Hastad & Lacy (1989, p. 255) boys and girls; Johnson & Nelson (1979, p. 217) boys, girls, men and women; McCloy & Young (1954, p. 81) boys; New York (1958, pp. 51-60) boys and girls; New York (1966, pp. 45-62) boys and girls; New York (1977, pp. 34-42) boys and girls; New York (1984, pp. 34-42) boys and girls; North Carolina (1977) boys and girls.

NOTE 1: Kirkendall, et al. (1987), recommend a time limit of 30 seconds and using the best of three trials (p. 122).

NOTE 2: Johnson (1934), recommends the use of two parallel lines 1.83m (6') apart.

NOTE 3: Neilson and Jensen (1972), recommend use of three parallel lines 1.52m (5') apart and a time limit of 20 seconds (pp. 182-183).

NOTE 4: Johnson and Nelson (1986), recommend use of five parallel lines 3' apart and the awarding of one point for each time they cross a line (pp. 216-217).

REVIEW

J. L. HAUBENSTRICKER, Ph.D.
Professor of Physical Education
Michigan State University
East Lansing, MI 48824

This test was originally proposed by Edgren (1934) as a "coordination test," part of a four item general athletic test to assess the basketball playing ability of college males. The test was inadequately described and little information was provided regarding its psychometric characteristics. Although Edgren reported that correlations between the four individual items and basketball playing ability ranged from .50 to .72, he did not specify the values for the individual tests. No evidence concerning the reliability or objectivity of the test was provided.

The test was devised to assess "the ability of an individual to shift his body from left to right similarly to the way a basketball player is forced to do when guarding an opponent" (Edgren, 1934, p. 171). Although the examinee was to shift laterally in a sidestepping manner across an eight foot lane 10 times (5 to the right and 5 to the left), the starting position was not specified. The examinee's score was the time required to complete the 10 lateral shifts.

The potential of Edgren's Side Step Test as a measure of agility was recognized by other investigators. McCloy and Young (1954) proposed a modification of Edgren's test in which three parallel lines four feet apart are marked on the floor, with the examinee straddling the middle line to start the test. On signal, the examinee alternately sidesteps to the right and to the left outside lines without crossing the feet. The score is the number of trips from the center line to an outside line and back to the center in 10 seconds. McCloy and Young reported a test-retest reliability coefficient of .982 and a validity coef-

ficient of .704 with basketball playing potential. Seils (1954), using McCloy's modification, obtained within day reliability of .956 with primary grade school children. He found that the test scores were unrelated to height and weight, but that they were moderately related to a measure of skeletal maturity (r = .55, boys; r = .43, girls). Sills and Everett (1953) reported that scores from McCloy's Side Step Test could discriminate endomorphs, mesomorphs, and ectomorphs from each other.

The Side Step Test is a valid measure of agility as the term is generally defined. McCloy and Young (1954) defined agility as "the ability to change the direction of the body or of parts of the body rapidly" (p. 75). However, it is limited to such changes in a lateral direction. Bosco and Gustafson (1983) reported a factor analysis study of agility tests by Jennett which identified at least six factors. Thus, agility cannot be completely assessed by a single test such as the Side Step Test.

Adaptations of the Side Step Test have been used in basketball tests for high school boys (Johnson, 1934) and in state physical fitness tests (Barrow & McGee, 1971) where agility was considered an important component of fitness. Johnson reported a reliability coefficient of .870 and a validity coefficient of .561. Modifications of the Side Step Test include the number of lines (2 or 3), the distance between the outside lines (6 ft. to 12 ft.), the length of the test (10 sec. or 30 sec.), and the scoring procedures.

An attractive feature of the Side Step Test is that it requires little space to administer. Moreover, when instructions are followed carefully, the test can be administered to relatively large groups of high school or college students where pairs of examinees score each other in response to start and stop signals from the tester. Trained assistants would be required when testing younger examinees. The test also is less dependent on running ability than many other tests of agility such as the Right Boomerang Run, the Dodging Run, the Auto Tire Test, the Loop-The-Loop Test (McCloy & Young, 1954), and the Shuttle Run (Kirkendall, et al. 1987). The test is relatively safe to administer providing caution is taken to use a non slip surface and appropriate shoes.

A potential shortcoming of the Side Step Test is that it may give the taller examinee an unfair advantage, because he/she needs to take fewer steps to cross the side lines than the shorter examinee (Johnson and Nelson, 1969). It is also limited as a measure of agility in that it only measures lateral movement.

SUMMARY

Major Strengths:

1. Consistently high reliability across a broad age range.

2. Validity as a measure of agility and as a moderate predictor of basketball playing ability.

3. Relative ease of administration.

4. Its potential for mass testing.

Major Weaknesses:

1. Undocumented objectivity.

2. Outdated and inadequate norms for various age groups.

3. Lack of uniformity in test format, duration, and scoring procedures.

4. Its specificity as a measure of agility (lateral movement).

In summary, modifications of the Edgren Side Step Test may be adequate for use in research and/or teaching settings. The test would be most effective when combined with tests measuring other aspects of agility or when studying activities in which lateral movements are of primary interest.

REVIEW REFERENCES

Barrow, H. M., & McGee, R. (1971). *A practical approach to measurement in physical education.* Philadelphia: Lea and Febiger.

Bosco, J. S., & Gustafson, W. F. (1983). *Measurement and evaluation in physical education, fitness, and sports.* Englewood Cliffs, NJ: Prentice-Hall.

Edgren, H. D. (1932). An experiment in the testing of ability and progress in basketball. *Research Quarterly,* 3:159-171.

Johnson, L. W. (1934). Objective tests for high school boys. Unpublished master's thesis, State University of Iowa.

Johnson, B. L., & Nelson, J. K. (1969). *Practical measurements for evaluation in physical education.* Minneapolis: Burgess.

Kirkendall, D. R. et al. (1987). *Measurement and evaluation for physical educators* (2nd ed.). Champaign, IL: Human Kinetics.

McCloy, C. H., & Young, N. D. (1954). *Tests and measurements in health and physical education.* New York: Appleton-Century-Crofts.

Seils, L. G. (1951). The relationship between measures of physical growth and gross motor performance of primary-grade school children. *Research Quarterly,* 22:244-260.

Sills, F. D., & Everett, P. W. (1953). The relationship of extreme somatotypes to performance in motor and strength tests. *Research Quarterly,* 24:223-228.

HEXAGON OBSTACLE TEST

Reference.
Arnot, R., & Gaines, C. (1986). *Sports Talent.* New York: Penguin Books, pp 144-146.

Additional Sources.
None.

Purpose.
To measure the ability of an examinee to maintain balance and to coordinate the body while changing directions of the body quickly and accurately.

Objectivity.
Not reported.

Reliability.
Not reported.

Validity.
Not reported.

Age and Sex.
Females and males, age 10 - adult.

Equipment.
A stopwatch, a tape measure, marking tape (5.08cm or 2" wide), and any safe suitable material (e.g., styrofoam) to construct the sides of the hexagon. Each side of the hexagon should be 66.04cm (26") in length, 5.08cm (2") in width, and labeled A, B, C, D, E, and F in a clockwise pattern. Side A block should be 33.02cm (13") high, side C block 25.40cm (10") high, side E block 35.56cm (14") high and sides B, D, and F blocks all 20.32cm (8") high (Figure 2-14a).

Space Requirements and Design.
A clear, level area approximately 3m (10') square with the hexagon marked off in the center.

Directions.
The examinee stands in the center of the hexagon facing side F. On the command, "Ready, Go," the examinee jumps with both feet over side A and then back into the center of the hexagon. The examinee continues jumping over each side and jumping back to the center of the hexagon in the following order: A, B, C, D, E, and F (Figure 2-14b). This sequence counts as one revolution and three such revolutions are required. Throughout the test, the examinee must continuously face side F and jump off both feet. The stopwatch is started on the signal, "Ready, Go," and is stopped when the examinee lands in the center of the hexagon after jumping side F for the third time. Three such trials are given.

Scoring.
The score is the best time of the three trials measured to the nearest tenth of a second. To derive a motor learning score, five trials are allowed and the difference in times between the first and fifth trials is used as the score.

Norms.
Arnot & Gaines (1986, pp. 145-146, 167) men and women.

NOTE: This test can also be administered with just the marked off hexagon on the floor (i.e., without the blocks). The score is the average time of three trials. A .5 second penalty is added each time the examinee lands on a line or fails to jump next to the proper line.

REVIEW

RICHARD TRIMMER, Ph.D.
Professor of Physical Education
Chico State University
Chico, CA 95929

The directions provide a clear list of equipment, but what are the uses for the tape measure and marking tape? The use for these items are not made clear in the write up, but are probably clarified in the text by Arnot and Gaines. Another confusing point is, are the ends of the hexagon to be placed end to end? The reviewer assumes the 2" tape is used to mark the boundaries, but it is not clear where to begin measurement in setting up the blocks. Unless a picture is included, it is very difficult to set up this test. When using just the markings and not the blocks, are the lines the same length as the blocks?

The basic set up for the test is unclear (Note: The reviewer did not have access to a copy of the text which may have included a picture). However, if there is not a picture, and the instructions are not more clearly defined, then what is presented here is inadequate. The reliability and objectivity of this test are questionable. As to validity, it is difficult to envision a sporting event where this series of movements is appropriate. As far as motor learning, quickness, and explosive power, the reviewer can see a possibility for this test.

There are many sports related agility drills/tests that are used, and quite honestly, this reviewer would not recommend the Hexagon Obstacle as an agility test, even if the directions were clear.

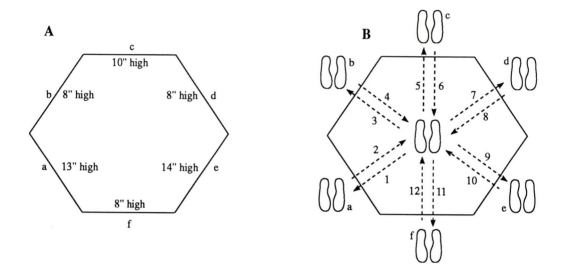

Figure 2-14. Hexagon Obstacle Test. (a) Hexagon design: all sides 26" and (b) movement pattern.

QUADRANT JUMP TEST

Reference.
Johnson, B. L., & Nelson, J. K. (1979). *Practical measurements for evaluation in physical education*. Minneapolis: Burgess Publishing, pp 228-230.

Additional Sources.
None.

Purpose.
To measure the ability of an examinee to jump rapidly from one area to another.

Objectivity.
r = .96 by Malone (1969) cited in Johnson and Nelson (1986 p. 228).

Reliability.
r = .89 test-retest method.

Validity.
Face validity was accepted.

Age and Sex.
Females and males, age 10 - college.

Equipment.
Marking tape, a stopwatch, and tape measure.

Space Requirements and Design.
A clear, level area approximately 2m (6') square with two lines, 1m (3') in length, intersecting each other at right angles marked in the center of the area. Another small line is marked off perpendicular to and at the end of one of the lines. This is the starting line and from this vantage point, the four quadrants are marked off as: (1) in the lower left, (2) in the upper right, (3) in the upper left, and (4) in the lower right (Figure 2-15).

Directions.
The examinee assumes a standing position behind the starting line. Upon the signal, "Ready, Go," the examinee jumps with both feet into quadrant 1, then into quadrant 2, then into quadrant 3 and then into quadrant 4 and then back to quadrant 1. The pattern is continued for 10 seconds. Both feet must land in the proper quadrant; a .5 point penalty is given each time the feet land on a line or in the wrong quadrant. Any examinee who stops or who could obviously do better, should be retested. A total of two trials are given.

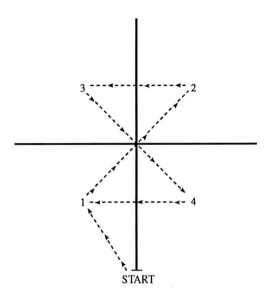

Figure 2-15. Quadrant Jump.

Scoring.
The score is the number of times the feet land in the proper quadrant minus the total of .5 penalties during the best of two trials.

Norms.
Johnson & Nelson (1986, p. 229) men and women.

REVIEW

ELIZABETH J. SCHUMAKER, D.P.E.

Associate Professor
Physical Education
Stetson University
DeLand, FL 32720

When this test was administered to a group of examinees by physical education/teacher education majors, the following problems were identified. The primary difficulty was consistency and objectivity in scoring. It was felt that considerable practice in scoring would be necessary for a tester to become consistent from trial to trial and examinee to examinee. There also were discrepancies between testers who were scoring the same examinee.

The floor surface also had an impact on the outcome of performance, especially when administered on a tile floor. This is often the type of floor found in all purpose rooms where many elementary physical education classes are held. The tile floor tended to be slippery and examinees were slowed by caution or they fell.

Examinees tended to focus intently on jumping in the correct quadrant and found they could not keep track of their own scores. This makes self scoring somewhat inconsistent with actual performance outcomes.

SUMMARY

Major Strengths:

1. The test does not require a lot of space.

2. The test is challenging and fun.

3. It would be useful to use as a formative or self testing activity.

Major Weaknesses:

1. The directions are not clear and create some confusion as to what is correct and what is incorrect procedure. The directions and scoring need to be more explicit. When an examinee stops or could obviously do better and is allowed to start over, this may create a bias towards those examinees who are allowed an additional trial. The scores of these examinees may differ significantly from those who took only two trials since performance improved with practice.

2. The best of two trials concept is affected by not allowing for practice. The second attempt was usually the best score. Three trials might give a clearer description of an examinee's ability to jump from square to square.

3. Questions were raised about the amount of time that should be allowed between trials.

This test could be used as a self testing activity or as a formative test. However, before it is used for research purposes, the validity and reliability should be updated. Questions were raised regarding intervening variables which would confound the jumping ability such as speed, endurance, and strength. The 10 second time factor makes other variables operable.

REACTIVE AGILITY TEST

Reference.
Chelladurai, P. et al. (1977). The reactive agility test. *Perceptual and Motor Skills,* 44:1319-1324, June (Part 2).

Additional Sources.
None.

Purpose.
To measure four types of agility: simple, temporal, spatial and universal.

Objectivity.
Not reported.

Reliability.
r = .59 to r = .97 using the Spearman-Brown Prophecy Formula and the odd-even and split half methods.

Validity.
Not reported.

Age and Sex.
College males.

Equipment.
An activator (i.e., on-off switch), a reaction mat, a control box, a set of three timers, and a light display containing 12 bulbs and switch plates (Figure 2-16).

Space Requirements and Design.
A clear, level area whose dimensions are adjustable (i.e., the distance between the mat and the bulbs and the distance between each of the 12 bulbs).

Directions.
The examinee assumes a standing position on the reaction mat and when ready, presses the activator switch which causes a randomly selected bulb on the display unit to light. The examinee then moves forward and touches the plastic plate in front of the bulb. The touch turns off the bulb. The examinee returns to press the activator switch to complete the trial. The apparatus enables the tester to manipulate the presentation of the stimulus. The temporal variations include: (a) lighting of a bulb instantaneously, (b) lighting of a bulb after a specified time of 1, 2, or 3 seconds, and (c) lighting of a bulb randomly between 0 and 3 seconds after pressing the activator switch. Spatial variations include: (a) lighting of the center bulb and (b) lighting of any of the 12 bulbs. Any or all of the temporal and spatial variations may be used. The following times may be derived from this test: (a) total time - the time required to leave the mat, run and touch the lit bulb and return to press the activator a second time; (b) forward time - the time required to leave the mat and run and touch the lit bulb; (c) total body reaction - the time between presentation of the stimulus and the examinee's departure from the mat; (d) movement time - the time required for the examinee to run and touch the lit bulb; and (e) return time - the time required to run from the bulb to the starter switch and press it. A total of 10 trials are given for each of the following four conditions in a random order, making a total of 40 total trials.

1. Simple - When the examinee pressed the activator, the center bulb lit up. Both temporal and spatial uncertainty were absent.

2. Temporal - The center bulb lit up 0 to 3 second(s) after the examinee pressed the activator. Temporal uncertainty was present.

3. Spatial - When the examinee pressed the activator, any one of the 12 bulbs lit up. Spatial uncertainty was present.

4. Universal - Any one of the 12 bulbs lit up 0 to 3 second(s) after the examinee pressed the activator. Both temporal and spatial uncertainty were present.

Scoring.
The score is the time measured to the nearest one-hundredth of a second to complete each of the four specified tasks. (The editor assumes that the mean of the 10 trials should be used as the score for each task.)

Norms.
Chelladurai et al. (1977, p. 1323) men.

REVIEW

BRENDA LICHTMAN, Ph.D.
Associate Professor
Health and Kinesiology
Sam Houston State University
Huntsville, TX 77341

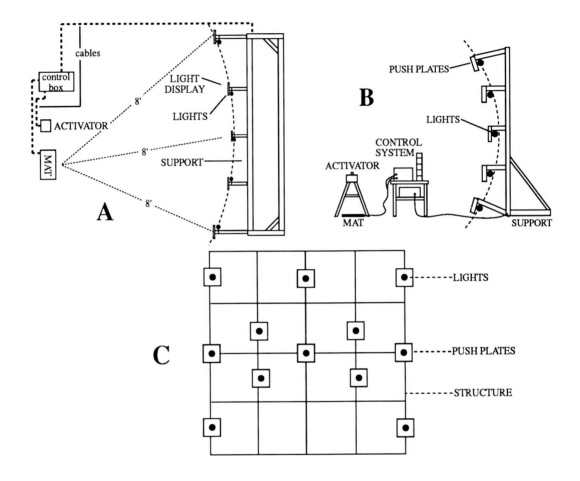

Figure 2-16. Reactive Agility Test: (a) top view, (b) side view, and (c) front view.

The scientific aspects of the Reactive Agility Test are incomplete in that no validation data was reported. Face validity could be questioned, as a procedure which purports to evaluate agility yet requires movement in one plane and demands only a single change of direction does not seem appropriate. The test claims to evaluate simple, temporal, spatial and universal agility, yet no evidence is presented to show these types of agility are distinct entities, and not merely aspects of the same construct. Correlational analyses would need to be performed to ascertain whether this is the case. Reliability across the different reactive situations ranges from poor to excellent. It is unclear whether the reliability coefficients evaluated total time for task completion, or assessed the reactive portion separately from the agility components. Even though objectivity is not provided, the timing devices should allow for consistency of measurement among testers. Since the procedures allow one to vary the spacing between the 12 lights and the distance the examinee must traverse, the tester can adapt the action to meet her/his unique situation. Such adaptability does have a drawback if comparative information is desired or if norms will eventually be developed.

In light of the temporal and spatial parameters, it would be interesting to determine whether changes in the time to complete the agility portion of the task is a function of the degree of uncertainty present. Choice reaction time literature would suggest that the reactive component would be affected much more than the agility component.

The Reactive Agility Test lacks practicality as few public school settings would have the necessary apparatus. In a human performance laboratory setting, most colleges would own the required equipment, but many professionals would not know how to set up the electrical circuitry. While the concept of reactive agility appears to relate to the decision making process and subsequent required movements in certain sports, interest would most likely be generated within a research paradigm rather than a field setting.

SUMMARY

Major Strengths:

1. By separating reaction time from movement time, the time it takes to complete the agility component can be totally divorced from the reactive aspect.

2. Even though no objectivity coefficient is provided, the nature of the measurement process should not result in this test quality being suspect.

3. While 10 trials would seem adequate for eliminating any potential effect due to learning, the suggested (by the editor) averaging over the 10 trials seems to defeat this very purpose.

Major Weaknesses:

1. The test purports to measure four types of agility, yet, logical validity would suggest what is really being evaluated is movement in one plane (forward and back with only one change in direction) which is preceded by four different kinds of reactive situations. Reaction/movement time literature would suggest that only the reaction time portion of the response time should be affected.

2. Validity is not reported.

3. With a range of almost .40 in the reliability coefficients, there seems to be some question regarding the consistency with which reactive agility is measured under each of the four conditions.

4. The equipment seems rather elaborate for a teaching situation and would require some knowledge of electrical circuitry for proper set up.

5. The time required to complete the 40 trials could not be justified in a teaching setting.

6. With the adjustable spatial dimensions, norms would not be especially pertinent.

Unacceptable test: rather than evaluate four types of agility, this test measures speed of movement, with only one change of direction, under four different reactive situations. Thus, the agility component of the test remains constant, but the reactive portion varies. No validity is provided. Furthermore, one must question whether a test requiring only one change of direction per trial would be an effective assessment of agility. While the equipment requirements are not unusual in a research setting, most schools would not have, nor would they probably choose to purchase, the apparatus for use in a teaching situation. Ten trials would most likely eliminate any potential learning, but the averaging across all trials for a given reactive situation (which the editor suggested), would defeat this purpose.

SQUAT THRUST OR BURPEE TEST

References.

Burpee, R. H. (1931). Differentiation in physical education. *Journal of Physical Education,* 28:130-136, March.

Burpee, R. H. (1940). *Seven quickly administered tests of physical capacity.* Bureau of Publications, Columbia University.

Weiss, R. A., & Phillips, M. (1954). *Administration of tests in physical education.* St. Louis: C. V. Mosby, pp 131-132.

Additional Sources.

Bosco & Gustafson (1983, pp. 114-115); Clarke & Clarke (1987, p. 166); Johnsen & Nelson (1986, p. 227); Kirkendall et al. (1980, p. 244); Kirkendall et al. (1987, p. 122); Miller (1988, pp. 124-125); Safrit (1986, pp. 319-320).

Purpose.

To measure the ability of an examinee to change positions of the body.

Objectivity.

$r = .99$ by Recio cited in Johnson and Nelson (1986, p. 137).

Reliability.

$r = .79$ to $r = .89$ for grades 5 - 11, New York State (1977, pp 32-33).

Validity.

Not reported.

Age and Sex.

Suitable for females and males, age 8 - adult.

Equipment.

Stopwatch.

Space Requirements and Design.

A clear, level area approximately 3m (10') square with the examinee in the center.

Directions.

The examinee starts from an erect standing position with the arms at the sides. On command, "Ready, Go," the examinee goes into a squat position by bending at the hips and knees and placing the hands flat on the floor in front of the body. The examinee then kicks both legs out behind and assumes a front leaning rest position with the body in a straight line and the legs fully extended. The examinee then returns her/his legs to the squat position, followed by standing erect with the hips and knees straight (Figure 2-17). The examinee receives one practice trial prior to being tested. Three trials are given with a 10 second time limit for each.

Scoring.

The score is the number of repetitions executed. One point is scored for each complete squat thrust while one-fourth point is given for each quarter movement of a squat thrust. For example, if the examinee completed three squat thrusts and finished in the squat position prior to the front leaning rest, 3 and 1/4 points would have been earned. One-half point is earned if the examinee is in the front leaning rest position and three-fourths of a point is earned if the examinee is in the squat position following the front leaning rest position.

Norms.

Barrow & McGee (1979, p. 210) boys and girls; Clarke & Clarke (1987, p. 166) time limits of 10 and 30 seconds for girls; Johnson & Nelson (1986, pp. 227, 382) boys, girls, men and women; McCloy & Young (1954, pp. 177-180) time limits of 10, 20, 30 and 60 seconds for boys, girls and women;

Metheny et al. (1945, p. 309) time limits of 10 and 30 seconds for girls; Miller (1988, p. 124) for boys and girls; New York (1977, pp. 34-42) boys and girls; O'Connor & Cureton (1945, p. 314) time limits of 10 and 30 seconds for girls.

REVIEW

DOYICE J. COTTEN, Ed.D.

Professor of Physical Education
Georgia Southern University
Statesboro, GA 30460

Agility is defined as the ability to change body position and direction quickly. While most agility tests consist of runs that involve changing directions, some involve changing the position of the body. The Squat Thrust (Burpee) Test involves rapidly moving the body from the vertical to the horizontal position and back again.

At first glance, the Squat Thrust appears to possess logical validity since it fits the definition of agility. In actual practice, however, it is easy to

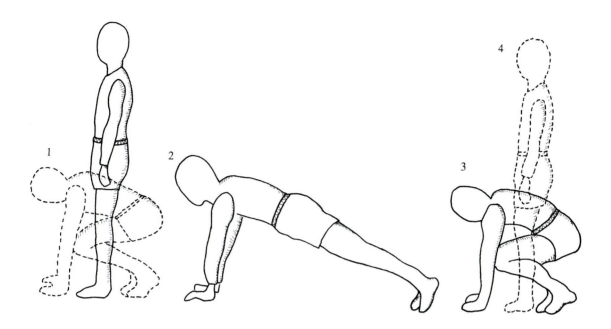

Figure 2-17. The four positions of the squat thrust.

see that significant variations in form occur when the test is performed at maximum speed. Because of the speed at which the task is performed, it is very difficult to make certain that the directions are followed accurately. As a result, scores are likely to reflect differences in form instead of the ability to change body position rapidly.

The validity of the test has been reported as .34 for females and .55 for males when compared with general athletic ability. These are not only low, but are also compared with a questionable criterion measure. Since agility is a component of general athletic ability, it makes little sense to use athletic ability as the criterion. Another point to consider is that the Squat Thrust has not correlated highly with other common tests of agility.

Reported reliability figures are satisfactory for this type of test; however, the reported objectivity figure (.99) raises a question. It is easy to see from the directions that the tester must check for several components of form. The examinee must go to the squat position, must keep the body straight in the front leaning rest position, and must return to a completely upright position each repetition. It is difficult to imagine two

testers judging correct executions and scoring the test identically. In general, when more judgement is required in scoring, lower objectivity results.

The test can be administered in any open area and requires no equipment other than a stopwatch. On the surface, the test appears easy to administer. In actual practice, however, accurate administration is difficult because the tester has to observe the form while the repetitions are occurring very quickly. The test is often administered by dividing the class in half and having individuals count for their partners. This procedure will result in scores that are neither valid, reliable, nor objective. One tester should test all examinees one at a time to maximize accuracy and consistency of measurement.

The ages recommended are satisfactory and the number of trials is more than adequate. The test can be used as a drill or as a conditioning exercise. The test cannot be self administered easily, however, it is completely safe. Because of its lack of objectivity, the test is not precise enough for use in research.

NOTE: The duration of this test is sometimes lengthened and the test used to measure endurance. While the test does provide a strenuous workload for measuring endurance, it has the same problem as when measuring agility. That is, it is difficult to keep the form consistent, particularly as the examinee becomes fatigued. It is also difficult to standardize the workload.

SUMMARY

Major Strengths:

1. The test requires no special equipment.
2. The test can be used as a conditioner (particularly if the time is lengthened.)

Major Weaknesses:

1. The validity of the test is very questionable.

2. The test, at best, measures only one aspect of agility.

3. The test is very difficult to administer accurately because it requires checking many aspects of form while the examinee is moving rapidly.

The Squat Thrust or Burpee Test is an unacceptable test. It is inadequate for research because of the validity and precision problems mentioned earlier. For class purposes, it can be used if the tester is aware of its limitations and uses great care in administering the test.

Chapter 3

BALANCE

DYNAMIC BALANCE TESTS

BALANCE BEAM WALK TEST

Reference.
Jensen, C. R., & Hirst, C. C. (1980). *Measurement in physical education and athletics.* New York: Macmillan Publishing, p 165.

Additional Sources.
Barrow et al. (1989, p. 128); Bosco & Gustafson (1983, pp. 120-121); Hastad & Lacy (1989, p. 266); Miller (1988, p. 138); Safrit (1986, p. 334); Safrit (1990, pp. 504-505).

Purpose.
To measure the dynamic balance of an examinee while walking on a regulation balance beam.

Objectivity.
Not reported.

Reliability.
Not reported.

Validity.
Not reported.

Age and Sex.
Not reported, but suitable for age 6 - adult.

Equipment.
A regulation balance beam with adequate mats positioned around and under the beam.

Space Requirements and Design.
A clear, level area approximately 3m x 9m (10' x 30') with the balance beam placed down the center of the 3m width.

Directions.
The examinee assumes a standing position on one end of the beam. The examinee then walks slowly the length of the beam, pauses five seconds, turns around and walks back to the starting end of the beam. A total of three trials are given.

Scoring.
The score is a "Pass" if the examinee successfully completes the balance task or a "Fail" if the examinee is unsuccessful in completing the task.

Norms.
Not reported.

NOTE: In order to make the test more difficult, a beam (2" x 12') may be substituted for the regulation beam. The criteria to be used in deciding what is a "Pass" and what is a "Fail" are not stated.

REVIEW

MARK J. MEKA, M.S.

Assistant Professor
Health and Physical Education
Lake Tahoe Community College
South Lake Tahoe, CA 95702

The Balance Beam Walk Test does measure dynamic balance and, from a scientific stand point, is a valid test that could be used in a very generic or basic type of screening. However, certain variables have to be taken into account which are not described in the literature. For example, the raised beam can affect some examinees' success as opposed to a beam on the floor. In addition, whether or not the examinees wear shoes may have an effect on their performance.

The test does show consistency in test administration since only one tester is needed to administer and evaluate the test. Furthermore, the directions are simple and easy to follow. The equipment and space requirements seem reasonable. Many facilities have a balance beam, or reasonable access to one.

The time factor is not a problem since most examinees complete the test in a matter of seconds. The three trials are adequate. Most examinees should need only one trial. The test is suitable for different age levels, not however, for the different ability levels at each age. The gender of the examinee may play a part in performance at specific age levels. The test is basically safe, if adequate mats are placed as described, however, examinees could slip and injure themselves on the beam itself.

The scoring is objective but too generic for research purposes. Examinees could evaluate themselves if necessary.

SUMMARY

Major Strengths:

1. Ease of administration requiring only one tester to supervise the test.
2. Many examinees can be tested in a very short amount of time.
3. The space and equipment needs are minimal.

4. The scoring is simple and easy to assess.

Major Weaknesses:

1. The test is too basic for extended research and/or conditioning, unless a narrower beam is used.

2. Gender discriminations could occur since many males have a more aggressive exercise history.

3. Beam height could be a factor for some examinees.

4. Even though the scoring is simple, it would not be adequate for research purposes.

The Balance Beam Walk Test, as described, is unacceptable for research but could be used as a very basic screening assessment for special or adapted physical education students. Modifications could be made, such as using a narrower beam on ground level, or developing a more comprehensive scoring system which assigns points 1 to 5 for performance.

BASS DYNAMIC BALANCE TEST

Reference.
Bass, R. I. (1939). An analysis of the components of tests of semicircular canal function and of static and dynamic balance. *Research Quarterly,* 10(2):33-52.

Additional Source.
Bosco & Gustafson (1983, pp. 121-122).

Purpose.
To measure the dynamic balance of an examinee while leaping from one location to another.

Objectivity.
Not reported.

Reliability.
r = .95.

Validity.
r = .69 with motor judgement and r = .74 with rhythm judgement.

Age and Sex.
Suitable for females and males, age 10 - college.

Equipment.
A stopwatch, protractor, tape measure and marking tape, chalk, or a felt tip marker.

Space Requirements and Design.
A clear, level area approximately 6m (20') square with 11 circles 21.59cm (8.5") in diameter. The first circle is drawn 45.72cm (18") forward of the starting circle (X). All the other circles are laid out 83.82cm (33") from the previous one. Circle 2 is located to the right of circle 1 at an angle of (112.5 degrees) from a straight line through the centers of circles X and 1. Circles 3 and 4 are located to the left of 2 on a straight line at an angle of (56.25 degrees) formed by a straight line through circles 1 and 2. Circle 5 is located to the right of 4 at an angle of (67.5 degrees) from a straight line through the centers of circles 2, 3 and 4. Circles 6 and 7 are located to the left of 5 on a straight line at an angle of (67.5 degrees) from a straight line through circles 5, 6 and 7. Circle 9 is located to the left of 8 at an angle of (22.5 degrees) from the line through circles 7 and 8. Circle 10 is located

directly forward of 9 at an angle of (90 degrees) from a straight line through circles 8 and 9 (Figure 3-1).

Directions.
The examinee stands in circle (X) with the right foot and begins the test by leaping into circle 1 with the left foot, circle 2 with the right foot, and so on alternating feet. The examinee must leave the floor completely when leaping from circle to circle and land on the ball of the foot within each circle. The examinee must remain within each circle for five seconds. It is an error if the examinee: (1) permits the heel to touch the floor, (2) hops upon the supporting foot, (3) slides or wriggles the supporting foot while within a circle, (4) touches the circle's boundary lines or the floor outside the circle with the supporting foot, (5) touches the floor with the other foot, or (6) touches the floor with any other part of the body. Each of these errors counts as a penalty point. The tester should start the stopwatch when the examinee leaps from the starting circle and count out loud when the examinee alights in each circle. If the examinee leaps to the next circle before the count of five, there is no penalty and the tester simply starts another five count when the examinee alights in the next circle. If the examinee remains in a circle longer than the count of five, the additional seconds are deducted from the total time used to cover the 10 circles.

Scoring.
The score = 50 + (the number of seconds required to take the test) - (3) (the number of errors made).

Norms.
Simons et al. (1990, p. 104) girls.

REVIEW

JEANNE WENOS, P.E.D.

Assistant Professor
Physical Education
Western Washington University
Bellingham, WA 98225

Dynamic balance has been defined as the ability of the body to perform purposeful movements while overcoming the effects of gravity

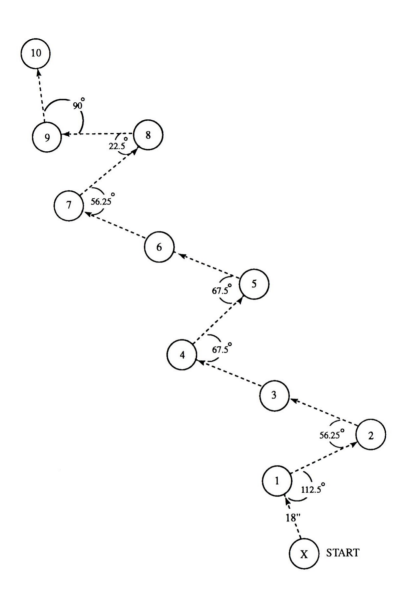

Figure 3-1. Bass Dynamic Balance Test with circles 8.5" in diameter and 33" apart.

(Kirchner, 1988; Keough & Sugden, 1985). It can involve a change of positions that reflect either a single change or a series of changes. In terms of face validity, and based upon this discussion, the Bass Test, which evaluates a series of dynamic to static movements, is a valid measure of dynamic balance. Content validity coefficients have been reported on two judgments: for a motor judgement $r = .69$ and for a rhythm judgement $r = .74$.

The Bass Test is reported to have a reliability coefficient of .95, meaning that a set of balance measurements on a given group remains the

same over repeated measurements. This test was administered to 20 examinees by two novice testers and was found to have an inter rater reliability coefficient of .89. This is a reasonable measure of objectivity, indicating that the test measures balance consistently when given by different testers.

The test can be administered in a space such as a classroom or part of a gymnasium. Some initial learning is required by the examinee to understand and establish the rhythm involved and by the tester, who must evaluate the examinees' rhythm as they proceed from target to target. One must simultaneously observe the examinee for errors while looking at a stopwatch for the total time spent on each target. The job is complicated by the fact that the tester must count the examinee's time on target out loud in seconds. The tester can easily miss an error when several are made by the examinee in rapid succession. Although examinees could be asked to count their own errors, it is not recommended because there is apt to be a lack of objectivity on the part of the examinees while they are performing. For these reasons, although only one tester is indicated, two are necessary.

Test set up is not only time consuming, but it is a tedious job to measure the angles and ensure that the target patterns are the correct size. One can feasibly test 25 or 30 examinees in one class period since a single trial requires approximately one minute. It is unclear how many trials are recommended.

The Bass Test can be utilized as a drill to enhance dynamic balance. Although one could not accurately measure one's own time on each target, it would be possible to roughly estimate the total amount of time taken to complete the test.

The Bass Test is appropriate for use within a wide age range and does not appear to discriminate, in terms of age, among its users. However, it cannot be used readily by certain disabled populations, including those who are blind or have limited vision, or those who have moderate to severe spasticity involving the lower limbs (who also benefit from measures of dynamic balance). It may be inappropriate, as well, for use with the moderately and severely retarded.

The test was initially conducted using cut out circular target patterns that were taped to the floor. To avoid injury, the slippery targets were eliminated and exchanged for patterns made solely of tape applied directly onto the gym floor.

With adequate practice, the administration of the Bass Test may be of sufficient precision to be used for research purposes. It's precision does not equal another measure of dynamic balance, the stability platform, because quantification of the Bass Test relies on human judgement.

SUMMARY

Major Strengths:

1. It is administered in a relatively small space.

2. The test equipment is minimal; little or no expense is involved.

3. The test itself takes approximately one minute to complete; therefore an entire class can be tested in a single class period.

4. The test is reliable.

5. Some self evaluation is possible, making the test suitable for use as a dynamic balance drill.

Major Weaknesses:

1. The test is time consuming and tedious to set up.

2. Some experience is required of the testers, and for best results, there should be orientation for the examinees.

3. Human judgement is the basis for quantification of scores.

4. Norms are not provided.

5. Impractical for use with certain types of disabling conditions.

This is an acceptable test that is adequate for research and/or teaching with the following qualifications: examinees receive an orientation to the test, more than one tester is used, and the testers receive training and experience before using this test for research. If used for research, one must consider the effect that the presence of two testers might have on an examinee's performance. Also, it must be used in conjunction with other balance measures since norms are not available. This test could be utilized as a self test for dynamic balance or by teachers on a criterion reference basis.

HEXAGON RAIL WALKING (FLEISHMAN'S) TEST

Reference.
Fleishman, E. A. (1964B). *The structure and measurement of physical fitness.* Englewood Cliffs: Prentice Hall, pp 86-89.

Additional Sources.
None.

Purpose.
To measure the ability of an examinee to maintain balance while walking backward on a narrow support.

Objectivity.
Not reported.

Reliability.
Not reported.

Validity.
Not reported.

Age and Sex.
Not reported, but suitable for females and males, age 8 - adult.

Equipment.
A rigid hexagon rail constructed of boards 1.90cm wide x 8.89cm high x 60.96cm long (.75" wide x 3.5" high x 24" long).

Space Requirements and Design.
A clear, level area approximately 3m (10') square with the hexagon positioned in the center.

Directions.
The examinee assumes a standing position on the hexagon rail. The feet must be positioned and maintained on one board segment at a time. The long axis of each foot must be kept parallel to the length of the segments on which they are placed. The examinee begins the test when ready by walking backward, placing one foot at a time on one new segment. The test is terminated when the examinee falls off the hexagon, steps on two board segments at one time, or fails to keep the feet parallel to the segments.

Scoring.
The score is the number of segments the examinee steps on before the test is terminated.

NOTE: To lessen the chances of the rail being overturned, the hexagon could be attached to a piece of plywood. In a further attempt to prevent injury, and to standardize the test, it is recommended that the tester use a stopwatch to establish a cadence, thus requiring the examinee to maintain balance on each segment for a specified time.

Norms.
Fleishman (1964B, p. 93) men.

REVIEW

JOHN DAGGER, Ph.D.

Assistant Professor
Physical Education
University of Illinois at Chicago
Chicago, IL 60680

The Rail Walking Test (RWT) described above purports to measure backward walking balance on a narrow support. It was taken from a classic text by Fleishman (1964) describing research to identify the components of "physical proficiency." As such, the RWT was designed to present a unique challenge to the examinee, which would measure a central balance trait with high inter subject variability. Although there is evidence that this test was successful in obtaining the variability, several aspects would caution the potential tester in selecting the RWT for broad application.

On a practical level, the test is easily administered and scored, requiring a minimal amount of time or training. The construction of the test apparatus is rather straightforward, presenting no real technical or fiscal restraints. The addition of the stabilizing plywood base removes any exceptional safety concerns. This balance task is unique and very challenging, one which would be motivating to and appropriate for children in a physical education body management curriculum. As a test, however, the documentation of procedures is inadequate. The test constructor failed to specify the number of trials to be given. The first obvious question is whether the examinee should be given a practice trial, seemingly necessary, especially to ensure young children's understanding of the task.

The lack of normative data across age levels would also limit the applicability of test results to locally derived norms, and then the interpretation of such information (e.g., the diagnosis of an examinee by comparison to the group mean) would necessarily be so circumspect as to only identify examinees with already obvious neuromotor problems. Of further concern is the assertion of appropriateness for all ages over eight. On this point, one must consider the fixed size of the balance apparatus in relation to the varying body segment lengths of differing aged children. Motor learning literature has suggested that, even in the case of linear positioning tasks, movement and its control is defined by angular parameters (Horgan & Horgan, 1982). Thus, requiring a child with a short limb length to step around the frame may be a much different task than that required of an adult with much longer limb length.

Because this test was originally one of 12 items measuring balance and 30 items measuring speed, flexibility, balance, and coordination for factor analysis, much of the quantitative evaluative information is missing from its description. Although the administration and scoring procedures are quite objective, there is little reason to assume high validity or reliability. In fact, results of a single unrehearsed trial on this item could be expected to be quite unreliable. Not only is the movement challenge complex, requiring rotation across the sagittal plane while walking backward, but the support structure is markedly narrower and more challenging than what is currently in common use, further increasing the complexity of the task. Inter subject variability obtained in Fleishman's original study, in which 204 approximately 18 year old Navy recruits produced a mean score of 15.34 steps (SD = 14.96) would support speculation about low reliability. Many tests, attempting to measure a balance, have obtained higher reliability by adding trials or items or both (Bruininks, 1978), again raising the question of number of trials. The instability of balance test performance over practice trials is well accepted, which is one contributing reason for its frequent use in motor learning research (Baumgartner & Jackson, 1987). Clearly, further work is needed to establish reliability and validity of this test.

It is impossible to examine the question of test validity without questioning the application of test results. Certainly, there remains a lively debate as to the validity of interpreting any performance in terms of a general motor ability trait (Hensley & East, 1989). If it may, in fact, be assumed that a motor ability balance performance predicts performance or learning of other tasks, then the RWT should demonstrate that it represents a balance trait. Factor analysis (Fleishman, 1964) failed to support this. In an analysis of 30 items, the RWT was one of 12 balance items investigated, and it was the only item which would be one of dynamic balance considered today. The only factor, on which it loaded heavily, was the balance factor, but it ranked fifth out of six items selected in variance accounted for by the factor and it failed selection in a factor identified as balance with eyes open. Additionally, no predictive validity data were developed.

SUMMARY

Major Strengths:

1. Materials are readily available and it can be safely and efficiently administered.

2. It is very objective in its scoring (yielding high inter and intra scorer reliability) and may be used in a self monitoring goal setting activity format.

3. The unique challenge it yields is particularly appropriate to elaborative balance practice as recommended by Battinelli (1984).

Major Weaknesses:

1. A lack of any reliability information or data from repeated trials to identify a learning curve.

2. An attending lack of norm referenced information.

3. A failure to establish either construct or predictive validity.

Although the validity of the RWT as a marker of specific or general neurophysiological readiness has not been established, intuitively, the RWT would seem to possess face validity, making it acceptable as a learning or training task to promote the development of skilled dynamic balance within a body management curriculum.

REVIEW REFERENCES

Battinelli, T. (1984). From motor ability to motor learning: The generality/specificity connection. *The Physical Educator,* 41, pp 108-113.

Baumgartner, T. A., & Jackson, A. S. (1987). *Measurement for evaluation in physical education* (3rd ed.). Dubuque, IA: Wm. C. Brown.

Bruininks, R. H. (1978). *Bruininks-Oseretsky test of motor proficiency,* Circle Pines, MN: American Guidance Service.

Fleishman, E. A. (1964). *The structure and measurement of physical fitness*. Englewood Cliffs: Prentice Hall.

Horgan, J. S., & Horgan, J. S. (1982). Measurement bias in representing accuracy of movement on linear-positioning tasks. *Perceptual and Motor Skills,* 55, pp 971-981.

Hensley, L. D., & East, W. B. (1989). Testing and grading in the psychomotor domain. In Safrit, M. J., & Wood, T. M. (Eds.), *Measurement concepts in physical education and exercise science.* Champaign, IL: Human Kinetics Books, pp 297-321.

LINE WALK TEST

Reference.
Powell, R. L. (1984). Dynamic balance testing. *National Strength and Conditioning Association Journal*, 6(4):42D.

Additional Sources.
None.

Purpose.
To measure the visualization abilities of an examinee by testing balance.

Objectivity.
Not reported.

Reliability.
Not reported.

Validity.
Not reported.

Age and Sex.
Not reported, but suitable for females and males, age 8 - adult.

Equipment.
Marking tape, tape measure, and stopwatch.

Space Requirements and Design.
A clear, level area that would allow for a 6m (20') long line to be marked.

Directions.
The examinee assumes an upright position on one end of the 6m (20') line. The examinee is asked to concentrate on the line and then to close the eyes. On command, the examinee walks heel to toe down the line until he/she thinks the line has ended. A 20 second time limit is given.

Scoring.
The score is from a rating of 1 to 5 based on performance. One point is awarded if the examinee does not lose balance and gets within 1 to 2 feet of the end of the line. Two points are awarded if the examinee experiences some balance problems but walks close to the end of the line. Three, four or five points are awarded if the examinee indicates increasingly greater difficulty with balance and does one or more of the following: uses arms for balance, walks off the line, loses balance or opens eyes.

Norms.
Not reported.

REVIEW

REGINALD T-A. OCANSEY, Ph.D.

Assistant Professor
Physical Education
State University of New York,
College at Brockport
Brockport, NY 14420

The test incorporates some physical components of dynamic balance (i.e., Line Walk) however, it does not directly measure dynamic balance. Whereas the Line Walk is a logical component in the measurement of dynamic balance, it may not be directly relevant when the purpose of the test is to measure visualization abilities. In addition, the test constructor did not report the test's objectivity, reliability or validity.

The test requires very minimal space and equipment and does not require the active participation of another individual. It can be administered in any clear open area that allows for a 20 foot line. The test components and procedures are thoroughly described and can be administered easily by one tester.

The amount of time required for the administration of the test is very minimal. The duration of the test for one examinee is 20 seconds. No trial is required prior to participation. In fact, the test can be used for training or conditioning purposes through practice repetitions. Therefore, trials may positively influence test data.

The test is both physically and psychologically safe. The test is not gender or age specific. There is no information regarding age, sex, or norms.

The scoring system requires subjective judgments from the second to the fifth points on the five point rating scale. The subjectivity of the scoring procedure may impose a limitation for self scoring. An examinee may be able to self score the first rating only and not the other points on the five point scale. This is because the first point has a clearly defined standard. Some form of training will be necessary for testers on the other points of the rating scale in order to ensure reliability and objectivity of test data.

SUMMARY

Major Strengths:

1. The test is easy to administer.

2. The test requires very minimal use of human, equipment, facilities, and temporal resources for administration.

3. The test is economically feasible.

4. The test requires very minimal personnel to administer.

5. The tester may require very minimal training.

Major Weaknesses:

1. The test lacks important information for judging objectivity, reliability, and validity.

2. The relationship between the test's purpose (measuring visualization abilities) and dynamic balance lacks clarity.

3. The subjective nature of some aspects of the scoring system may impose serious limitations upon the objectivity and reliability of the test data.

The test is not suitable for research purposes. It is clearly a diagnostic test and more suitable for assessing visualization abilities rather than dynamic balance. Since this test is intended to measure visualization abilities, "Visualization Abilities Testing" may be the appropriate description rather than Dynamic Balance Testing.

Dynamic balance is the ability to maintain equilibrium while in motion (Safrit, 1990). The Line Walk logically represents a component of dynamic balance as in the Balance Beam Walk (Jensen & Hirst, 1980). The Balance Beam Walk and Line Walk both possess the logical content that describe the ability to maintain equilibrium while moving. Thus, it appears that modifications can be made in the Line Walk to measure dynamic balance directly. For example, the Line Walk can be considered as a lower level progression to the Balance Beam Walk. The Line Walk-Balance Beam Walk continuum suggests that the Line Walk may be modified to take on some of the physical characteristics of the Balance Beam Walk Test. However, there must be a time limitation to prevent an excessively slow walk. Also, clear penalties should be identified for all errors that occur throughout the test.

With appropriate modification and validation, the Line Walk can be utilized for assessing dynamic balance and also, for prescriptive or intervention purposes in physical activity settings.

MODIFIED BASS DYNAMIC BALANCE TEST

References.

Johnson, B. L., & Leach, J. (1968). A modification of the bass test of dynamic balance. Unpublished study, East Texas State University.

Johnson, B. L., & Nelson, J. K. (1986). *Practical measurements for evaluation in physical education*. Edina, MN: Burgess, pp 242-243.

Additional Sources.

Hastad & Lacy (1989, pp. 264-265); Jensen & Hirst (1980, pp. 165-167); Kirkendall et al. (1980, pp. 251, 254); Kirkendall et al. (1987, pp. 129-130); Miller (1988, pp. 137-138); Safrit (1986, pp. 332-333); Safrit (1990, pp. 502-503).

Purpose.

To measure the ability of an examinee to leap accurately and to maintain balance after leaping from one location to another.

Objectivity.

r = .97.

Reliability.

r = .75 by test-retest method.

Validity.

Face or content validity is accepted.

Age and Sex.

Females and males, high school through college.

Equipment.

A stopwatch, 1.90cm (3/4") wide marking tape, and a tape measure.

Space Requirements and Design.

A clear, level area approximately 2m x 7m (6' x 20') with 11 pieces of marking tape 1.90cm x 2.54cm (.75" x 1") arranged as illustrated (Figure 3-2).

Directions.

The examinee stands on the starting tape marker with the right foot. When the examinee feels ready, he/she leaps and alights on marker 1 on the ball of the left foot. The examinee holds this balanced position for five seconds. The examinee then leaps and alights on marker 2 on the ball of the right foot for five seconds. The examinee continues alternating feet for each successive tape marker until the test is completed.

The examinee must hold the balanced position at each marker for five seconds. Penalties are classified into landing errors and balance errors. Five points are deducted for committing a landing error. It is a landing error if the examinee: (1) fails to stop upon alighting, (2) touches the floor with any part of the body other than the ball of the supporting foot, and (3) fails to cover the tape marker completely with the ball of the foot. If a landing error is committed, the examinee can reposition the foot to begin the five second balance. It is a balance error if the examinee (1) touches the floor with any part of the body other than the ball of the supporting foot or (2) moves the foot while in the balanced position. One point is deducted for each of the five seconds remaining when the examinee commits either of the balance errors. Whenever balance is lost, the examinee must stand back on the appropriate mark and leap to the next tape mark. The tester should use the stopwatch to assist in counting the five second periods aloud at each marker.

Scoring.

The score is 5 points for each tape marker the examinee successfully lands on plus 1 point for each second (up to a maximum of 5 seconds) balance is maintained at each marker.

Norms.

Harrison & Bradbeer (1982, pp. 24-25) boy and girl athletes; Johnson & Nelson (1986, p. 243) women; Kirkendall et al. (1980, p. 253) women; Kirkendall et al. (1987, p. 130) women.

REVIEW

MARY L. DAWSON, Ph.D.

Associate Professor
Health, Physical Education and
Recreation
Western Michigan University
Kalamazoo, MI 49008

Based on the reliability (r = .75), calculated by the test-retest method and the validity, face or content, some concerns arise regarding the scientific aspects of the Modified Bass Test of

Dynamic Balance. First, the name of the test is misleading in that it indicates only dynamic balance is being measured. However, after reading about the test and its purpose, it becomes obvious that two variables are measured: dynamic balance and accuracy of movement. Second, one must question the relationship between the two variables being measured: movement accuracy and dynamic balance. If these two variables have a high correlation coefficient there would be less concern regarding the interpretation of individual scores. However, if they are not related then individual scores on this test will be difficult or impossible to interpret. Third, these variables are integral parts of one another and are commonly observed in activities such as gymnastics, dance, and figure skating and are important to the functional and aesthetic components of these sports.

The low to moderate reliability coefficient may be a result of the composition of the test, the scoring of the test, or a combination of these factors. First, the score is a combination of movement accuracy and dynamic balance ability. If one or both of these variables is altered or changed to a small degree from trial to trial, scores would change. The score will not reflect which variable changed; one or both. Second, the methods used to score dynamic balance and movement accuracy are different. Movement accuracy is measured by an all or none concept. Five points are awarded if the ball of the foot completely covers an area marked on the floor. If any part of the mark is not covered or any other landing error is detected, zero points are awarded. The points awarded for the dynamic balance portion of the test can be any number from zero to five. One point is awarded for every second that the examinee is able to balance with the ball of the foot remaining on the marked area.

The high test objectivity, r = .97, reflects that the directions for administrating and scoring the test are easy to understand, follow, and interpret. In addition, a well defined scoring procedure is outlined for adding and subtracting points under a variety of situations. To enhance the objectivity, two testers should administer the test; one tester to count the points given to the dynamic balance portion of the test and one tester to look for errors in landing. Thus, each tester is able to concentrate on a reasonable number of observations throughout the duration of the test. The second individual required to help administer the test could be a student since that individual in no way interacts with the examinee. Since the test consists of points awarded for two different variables, it would be hard for the examinee to use the test for self evaluation.

Equipment and facility needs for the test are minimal. A flat surface approximately 6' x 20', stopwatch, floor marking tape, and tape measure are all that are needed. The testing site is easy to set up and requires a minimal amount of time. The test does not specify the number of trials that

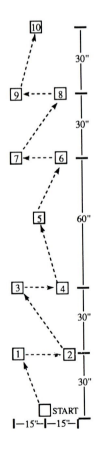

Figure 3-2. Modified Bass Dynamic Balance Test.

should be given for practice or for the test. However, the testing site is constructed in a manner that requires the examinee to repeat the movement accuracy task and the balance task 10 times alternating feet. Therefore, to a certain degree, trials are built into the repetitive cyclic nature of the test. The testing set up and administrative needs tend to allow only one examinee at a time to be tested. However, if the tester(s) is organized, a large number of examinees can be tested in a short amount of time.

The test was intended for college age women. However, the test is within the motor development ability of junior and senior high school, male and female students. With modification to the distance required for the dynamic aspects, the test could be used with younger examinees. Johnson and Nelson (1986) provide norms for college age women; norms need to be developed for other genders and age groups.

SUMMARY

Major Strengths:

1. A high degree of objectivity reflecting the test's standardized directions, scoring, and site preparation make the test appealing as a field test.

2. Equipment needs and physical site requirements make this test practical for many situations.

3. The time requirements for administering and preparing the test are minimal.

Major Weaknesses:

1. The reliability is moderate and would not be acceptable in most research settings.

2. Due to the moderate reliability, the validity of the test would be questionable.

3. The test measures more than one variable.

4. Norms were established for college age women on a small sample size, n = 100.

Because the test measures more than one variable and the reliability is moderate, r = .75, this test would not be appropriate for research purposes. However, the test could be used as a screening device or field test with the understanding that the scores represent both movement accuracy and dynamic balance. The score cannot be used as a measure of one variable exclusive of the other. Also, the norms are based on a small sample of college age women from a single institution. Therefore, the ability to generalize the reported norms to other settings is questionable.

STATIC BALANCE TESTS

BASS STICK TESTS

References.

Bass, R. I. (1939). An analysis of the components of tests of semicircular canal function and of static and dynamic balance. *Research Quarterly,* 10(2):33-52.

Johnson, B. L., & Nelson, J. K. (1986). *Practical measurements for evaluation in physical education,* Edina, MN: Burgess, pp 238-240, 443-444.

Additional Sources.

Bosco & Gustafson (1983, pp. 118-119); Hastad & Lacy (1989, pp. 261-263); Jensen & Hirst (1980, pp. 160-161); Kirkendall et al. (1980, pp. 325-327) variation; Miller (1988, pp. 136-137); Safrit (1986, pp. 330-331); Safrit (1990, p. 499); Verducci (1980, pp. 257-258).

Purpose.

To measure the static balance of an examinee while standing on the ball of the foot on a narrow surface.

Objectivity.

Not reported.

Reliability.

$r = .90$ for foot crosswise and $r = .86$ for foot lengthwise.

Validity.

$r = .49$ for crosswise and $r = .50$ for lengthwise and ratings of general motor ability in women.

Age and Sex.

Suitable for females and males, age 10 - college.

Equipment.

A stick .39cm x .39cm x 30.5cm (1" x 1" x 12"), adhesive tape, and a stopwatch.

Space Requirements and Design.

A clear, level area approximately 2m (6') square with the stick and the examinee in the center.

Directions.

The examinee places the supporting foot perpendicular (crosswise) to the stick with the ball of the foot resting on top of the stick. On command, the examinee lifts the opposite foot from the floor and attempts to balance on the stick up to a maximum time of 60 seconds. If any part of the non supporting foot or either the heel or toe of the supporting foot touch the floor, the trial is terminated and the time recorded. Up to three practice trials and a total of three legal trials are given for each foot. The second count should be given aloud during each of the trials.

The above directions are also used to measure static balance with the supporting foot parallel (lengthwise) to the stick instead of perpendicular.

Scoring.

The score is the total time for all three trials with the foot crosswise and for all three trials with the foot lengthwise.

Norms.

Johnson & Nelson (1986, pp. 239-240, 444) boys, men and women; Kirkendall et al. (1980, pp. 328-330) boys and girls (variation); McCaughan (1975, p. 16) boys (variation); Miller (1988, p. 135) men and women; Ostyn et al. (1980, p. 110) boys.

REVIEW

HERBERTA M. LUNDEGREN, Ph.D.

Professor of Physical Education and Leisure Studies
The Pennsylvania State University
University Park, PA 16802

The Bass Balance tests are among the oldest tests in the literature whose purpose it is to measure static and dynamic balance. Because of their longevity they have been used extensively, with recent use being less widespread partially because researchers have questioned what the components of balance are and whether its components can be measured separately. In the early days of the move in physical education to include testing of motor and physical performance factors in program planning, it was believed that in the area of balance one could test for something called static balance in which movement is not involved, and dynamic balance, which involves maintaining equilibrium while moving from place to place. Easy as it would be to test for and categorize the ability to achieve balance as though it were comprised of independently testable factors, that is not true. The basic constituents of each are the same, but manifest themselves in the task differently. The semicircular canals of the inner ear, proprioceptors in the muscles and joints, pressure receptors on the soles of the feet, the eyes, and the location of the center of gravity of the body during the assumption or maintenance of a certain position all contribute to being "balanced" or "in equilibrium." In the Bass Stick Test, then, what is being measured? The purpose given is "to measure static balance while standing on the ball of the foot on a narrow surface." Such a specific description narrows the possibility of generalization of the skill to a range of situations. All the components of balance mentioned here are probably involved in this particular test. Further, it has been shown in various studies that performance on this type of test improves with training. The statistics on the test show that it has satisfactory reliability, that is, it tests the same thing consistently. However, the validity correlations are more moderate and if one is using the test as a verification of motor abilities of women then some caution should be shown in interpretation of the data. The results of this test would probably be helpful in pinpointing skill abilities used in certain sports, such as balance beam, and with modern dancers.

SUMMARY

Major Strengths:

1. This test is easy to use, takes up very little space, and does not take much time to give.

2. The results are known immediately.

3. It is usable over a wide range of ages.

Major Weaknesses:

1. It specifically prohibits generalization to other balance situations.

2. No mention is made of what the arm position should be, whether the eyes should be open or closed or whether the gaze should be focused on a spot during the test performance; so, the tester assumes these factors should be allowed to float and not be mentioned. Since these factors influence performance, it might be useful to control them for a set of trials given in order to see if performance varies.

This test is acceptable as a tool to measure specific static balance for use in both research and teaching. For example, if a study is designed to see whether static balance can be improved over the course of a program or season, then this test may well be used to document that change. It may be concluded from all of this that balance is specific to the activity, and being able to perform the skill of the given activity is the best test.

BOARD BALANCE TEST

Reference.

Fleishman, E. A. (1964B). *The structure and measurement of physical fitness.* Englewood Cliffs: Prentice Hall, pp 88, 93.

Additional Sources.

None.

Purpose.

To measure the ability of an examinee to maintain balance while standing on a movable support.

Objectivity.

Not reported.

Reliability.

Not reported.

Validity.

Construct validity was established.

Age and Sex.

Suitable for females and males, age 13 - adult.

Equipment.

A stopwatch and a teeter board constructed of wood 2.54cm thick x 30.48cm wide x 60.96cm long (1" x 12" x 24") supported in the middle by a board 5.08cm wide x 10.16cm high x 30.48cm long (2" x 4" x 12") whose bottom edge has been planed off to a 2.54cm (1") width.

Space Requirements and Design.

A clear, level area approximately 2m (6') square with the teeter board positioned in the center.

Directions.

While placing one hand on the tester's shoulder, the examinee assumes a balanced standing position on the teeter board. When the examinee feels properly balanced, he/she removes the hand from the tester's shoulder and tries to maintain balance for as long as possible. The tester starts the stopwatch when the examinee's hand is removed from the shoulder and stops the stopwatch when either end of the teeter board touches the floor or the examinee falls off the board.

Scoring.

The score is the number of seconds the examinee maintains the desired position.

Norms.

Fleishman (1964B, p. 93) men.

NOTE: The number of trials is not stated nor is the exact positioning of the feet on the teeter board standardized.

REVIEW

WILLIE S. SMITH, Ed.D.

Associate Professor
Physical Education
North Carolina Central University
Durham, NC 27707

The procedure as described in the test purpose is generally accepted as an adequate measure of static balance, although the precise foot placement and body position to be held while executing the test are not furnished. Test validity could be improved by specifically describing the requirements for each of these. While the establishment of construct validity is indicated, statistical validity measures are not reported. The same is true for the test's reliability and objectivity, as statistical measures for these characteristics are also unreported. The test requires active involvement by a tester who hand scores the examinee's performance with a stopwatch and thus, the performance outcome could be significantly affected as it is largely dependent upon the tester's overall scoring precision.

Test administration considerations such as facility and/or space requirements are set as are essential equipment specifications. Viewed together, these administrative concerns pose little or no problem, although the teeter board with dimensions as specified may not be within the current equipment inventory of most facilities. The test is quite easy to administer, but precision in using the stopwatch is necessary. This test is administered by a single tester, it can be quite a time consuming process especially with large groups and when examinees hold their balance for lengthy periods. Although information on the number of trials to be administered is not provided, the test could be useful in serving as a motivational tool with results allowed to be used only as a rough indication of an examinee's balance. In this respect it is quite suitable for use among the age and ability levels intended. The test is quite safe and lacks any difficult task requirements. While scoring objectivity is dependent upon the precision and accuracy of the tester, this factor limits the ease by which the test could be used for self evaluation purposes. As constructed, the test is not viewed to be of suitable precision for research purposes. Test norms are unfurnished for the intended age groups and sexes.

SUMMARY

Major Strengths:

1. The test is quite easy to administer and can be used with females as well as males of most age levels.

2. It is safe and free of difficult task assignments.

3. Mass testing poses no problems especially when assistants are thoroughly familiarized with testing procedures.

4. The test can be a useful motivational tool and can provide rough estimates of the static balance ability of examinees.

Major Weaknesses:

1. The precise foot placement and position the examinee is expected to hold while balancing are not clearly defined.

2. Technical material on validity, reliability, objectivity, and norms is not furnished.

3. Practical matters in preparing examinees for the test such as type of clothing and whether footwear is to be worn or removed are not addressed.

4. Availability of a teeter board constructed to the specifications outlined may pose a problem.

5. Information on test demonstration and test trials is not furnished.

6. The test could be quite time consuming, especially if large numbers of examinees hold their balance for lengthy periods.

7. Scoring precision is dependent upon the accuracy of the tester.

This test is deemed inadequate for research or for teaching purposes because correlation coefficients on validity, reliability, objectivity, and norms are not furnished. These standards need to be given for sex and age groups intended to be tested. Additionally, some provision should be made for the examinee to see a demonstration of the test and perform trials prior to testing. The precise foot placement and balancing position to be held by the examinee should, also, be clearly defined. In general, however, the test could prove useful as a motivational tool for examinees and their resulting performances could be viewed as rough indicators of their static balance ability.

FLAMINGO BALANCE TEST

Reference.
Committee of Experts on Sports Research (1988). *Eurofit: handbook for the eurofit tests of physical fitness*. Rome, Italy, pp 16, 42-43.

Additional Sources.
None.

Purpose.
To measure the static balance of an examinee while standing on one leg.

Objectivity.
Had to be high to meet their criteria, but an exact figure is not reported (Committee, 1988, p. 16).

Reliability.
Had to be high to meet their criteria, but an exact figure is not reported (Committee, 1988, p. 16).

Validity.
Had to be high to meet their criteria, but an exact figure is not reported (Committee, 1988, p. 16).

Age and Sex.
Females and males, age 6 - 18.

Equipment.
A metal beam 3cm wide, 4cm high and 50cm long (1.2" x 1.6" x 19.7") which is covered with padding a maximum thickness of 5mm (.2"), two beam supports 2cm wide and 15cm long (.8" x 5.9"), and a stopwatch.

Space Requirements and Design.
A clear, level area approximately 3m (10') square with the beam on its supports positioned in the center.

Directions.
The barefoot examinee stands with the preferred foot on the beam and the other leg bent backward so that the top of its foot can be gripped in the hand on the same side of the body. The other hand, on the same side of the body as the preferred foot, is rested on the forearm of the tester who is positioned in front of the examinee (Figure 3-3a). When the examinee feels ready, he/she removes the hand from the tester and the stopwatch is started (Figure 3-3b). The examinee tries to maintain the balanced position for one minute. Each time the examinee lets go of the free leg or touches the floor with any body

part, the stopwatch is stopped. After each such instance, the same procedures used in beginning the test are repeated until one minute has elapsed. One practice trial and one legal trial are given.

Scoring.
The score is the number of attempts needed to remain balanced on the beam for one minute. If the examinee makes 15 attempts during the first 30 seconds, the test is terminated and a score of zero is recorded.

Norms.
Not reported.

REVIEW

SHERRY L. FOLSOM-MEEK, Ph.D.

Assistant Professor
Physical Education
University of Missouri
Columbia, MO 65211

Although this test purports to measure one foot static balance, no validity figures are available. Because the test is from a book of physical fitness tests, it appears that the test constructors consider static balance to be a measure of physical fitness. In recent motor development and physical education literature, static balance is classified as a test of motor fitness, not physical fitness. Although static balance requires strength, it is primarily a measure of the integrity of sensory input systems (visual, vestibular, proprioceptive, and tactile) and sensory motor integration. Measurement in the Flamingo Balance Test (number of attempts required to balance for 1 min.) is different from more common measures of static balance - time in balance and amount of sway. The test position is unusual, requires hyperflexion of the knee, and is similar to that of the now contraindicated quadriceps stretching exercise. This hyperflexion of the knee could cause stretching of ligaments and the joint capsule, possibly resulting in damage.

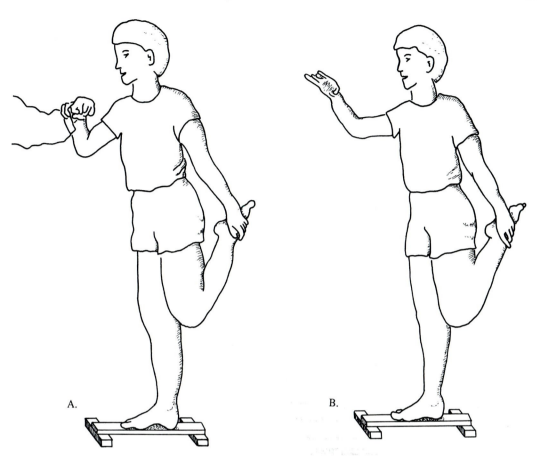

Figure 3-3. Flamingo Balance Test: (a) starting position and (b) balance position.

Reliability and objectivity figures are not included with the test description. Test directions are clear in regard to: (a) when to begin timing, (b) which trial counts, and (c) when to stop timing. The barefoot protocol eliminates the effect various types of shoes may have on the results of other balance tests. Test directions are not clear in regard to the following areas: (a) if eyes are open or closed, (b) what eyes should focus on if protocol is eyes open, (c) position of examinee's free arm after letting go of tester's arm, (d) position of thigh - vertical or flex hip so thigh tilts forward, (e) lateral position of nonsupport leg in relation to support leg, (f) how to determine "preferred" foot, and (g) whether tester can demonstrate test position. Lateral position of the nonsupport leg affects examinee's posture. Three lateral positions in relation to the support leg are possible: (a) not touching, (b) touching, and (c) pressing. Pressing usually occurs when the examinee requires greater proprioceptive and tactile feedback and results in a comma like posture.

It appears that a separate room is needed to administer the test. Although the size of the balance beam is standardized, it is very narrow (3cm wide) when compared to most balance beams. The ratio of width to height (3cm to 4cm) may frighten younger children and handicapped children and youth if they are gravitationally insecure.

The test would be difficult to administer because the tester is measuring the number of times the examinee loses balance during one minute. In addition to helping the examinee position herself/himself after losing balance and starting and stopping the stopwatch, the tester is responsible for counting the number of times the examinee loses balance. This test requires more time than other balance tests to administer; a minimum of two minutes is required for practice and legal trials. Most static balance tests measure for 10 to 15 seconds. One practice trial and one legal trial are allowed; the practice trial should allow for learning test position and requirements. The test is not suitable for use as a drill or for self evaluation because a one to one relationship between tester and examinee is required.

There is a wide age range stated for the Flamingo Balance Test, with no accompanying norms by age or gender. Generally, balance improves with age until age 12 and levels off, and girls outperform boys until age eight with similar abilities by gender after age eight. The test position may be difficult for younger children in the age range; it is difficult for some young children to achieve an easier position - the 90 degree bent leg. The suitability of measuring balance of adolescents is questionable unless neurological dysfunction is suspected. With neurological dysfunction, examinees would have difficulty achieving the test position.

If the test is intended to discriminate among its users, then age related norms or criterion reference numbers by age should be included. In addition, the scoring criteria includes varying types of measurement. According to the test developers, an examinee would score zero if he or she made 15 failed attempts during the first 30 seconds. However, the examinee could also score zero if he/she did not lose balance during the one minute time period. Differing types of measurement limit suitability of the test for research purposes.

There are several potentially dangerous aspects to the test. First, with extreme lateral swaying, an examinee could fall off the beam. Second, if the thigh is to be in a vertical position and the quadriceps are tight, then the pelvis may be tilted in an anterior direction; this position could cause low back strain.

SUMMARY

Major Strengths:

1. The balance beam is standardized.

2. Protocol is barefooted.

3. Both practice and legal trials are allowed.

Major Weaknesses:

1. The test encompasses a wide age range with no norms by age or gender and no criterion reference numbers by age.

2. The test position is unusual and is not clearly described.

3. The types of measurement within the scoring system differ.

The test is unacceptable for research and teaching for the following reasons: the balance beam may threaten the internal validity of a study due to reactive measures associated with testing, the differing types of measurement make scoring for research purposes inadequate, many younger examinees may not be able to achieve the test position, and for many examinees the test position may require more than one practice trial. Use of the test in school environments is impractical because it is too time consuming and requires a one to one tester/examinee ratio.

HAWAII BALANCE ON ONE FOOT TEST

Reference.

(Hawaii) Aizawa, H. M. (1989). Memo to district superintendents, principals, and physical education department heads. August 31. Honolulu, HI: Department of Education, pp 16, 19-20.

Additional Sources.

None.

Purpose.

To measure the ability of an examinee to maintain balance while standing.

Objectivity.

Not reported.

Reliability.

Not reported.

Validity.

Not reported.

Age and Sex.

Females and males, grades K - 3.

Equipment.

A stopwatch and a balance beam 5.08cm (2") wide and ". . . as long as possible" (Hawaii, 1989, p. 16). Since no other dimensions are stated, it is assumed that the beam is positioned directly on the floor.

Space Requirements and Design.

A clear, level area large enough to position the balance beam down the center.

Directions.

The examinee stands on the balance beam with one foot. It is assumed by the editor that the examinee may stand on the beam with the preferred foot. The tester starts the stopwatch when the examinee is balanced and stops the stopwatch when the examinee has maintained the balanced position for 180 seconds or the examinee's free leg touches: the beam, the standing leg, or the floor. The number of trials is not stated.

Scoring.

The score is the number of seconds the examinee is able to maintain the proper balanced position.

Norms.

Hawaii (1989, pp. 19-20) boys and girls.

REVIEW

MARY LOU VEAL, Ed.D.
Assistant Professor
Exercise and Sport Science
University of North Carolina at
Greensboro
Greensboro, NC 27412-5001

No information is reported on objectivity, reliability, or validity. The test is designed to be administered to one examinee at a time.

This test is very simple to administer since the only requirements are a 2" balance beam of unspecified length and a stopwatch. It could be used in practice situations for large numbers of children, provided there were sufficient numbers of the balance beams. Since the test instructions specify a maximum time limit of three minutes, examinees could be given an ample number of trials, although the number of trials is not specified.

Scoring for the test begins when the examinee is balanced but this may be difficult to determine with young children. The test is ended when the free leg touches the beam or when three minutes have elapsed. Because of the imprecise directions for starting the stopwatch, the test is not appropriate for research purposes, but it could be used in a school situation to diagnose balance problems in young children. Norms for the test are provided with the directions.

SUMMARY

Major Strengths:

1. The test is easy to administer.

2. There are few requirements for equipment and space.

3. The test is appropriate for young children.

Major Weaknesses:

1. No information on objectivity, reliability, or validity.

2. Directions for starting the stopwatch are imprecise.

The Hawaii Balance On One Foot is an acceptable test for teaching young children but is unacceptable for research because of the imprecise
directions for starting the stopwatch. While
there is face validity to the test as a diagnostic
tool, the absence of information on reliability
and validity weakens its use as a testing and
research tool.

ONE FOOT BALANCE TEST

Reference.

Fleishman, E. A. (1964B). *The structure and measurement of physical fitness,* Englewood Cliffs: Prentice Hall, pp 115, 128, 170-171.

Additional Sources.

None.

Purpose.

To measure the ability of an examinee to maintain balance while standing.

Objectivity.

Not reported.

Reliability.

r = .82 test-retest method.

Validity.

Construct validity was established.

Age and Sex.

Suitable for females and males, age 13 - adult.

Equipment.

A stopwatch, a wooden rail 3.81cm high x 1.90cm wide x 60.96cm long (1.5" x .75" x 24") attached to the middle of a wooden platform 2.54cm thick x 15.24cm wide x 60.96cm long (1" x 6" x 24").

Space Requirements and Design.

A clear, level area approximately 2m (6') square with the platform positioned in the center.

Directions.

The examinee assumes a standing position with the preferred foot placed on and parallel to the rail. The other foot is kept on the floor for increased stability. The examinee then places the hands on hips and lifts the other foot assuming a balanced position. When properly balanced, the examinee closes the eyes and says, "Go," and the tester starts the stopwatch. The tester stops the watch when the examinee: touches the floor or the platform with any body part, removes a hand(s) from the hip(s), or opens the eyes. One practice trial with the eyes open and two legal trials with the eyes closed are given. A maximum of 20 seconds is allowed for each trial.

Scoring.

The score is the total number of seconds the examinee maintains the desired balanced position during the two trials.

Norms.

Fleishman (1964B, p. 115) boys and girls.

REVIEW

EUGENE R. ANDERSON, Ph.D.

Associate Professor
Health, Physical Education and
Recreation
University of Mississippi
University, MS 38677

The One Foot Balance Test would appear to have empirical or logical validity in that we can assume standing on one foot with the eyes closed would be an indicator of an examinee's sense of balance. Although the test does indicate that construct validity was established, how this was done was not specified. The objectivity of the test should be fairly easy to establish and should be done by those selecting this test for use. The test's reliability (r = .82), although acceptable, would be considered marginal at best. An advantage that this test has is that one examinee's performance is not influenced by the performance of another.

The nature of the test and the equipment utilized lend themselves to a variety of facilities. Any large area, the size of a classroom or gym, could be used for testing. The test can be administered easily, and require only one tester. It is recommended that the immediate area surrounding the apparatus be padded for those examinees with poor balancing abilities. It is important to note that the test can be completed with two 20 second trials. This eliminates the prospect of an examinee balancing for an indefinite period of time.

The test was constructed to be suitable for a wide range of ages. It may be used for learning without any ill effects for the examinees. Although the measure (i.e., time) is objective, there may be some tester influence in the form of reaction time. As with most tests, modern electronics would be preferred over the use of stopwatches. Electronic timing devices would be more suitable for research purposes, however, use of the recommended equipment would be appropriate for a teaching/learning situation. Norms are available for both boys and girls, but they are somewhat dated.

SUMMARY

Major Strengths:

1. The test is easily administered and requires little equipment or space and few testers.

2. The equipment is relatively inexpensive.

3. The test can be administered in most educational settings without a great deal of prior experience.

Major Weaknesses:

1. The test would not be generally accepted as a sophisticated research tool.

2. The test lacks objectivity and validity and the method of testing used evaluates only one aspect of balance.

It can only be assumed that this test would not be a valid indicator of overall balancing ability.

PROGRESSIVE INVERTED BALANCE TEST

References.

Johnson, B. L. (1966). A progressive inverted balance test. Unpublished study, Northeast Louisiana University.

Johnson, B. L., & Nelson, J. K. (1986). *Practical measurements for evaluation in physical education*. Edina, MN: Burgess, pp 239-242, 378, 380.

Additional Sources.

None.

Purpose.

To measure the ability of an examinee to balance in an inverted position.

Objectivity.

Not reported.

Reliability.

r = .82 test-retest method.

Validity.

Face validity was accepted.

Age and Sex.

Females and males, age 9 - college.

Equipment.

A stopwatch and a tumbling mat.

Space Requirements and Design.

A clear, level surface approximately 3m (10') square with the mat in the center.

Directions.

The test consists of the five inverted balance stunts: Tripod Balance, Tip Up Balance, Head Balance, Head and Forearm Balance, and Handstand. The reader should refer to the directions for the individual tests in Johnson and Nelson (1986, pp. 239-240).

Scoring.

Scoring for the test can be done by either the long form or the short form. The method of scoring in the long form consists of assigning weights to each of the balances as follows: Tripod = 1, Tip Up = 2, Head Balance = 3, Head and Forearm = 4, and Headstand = 5. The examinee, once balanced, tries to hold each balance for a maximum of five seconds. The amount of time achieved for each individual stunt is multiplied by the weight assigned to that particular stunt. The procedure is followed for each of the five individual stunts and then added to determine the examinee's total score. Seventy-five points is the maximum obtainable score. If the examinee cannot balance or does not make an attempt to balance for a stunt, a score of zero is recorded for that stunt.

Scoring for the short form is conducted the same as in the long form with the exception that the examinee selects only one of the five balance stunts. The maximum score of 25 points, however, can only be achieved if the examinee selects the Headstand and performs it for the full five seconds.

Norms.

Johnson & Nelson (1986, pp. 242, 380) men and women.

REVIEW

DALE E. DEVOE, Ph.D.

Associate Professor
Exercise and Sport Science
Colorado State University
Fort Collins, CO 80523

Balance is an important component which underlies many movement activities. Static balance involves the ability to maintain posture when the body is stationary. Because of the complexity of balance as a skill, concern should exist for considering a measure of balance as useful when testing various age ranges. Since static balance is specific to the position of the body there is a need for a variety of tests.

Strength would appear to have considerable influence on the scores generated from testing, especially with regard to the effects of fatigue. Administration of this test would be time consuming due to the number of trials and the difficulty in getting the examinees to achieve the correct position.

The descriptions of the five balance stunts and the scoring scales that are provided are adequate for suitable administration by experienced and inexperienced testers. Norms are published, based on the scores of college men and women. There is a need for norms for children and older adult. This test appears to be most appropriate for gymnastics. The test is acceptable as an assessment measure to be utilized by teachers.

SQUAT STAND (TIP UP) TEST

References.

Meyers, C. R. (1974). *Measurement in physical education.* New York: Ronald Press, p 296.

State Education Department (1958). *The New York state physical fitness test: For boys and girls grades 4-12.* Albany: State Education Department, pp 30-31, 51-60.

Additional Source.

Jensen & Hirst (1980, p. 162).

Purpose.

To measure the static balance of an examinee while in an inverted position.

Objectivity.

Not reported.

Reliability.

r's = .88, .95, and .95 derived from fifth, eighth, and eleventh grade males respectively while r's = .72, .92, and .98 were obtained from females in the same grades five, eight, and eleven, as cited in Meyers (1974), p. 296.

Validity.

Not reported.

Age and Sex.

Females and males, grades 5 - 11.

Equipment.

A mat and a stopwatch.

Space Requirements and Design.

A clear, level area approximately 2m (6') square with the mat in the center.

Directions.

From a standing position in front of the mat, the examinee assumes a squatting position with the feet slightly more than shoulder width apart. The fingers are placed on the floor between the feet. The fingers are pointed forward, and the inner knees rest against the elbows. The examinee then attempts to obtain a balanced position on both hands by slowly leaning forward until the feet are raised from the floor. The examinee tries to keep the head up and over the mat. If the examinee's balance is lost within five seconds, a second trial is given.

Scoring.

The score is the number of full seconds recorded with one trial greater than five seconds or the greater number of seconds of two trials.

Norms.

New York (1958, pp. 51-60) boys and girls; New York (1966, pp. 45-62) boys and girls.

NOTE: Jensen and Hirst (1980, pp. 161-162) recommend a modification of this test which requires the examinee to rest the forehead and hands on the mat in a tripod stance. Three trials should be given.

REVIEW

JOANNE ROWE, Ph.D.

Assistant Professor
Physical Education
University of Louisville
Louisville, KY 40292

The test is valid in that it does measure static balance. The test has reliability of .72 to .98 for females and males in grades 5, 8 and 11. This indicates consistency of measurement.

The test does not require a large space, therefore a classroom, gymnasium, or outdoor space would be appropriate. No equipment is needed except a stopwatch. It is suggested that when indoor space is used, a mat would add to the safety aspect. Administration of the test to individuals, as well as to large groups, is very easy. The number of trials is appropriate for the age group. More trials might possibly indicate testing of arm strength rather than balance ability.

The Squat Stand (Tip Up) Test can be used as a learning task and as a measure on pretest and posttest basis. The test could serve as a good lead up activity for learning the hand stand in gymnastics.

Although timing by another individual is preferred, examinees could time themselves by watching a stopwatch placed on the floor by their head or by counting seconds. This procedure would be satisfactory for practice only.

Norms are available for this test, but there is no indication of when and how they were established.

SUMMARY

Major Strengths:

1. A good indicator of static balance in an inverted position.

2. Easy to administer.

3. Very little equipment is needed.

4. Very little time is required to administer.

Major Weakness:

1. Has not been widely accepted by professionals as indicated byits infrequent use.

This is an acceptable test for measuring static balance in an inverted position. It is a good lead up to the skill of head stand.

STATIC VISUALIZATION TEST

Reference.
Powell, R. L. (1984). Dynamic balance test. *National Strength and Conditioning Association Journal*, 6(4):42D.

Additional Sources.
None.

Purpose.
To measure the visualization abilities of an examinee by testing balance.

Objectivity.
Not reported.

Reliability.
Not reported.

Validity.
Not reported.

Age and Sex.
Not reported, but suitable for females and males, age 8 - adult.

Equipment.
Any object the examinee will be able to see clearly and a stopwatch.

Space Requirements and Design.
A clear, level surface approximately 3m (10') square with the examinee in the center.

Directions.
The examinee assumes a standing position with feet 10cm to 15cm (4" - 6") apart. The examinee is asked to concentrate on an object that is placed at a distance. On command, the examinee closes her/his eyes and balances on one foot for a maximum of 10 seconds. The same procedure is repeated for the opposite foot. The longer the examinee maintains balance, the greater the indication of a strong visual system.

Scoring.
The score is derived from the number of seconds the examinee remains balanced. A rating of 1 to 5 is given based on the examinee's performance. The scoring criteria are:

1. The examinee remains balanced the full 10 seconds.

2. The examinee moves from side to side and uses the arms for balance.

3. The examinee holds the arms straight out and has difficulty balancing.

4. The examinee loses balance after 5 to 6 seconds.

5. The examinee loses balance under 5 seconds.

Norms.
Not reported.

NOTE: The exact distance the object is to be placed from the examinee is not given. The size of the object and the height is should be placed were also not given.

REVIEW

FRANK SMITH, Ph.D.
Dean, School of Education
St. Edward's University
Austin, TX 78704

It was stated that this test measures visualization abilities with respect to maintenance of static balance; however, during the balance phase, sensory stimuli are also provided by the vestibular apparatus, the joint receptors of the neck, and other proprioceptors and exteroceptive sensors throughout the body. No measures are taken to control the effect that these sources of input might have on the maintenance of static equilibrium. How then can it be assumed that the visualization techniques play any role in the observed results?

No evidence has been presented to demonstrate that the test will provide reliable/consistent results. Test scores could improve with replication due to the practice effect.

The vagueness of the directions and the subjectivity of the scoring system would make it difficult for multiple testers to elicit consistent results. These shortcomings will be discussed in more detail below.

The nature of the object that is to be used for visualization and its location in relation to the examinee is not clearly defined. The nature of the surface material needs to be defined more clearly (e.g., hard floor or carpet).

The tester should be provided with explicit verbal instructions to communicate with the examinee. There are no guidelines for the mental routine that the examinee should exercise once the eyes are closed. More importantly, no directions are given concerning the initial position of the arms or the non supporting leg. The subsequent actions of these limbs play a significant role in the scoring of the test.

The rating scale is based upon a confusing combination of both objective and subjective criteria. Ratings 1, 4, and 5 are founded on simple time increments, while ratings 2 and 3 require the tester to evaluate the behavior of the examinee. The test results are not very meaningful to the tester or the examinee since no norms are reported.

SUMMARY
Major Strengths:
1. The test attempts to measure the influence of visualization abilities upon static balance.

2. The test utilizes an accepted method for evaluating static balance, the stork stand.

Major Weaknesses:
1. No rationale is presented, nor is such rationale obvious, which would substantiate the validity, reliability, or objectivity of the test.

2. No control for the other factors which play a significant role in the maintenance of static balance is included.

3. Test directions and requirements are not clearly defined or stated.

4. The system of scoring is a confusing mixture of subjective and objective criteria.

5. Apparently no norms have been developed which give the test results meaning.

In its present form, the Static Visualization Test is unacceptable for research and/or teaching purposes. Not only is the test written in such a way that it would be difficult to administer and score, any results obtained would have little if any significance to the tester or examinee.

STORK STAND TEST

References.
Johnson, B. L., & Nelson, J. K. (1986). *Practical measurements for evaluation in physical education*. Edina, MN: Burgess, pp 237-238, 383.

Jensen, C. R., & Hirst, C. C. (1980). *Measurement in physical education and athletics*. New York: Macmillan, pp 159-160.

Additional Sources.
Bosco & Gustafson (1983, p. 113); Hastad & Lacy (1989, pp. 263-264); Kirkendall et al. (1980, pp. 250-251); Kirkendall et al. (1987, pp. 127-129); Miller (1988, pp. 134-135); Safrit (1986, pp. 330-332); Safrit (1990, pp. 500-501).

Purpose.
To measure the static balance of an examinee while supported on one foot.

Objectivity.
r = .99 by Knox (1969) as cited in Johnson and Nelson (1986, p. 237).

Reliability.
r = .87 standing on ball of foot (Johnson & Nelson, 1986, p. 237); r = .85 standing on flat foot (Jensen & Hirst, 1980, p. 159).

Validity.
Face or content validity.

Age and Sex.
Females and males, age 6 - college.

Equipment.
A stopwatch.

Space Requirements and Design.
A clear, level area approximately 2m (6') square with the examinee in the center.

Directions.
The examinee assumes a standing position on the dominant leg. The hands are placed on the hips and the foot of the nondominant leg is positioned on the inside of the knee of the dominant leg. On the signal, "Go," the examinee raises her/his heel from the floor and maintains that position as long as possible. The test is stopped when the examinee permits the heel to touch the surface, removes the hands from the hips, and/or moves the foot from its original position. Several practice trials and three legal trials are given.

Scoring.
The score is the number of seconds the examinee maintains the desired position. The best score of three trials is recorded.

Norms.
Johnson & Nelson (1986, p. 238) men and women; Kirkendall et al. (1980, pp. 252-253) men and women; Kirkendall et al. (1987, p. 128) men and women; Miller (1988, p. 135) men and women.

NOTE: Jensen and Hirst (1980) presents a variation of this test of maintaining balance while standing with the dominant foot flat on the surface.

REVIEW

JACQUELINE A. DAILEY, Ed.D.
Program Coordinator
Health, Physical Education and
Recreation
University of Wisconsin-Whitewater
Whitewater, WI 53190

While static balance may be simply defined, balancing tasks are very complex in nature, and they require the establishment of numeric validity to indicate the degree to which tests claiming to measure this ability actually do measure it. Just as important, this determination must be made objectively, not by professional judgement. That the Stork Stand is a measure of static balance, and not dynamic balance has been established as commonly defined in the literature. Whether it measures the static balancing abilities required of gymnasts, divers, tumblers, or wrestlers is open to conjecture. Reported stability coefficients must be viewed with a degree of skepticism as performance on this test can be significantly improved with practice over a very short time period. It seems to hold promise for the establishment of objectivity, if the tester follows exact administration and scoring procedures. Analysis of variance techniques are very helpful in obtaining this measure. No current objectivity coefficients have been reported.

As for the practical aspects of the test, neither space requirements, design, nor equipment seem to pose problems. Test directions, however, pose several problems for the tester. First, the dominant leg is not the one on which some examinees prefer to stand. Perhaps, preferred/favorite leg would be better here. Second, the non preferred foot is cited as being positioned on the inside of the knee of the dominant leg (Johnson & Nelson, 1986), but the figure accompanying the directions does not aid in this positioning. Other authors cite placing the non supported foot flat on the medial (inside) aspect of the supporting knee (Bosco & Gustafson, 1983); placing the toes of the nondominant leg against the knee of the dominant leg (Kirkendall et al, 1987); and holding the other foot so it touches the inside of the supporting knee (Safrit, 1986). Third, younger examinees might be better off using a flat foot with their eyes open. Fourth, if the eyes are closed, which is suggested by Fleishman (1964), then a different skill is probably being assessed. The tester is thus left to decide which conditions are suitable for the examinees being tested.

There is no time limit to this test, so administration could become very time consuming. Some suggestions have been advanced by test administrators to alleviate this problem: (a) partner testing, and (b) imposing a time limit. When to stop the watch, is not clear for the uninitiated tester, posing a fifth problem with the directions. It is difficult: (a) to watch for hands coming off of the hips, (b) to establish whether the heel comes down, and/or (c) if the foot moves, and (d) to keep the eyes on the second hand of the stopwatch. There is no mention in the test directions of the role of the non supporting foot (see Safrit, 1986, p. 330). Should it be watched as well? Practice for the examinee, and the tester should improve the performance of both considerably.

Since the Stork Stand is a field test of static balance, it obviously is not intended to meet the scientific rigor demanded of the researcher. Research is needed, however, in establishing criterion levels of performance desired for other than college aged examinees. Some authors deem the test usable for 6 year olds, but how can this be verified, if no norms or criterion levels have been established for this age?

SUMMARY

Major Strengths:

1. This test of static balance requires no special equipment.

2. Significant improvement may be noted in a short period of time.

3. This test may be used to fulfill specific tumbling, diving, gymnastic, or wrestling instructional objectives.

4. This test is versatile in that static balance may be assessed with eyes open or closed, with the heel of the supporting foot down or up, and it can be easily adjusted for the group being tested.

Major Weaknesses:

1. Physical activities require activity specific types of balance, the validity of which must be statistically established.

2. This test is not reliable (stability) because of the learning effect, thus results cannot be used for prediction, for diagnosis, or for classification purposes.

3. Other factors that may be involved in static balance (e.g., strength and flexibility) have yet to be identified.

4. This test is not sophisticated enough for the laboratory researcher to use - the stabilimeter and the free standing Bachman ladder, which can be electronically scored offer much more promise.

This is an acceptable test for the practical assessment of abilities in specific activities requiring the maintenance of total body equilibrium while balancing in one spot, if used exactly as test constructors have instructed. Even though scores on this test are not absolutes, they do provide a framework for program planning, and due to the multidimensional nature of balance, they must not be the only measures taken. Adaptations will have to be made for examinees with physical and/or medical limitations.

COMBINATION DYNAMIC AND STATIC BALANCE TESTS

BALANCE STABILIZATION TEST

Reference.
Arnot, R., & Gaines, C. (1986). *Sports Talent.* New York: Penguin Books, p 176.

Additional Sources.
None.

Purpose.
To measure an examinee's dynamic and static balance.

Objectivity.
Not reported.

Reliability.
Not reported.

Validity.
Not reported.

Age and Sex.
Not reported, but suitable for females and males, age 8 - adult.

Equipment.
A stopwatch.

Space Requirements and Design.
A clear, level area approximately 3m (10') square with the examinee in the center.

Directions.
The examinee takes this test in socking feet. The examinee stands flat footed on the dominant leg with the foot of the other leg braced against the inside of the knee of the dominant leg. The examinee must keep her/his hands on her/his hips and her/his eyes open throughout the test. Once the examinee is in the above position, the tester starts the stopwatch and announces the time at five seconds. With the announcement, the examinee turns 180 degrees to the right by pivoting on the ball of the foot. After five more seconds have elapsed, the tester announces the time and the examinee turns back to her/his original position. The examinee continues turning back and forth every five seconds until the braced foot comes off the knee or until the hands come off the hips.

Scoring.
The score is the number of seconds, measured to the nearest tenth of a second, that the examinee is able to maintain the proper balanced position.

Norms.
Arnot & Gaines (1986, p. 176) men and women.

REVIEW

JIMMY H. ISHEE, Ph.D.

Associate Professor
Physical Education
University of Central Arkansas
Conway, AR 72032

This test purports to measure both commonly accepted types of balance; thus, static and dynamic balance requirements are included in a single test. Due to the specificity of balance, poor performance on this test may be attributed to either static or dynamic balance. Also, the complexity of the requirements for balance make it difficult to identify what is actually being measured. There are no indices of objectivity, reliability, or validity reported with the test. This is an obvious deficiency. The test is similar to other practical measures of balance noted in the literature; however, it is not appropriate to assume the test possesses the necessary psychometric characteristics of a good test simply because of similarity to other measures of balance. Investigations by the tester would be necessary to provide this additional information.

The test requires a minimum space and only a stopwatch to administer. The time to administer the test depends on the ability of the examinee, but is relatively short. If the examinee lacks muscular strength and endurance in the lower extremities, this could also be a confounding factor in the resulting score. The directions do not indicate the number of trials that should be performed, but the test could be used as a drill to promote balance and familiarize the examinee with the test. The normative data is available for interpretation purposes with an adult population.

SUMMARY

Major Strengths:

1. Practical in terms of time and equipment.

2. Provides normative data for adult.

Major Weaknesses:

1. Absence of reported objectivity, reliability, and validity.

2. Questionable interpretation due to confounding requirements of the test.

3. Absence of normative data for children and youth.

The Balance Stabilization Test is an unacceptable test for research and teaching purposes. No test should be employed in these settings until the scientific aspects of the test have been addressed. Lack of reported data in this area make the norms provided of questionable concern. Further investigations could possibly provide the necessary information for acceptance as a practical measure of static and dynamic balance.

DYNAMIC POSITIONAL BALANCE TEST

References.

Johnson, B. L., & Nelson, J. K. (1979). *Practical measurements for evaluation in physical education*. Minneapolis: Burgess, pp 235-238.

Johnson, B. L., & Fitch, J. (1968). Dynamic test of positional balance. Unpublished study, East Texas State University.

Additional Sources.

None.

Purpose.

To measure the ability of an examinee to land accurately and to maintain balance in various positions.

Objectivity.

r = .94.

Reliability.

r = .76 test-retest method.

Validity.

Face validity.

Age and Sex.

Females and males, age 10 - college.

Equipment.

A stopwatch, tape measure, and five small pieces of marking tape cut 2.54cm x 1.90cm (1" x .75") and one piece of tape cut 2.54cm x 30.48cm (1" x 12") to be used as the starting line.

Space Requirements and Design.

A clear, level surface approximately 3m (10') square. The starting line tape is placed on the floor in the center of and near one sideline of the square. The first small piece of tape (A) is placed 76cm (30") from the starting line. The second piece of tape (B) is placed in line with the starting line and point A with the distance from point A being 76cm (30"). The third (C) and fourth (D) pieces of tape are placed at a 90° angle to the right of and in line with point B, with a distance of 76cm (30") between each point noted. The fifth piece of tape (E) is placed at a 90° angle to the left of point D at a distance of 76cm (30") (Figure 3-4).

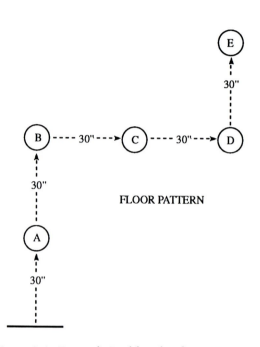

Figure 3-4. Dynamic Positional Balance Test.

Directions.

To begin the test, the examinee stands on the left foot behind the starting line and then leaps to point A and lands on the right foot.

(A) Stork Stand

At point A the examinee balances on the ball of the foot in a stork stand for a maximum time of five seconds (Figure 3-5a).

(B) Front Scale

The examinee then leaps to point B landing on the ball of the left foot and immediately lowering into a front scale. The trunk is lowered forward while the non supporting leg is raised parallel to the floor in the rear. The arms are extended horizontally to the sides with the head and chest held high while the supporting leg remains straight. The examinee balances on the ball of the foot (Figure 3-5b).

(C) Side Scale

The examinee then returns to an upright position while remaining on one foot and leaps to point C, landing on the left foot and going into a side scale. The body leans to the right side with the right leg being raised parallel to the floor. The left arm is extended along the side of the body with the hand placed on the thigh while the head is leaned close to the forward extended right arm. The examinee should keep the supporting leg straight and balance on a flat foot (Figure 3-5c).

(D) One Foot Balance - Upon returning to the upright position on one foot, the examinee leaps to point D, lands on the ball of the left foot and maintains a balanced position (Figure 3-5d).

(E) Knee Scale - From point D, the examinee turns and lowers the body to the floor to a position with the hands placed on each side of point E. The left leg is then drawn under the body and the knee is placed on point E. The hands, non supporting leg, and foot of the supporting leg are raised to obtain a balanced position on the left knee. After the attempt is made, obtain a balanced position on the right knee and repeat the procedure (Figure 3-5e).

Scoring.

Five points are received for each landing completed properly with the exception of point E where no points are awarded. Throughout the test, the tester should count the seconds aloud. Improper landings are a failure to stop upon landing from the leap or a failure to cover completely the piece of tape with the foot. The examinee may reposition after a landing error in order to attempt the five second balance phase of the test. A total of 20 points are possible during the landing phase. During the balance phase, one point is given for each second balance is properly maintained up to a five second maximum in each position. The loss of balance results when the examinee touches any part of the body to the floor excluding the point of support or when the examinee moves the supporting foot. When balance is lost, the examinee must step back on the point before leaping to the next point. A total of six balance positions provides for a maximum score of 30 points. The highest cumulative total for the test is 50 points with the best of three trials noted as the test score.

Norms.

Johnson & Nelson (1979, p. 235) men.

NOTE: A small mat for executing the Knee Scale would seem warranted.

REVIEW

MARY L. PUTMAN, Ph.D.

Assistant Professor
Health and Physical Education
Glassboro State College
Glassboro, NJ 08028

The Dynamic Positional Balance Test measures the ability to land accurately and maintain balance in various positions. The examinee is required to demonstrate dynamic and static balance. The accuracy of landing is observed at points A through D but is not a factor at point E. The static balance positions are learned skills, commonly used in gymnastics and dance, which require some degree of strength and flexibility to perform.

Balance is a "task specific" ability which infers that different motor skills require different types of balance. In this situation, face validity is specific to the skills of landing and positional (static) balance as they are used in this test. The interpretation and application of results are specific to these motor skills and should be used cautiously in evaluating an examinee's general ability to balance.

The coefficients for the psychometric qualities of objectivity (r = .94) and reliability (r = .76) are comparable to the scores reported for other measures of dynamic balance. The test constructors do not indicate whether the objectivity is intrajudge or interjudge objectivity. The reliability coefficient is within an acceptable range. Since balance is a learned ability, there is a tendency for the test-retest reliability to be less stable and produce a slightly lower coefficient. The test is identified as being appropriate for females and males, age 10 through college, but no reliability and objectivity coefficients are provided for the different age and gender groups.

The decisions and procedures involved in the test administration can be easily satisfied and do not require any specialized training on the part of a qualified tester. The equipment and facilities needed are accessible in most school based, and nonschool based, settings. The testing station must be accurately prepared, a process which is facilitated by a corresponding diagram and description. The use of a gymnastic mat for position E (knee scale) should be added to reduce the discomfort of a knee support position on a hard surface. The testing procedures provide for one tester, however, a timer and observer would contribute to the objectivity of the scoring procedure. The timer would be responsible for counting the length of each static balance while the observer would determine the accuracy of landing, the correct foot position (ball or flat foot), and the correct body position for each balance. A minimum of three to five minutes is required for each examinee to complete three trials.

The tester must determine the standards of acceptable performance for each static balance position as a component of the pretest procedures. The examinee will also need time to practice and become familiar with the different static balance positions. The test constructors have indicated that norms are available for college men. Local norms and/or criterion scores would need to be developed for other age and gender groups.

Performance of all motor skills requires some degree of balance. However, this test should be used in conjunction with instructional units in which balance is an important component of skill development. Gymnastics, diving, and modern dance classes, taught in either school based or nonschool based settings, exemplify appropriate application of this instrument. Research in the area of motor learning uses objective balance tests to qualify and quantify skill learning.

SUMMARY

Major Strengths:

1. The test constructors have done a conscientious job in developing a "task specific" measure of dynamic and static balance.

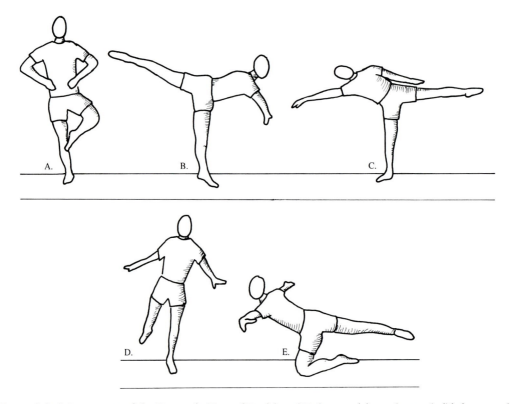

Figure 3-5. Movements of the Dynamic Test of Positional Balance: (a) stork stand, (b) front scale, (c) side scale, (d) one foot balance, and (e) knee scale.

2. The test requires a minimal amount of equipment and space which makes it adaptable to school based and nonschool based settings.

3. An individual with training in measurement and evaluation at the undergraduate level would have the expertise necessary to administer this test.

4. The face validity of this instrument is good as long as the application of the results remains within the parameters of motor skill comparable to those used in this measure of static and dynamic balance.

Major Weaknesses:

1. The skills used to measure static balance require a certain degree of strength and flexibility which could affect the face validity of this test.

2. The knee scale at point E satisfies the purpose of maintaining a positional balance but does not involve accuracy of landing. The test constructors fail to provide a justification for the inclusion of this fifth static balance position.

3. The test constructors do not provide gender and age specific norms and/or criterion scores for this test. Professionals interested in using this test do not have a baseline for comparison.

4. The directions clearly describe and illustrate the positions for each balance but do not provide standards for the quality of form expected of the examinee.

5. This is a task specific test and should not be used to provide a general measure of balance.

This is an acceptable test of static and dynamic balance when used within the limitation of the face (content) validity.

The interpretation and application of results must be reserved to instructional settings which emphasize comparable balancing skills. The specificity and objectivity of this test could make it an appropriate instrument for use in research studies.

NELSON BALANCE TEST

References.

Nelson, J. K. (1968). The Nelson Balance Test. Unpublished study, Louisiana State University.

Johnson, B. L., & Nelson, J. K. (1986). *Practical measurements for evaluation in physical education.* Edina, MN: Burgess, pp 247-249.

Additional Sources.

None.

Purpose.

To measure an examinee's static and dynamic balance with a single test.

Objectivity.

Not reported.

Reliability.

r = .91, r = .90, and r = .68 were derived for fourth, fifth, and sixth grade males, respectively as cited in Johnson and Nelson (1986, p. 247).

Validity.

Face validity was accepted and r = .77 correlated with the combined score of several standard balance measures as cited in Johnson and Nelson (1986, p. 247).

Age and Sex.

Females and males, age 9 - college.

Equipment.

Seven wooden blocks 5.08cm x 10.16cm x 20.32cm (2" x 4" x 8") with pieces of rubber glued to the bottom of each. Four of the seven blocks should be marked alike so they differ from the remaining three. A wooden balance beam 5.08cm x 10.16cm x 3.05m (2" x 4" x 10') supported edgewise by three triangular shaped braces is required (Figure 3-6a). A stopwatch, tape measure, and marking tape to indicate the position of the blocks on the floor are also needed.

Space Requirements and Design.

A clear, level area approximately 2m x 8m (6' x 25') with the balance beam positioned in the center. The seven blocks are positioned as illustrated in the accompanying figures (Figures 3-6a and 3-6b).

Directions.

The examinee begins the test at the end of the beam where four blocks are positioned. To begin the test, the examinee places the ball of the left foot on the first marked block and attempts to balance for 5 seconds. The tester reads aloud the seconds. If the examinee loses balance or leaves any of the other marked blocks before the 5 seconds have elapsed, the examinee must return to the block for the remainder of the 5 second period not completed. The examinee must step on each of the unmarked blocks, but not for any set time. The examinee alternates feet in stepping from one block to another as quickly as possible with all of the marked blocks requiring the examinee to balance for 5 seconds. The examinee first contacts the balance beam with the left foot and proceeds to walk heel to toe for half the length of the beam and then sidesteps to the right the remainder of the distance. If the examinee's balance is lost or any deviation in the walk across the beam occurs, the examinee must return to that point before continuing. After completion of the sidestep right, the examinee steps on the nearest unmarked block with the right foot and continues alternating feet until the three blocks have been stepped on. As the examinee steps off of the last block, the stopwatch is stopped and the first phase of the test is completed. The stopwatch is not reset, but started again at the moment when the examinee places the ball of the left foot on the first block and attempts to return to the starting point.

The above procedure is followed during the second phase of the test with the exception that the beam is contacted first with the right foot, a sidestep to the left is used on the second half of the beam, and the nearest block at the end of the beam is contacted with the left foot. The stopwatch is stopped at the time the examinee steps from the last block.

The examinee attempts to complete the test as quickly as possible with the least number of mistakes. One trial is given.

Scoring.

The score is the total time, measured to the nearest tenth of a second, needed to complete both phases of the test.

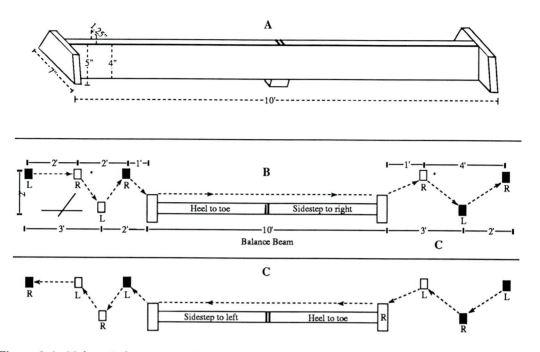

Figure 3-6. Nelson Balance Test: (a) balance beam, (b) movement pattern for phase 1, and (c) movement pattern for phase 2. NOTE: The dark blocks are the blocks on which the examinee must balance for 5 seconds.

Norms.

Johnson & Nelson (1986, p. 248) boys.

REVIEW

PERRY F. MILLER, Ed.D.

Professor
Health and Physical Education
Southwest Missouri State University
Springfield, MO 65804

The Nelson Balance Test is designed to measure static and dynamic balance with a single test. The test does require both, although it would seem to have more of the dynamic component. Because of the necessity to maintain one's position on the blocks and the beam in both the static and dynamic situations, face validity would seem acceptable.

Reliability coefficients of .91, .90 and .68 are given for fourth, fifth, and sixth grade boys, respectively. Because of the complexity of the test, the opportunity for only a single trial and the strong possibility of time penalties, acceptable consistency would be questioned. Several opportunities for prior learning experiences and/or the giving of up to three trials might improve the reliability factor considerably.

This is a complicated test to administer. Because of starting and stopping the clock, counting while the examinee is on certain blocks, and making sure the examinee is on the correct foot or performing the correct step, many opportunities for subjectivity exist. The objectivity would be questionable.

While facility and space requirements are simple, the specific equipment necessary to administer the test is not. A ground level balance beam and seven specially constructed painted wooden blocks are required. Of course, once this equipment has been obtained or constructed, subsequent test set up is simplified.

The administration of the test could create several problems. Each examinee will require a minimum of one to two minutes per trial, so trying to test a large group in a single class period could be difficult. Also, considerable preparation by both the tester and examinees are necessary to ensure that the testing will go smoothly. Some prior practice by the examinees should enhance their eventual performance. Because of this learning advantage, more than a single trial would be suggested if the examinees are going to have the opportunity to score their best.

The test routine would certainly be a good mechanism for drill to improve static and dynamic balance. However, the actual test would be difficult, if not impossible, to self administer because of the timing complexities.

Even though norms are given only for young boys, the test would seem to be applicable to any group.

SUMMARY

Major Strengths:

1. The test seems to be a valid measure of both static and dynamic balance.

2. Once the equipment for the test (the low balance beam and the blocks) has been obtained, it makes subsequent set ups relatively easy.

Major Weaknesses:

1. Questionable reliability levels.

2. The necessity of the specialized equipment for the test.

3. Because of complexity of the routine for the test, considerable prior practice or learning is necessary for the examinee to complete the test efficiently and correctly.

4. The subjectivity involved in the administration of the test.

Overall, this test is an acceptable test for research and/or teaching. The level of acceptability would be determined by the tester's experience and skill in administering the test and the examinees having the opportunity for more than a single trial.

SIDEWARD LEAP TEST

References.

Scott, M. G., & French, E. (1959). *Measurement and evaluation in physical education.* Dubuque: Wm. C. Brown, pp 320-322.

Johnson, B. L., & Nelson, J. K. (1979). *Practical measurements for evaluation in physical education.* Minneapolis: Burgess, pp 238-239.

Additional Sources.

Jensen & Hirst (1980, pp. 167-168); Miller (1988, p. 139); Safrit (1986, pp. 333-334); Safrit (1990, pp. 503-504).

Purpose.

To measure the ability of an examinee to land accurately and maintain balance during and after movement.

Objectivity.

Not reported.

Reliability.

r = .88 by using alternate trials and the Spearman-Brown formula. Riley derived coefficients for grades 1 - 6 that ranged from .68 to .80 by correlating odd and even trials and the Spearman-Brown formula as cited in Scott and French (1959, p. 321).

Validity.

Not reported, but face validity is obvious.

Age and Sex.

Females and males, age 10 - college.

Equipment.

A stopwatch, marking tape, tape measure, and small objects such as the cork heads cut off of old badminton birds.

Space Requirements and Design.

A clear, level area approximately 2m (6') square. Three 2.54cm (1") square pieces of tape are placed on the floor in a straight line 46cm (18") apart (Figure 3 = 7). Marks 7.6cm (3") apart are also placed on the floor on a line perpendicular to the above straight line and in line with the center square. These marks should be 61cm to 102cm (24" - 40") from the center square. Normally three or four marks will be sufficient to cover the range in height found in a particular group of examinees. A small cork is placed on each square on either side of the center square.

Directions.

The length of the examinee's leg, from the hip joint to the floor, is measured. The length of the leg is used to determine the mark on the floor that the examinee will use as a starting mark. The examinee then places the left foot on that starting mark and leaps sideward attempting to land on the center square with the right foot. Immediately following the landing, the examinee bends forward and pushes the cork off the square. The trial is deemed successful if the examinee places the foot completely over the center square, keeps the foot stationary on the center square, leans forward immediately to push the cork off the square, keeps the hands off the floor, remains balanced for five seconds and remains standing. Three trials to the right, three trials to the left and another three trials to the right, three trials to the left represent the proper sequence and number of trials.

Scoring.

The score is the total number of successful trials out of 12.

Norms.

Johnson & Nelson (1979, p. 239) men and women for their modification of the test.

NOTE: A modification of the Sideward Leap is presented by Johnson and Nelson (1979), in which two trials are given for each direction. Five points are awarded for covering the center square, five points are awarded for pushing the cork from the proper square within two seconds, and one point is awarded for each second that balance is maintained up to five seconds. The maximum score for the four trials is 60 points.

REVIEW

PAUL A. ANDERSON, Ph.D.

Assistant Professor
Physical Therapy
University of Maryland
Baltimore, MD 21201

The ability to interact safely within our world is necessary for the human being. Movement requires one to maintain balance while performing the physical tasks of daily living. The maturation

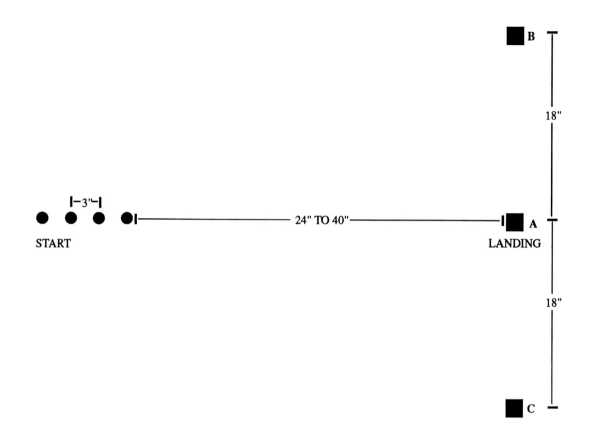

Figure 3-7. Sideward Leap Balance Test.

process refines the neuro and musculoskeletal systems which in turn improves balance. Thus the ability to measure balance provides a means of evaluating the motor system.

The test constructors state the test is face valid and this reviewer would agree. However, the test measures only one aspect of balance. This test measures balance to the left or right and with one or two feet involved. For most interactions within the world, balance is a forward or backward movement and involves both feet. This test might be useful for the athlete involved in a sport requiring left and right balance. Thus the validity would be for a very special population within our society.

The unclear test directions suggest two possible methods of performing the test. One could jump from one foot and land on the opposite foot or jump from two feet and land on two feet at the respective points on the floor. Both interpretations are feasible but because of the imprecise

use of the language, the intent of the test and the communication between the test constructors and prospective users fails.

This test is of a difficult motor skill and would need some motor learning. No mention is made of any practice trials permitted. For the measures to be truly representative of balance and not the learning of the motor task, a practice session would be appropriate. Then, instead of scoring 12 trials, one could have 9 trials of practice and score the remaining 3. The exact ratio of scored and unscored trials would have to be investigated.

A correlation coefficient of 0.9 or greater is the standard for reliability thus this test with a $r = 0.88$ is close to reliable but room for improvement exists. There is no reported measure for. objectivity. An intraclass correlation as reported by Shrout and Fleiss (1979) and comparison of more than two performances would give a better indication of objectivity.

Normative data exists for college men and women. Norms for youngsters ranging from the age of 10 to college age have not been established. The needed space and test directions appear to be adequate.

SUMMARY

Major Strength:

1. The space, directions, equipment, and face validity are fine.

Major Weaknesses:

1. The test examines only one small aspect of balance.

2. The test directions are not clear as to whether one or both feet are involved.

3. The test's directions do not permit any motor learning of the skill prior to the test.

4. The reliability could be improved.

5. The test needs more normative data.

Because the directions do not adequately describe the test's execution, the validity is questioned. Additionally, the unsatisfactory reliability makes the Sideward Leap Test unacceptable.

REVIEW REFERENCE

Shrout, P. E., & Fleiss, J. L. (1979). Intraclass correlations: Uses in assessing rater reliability. *Psychological Bulletin*, 86:420-428.

Chapter 4

CARDIORESPIRATORY ENDURANCE

BICYCLE/CYCLE TESTS OF CARDIORESPIRATORY ENDURANCE

ASTRAND-RYHMING TEST

References.

Astrand, P. O., & Ryhming, I. (1954). A nomogram for calculation of aerobic capacity (physical fitness) from pulse rate during submaximal work. *Journal of Applied Physiology*, 7:218-221.

deVries, H. A. (1971). *Laboratory experiments in physiology of exercise*. Dubuque: Wm. C. Brown, pp 89-93.

Additional Sources.

Baumgartner & Jackson (1991, p. 312-313); Bosco & Gustafson (1983, p. 137); Jensen & Hirst (1980, p. 113); Safrit (1986, p. 259); Safrit (1990, p. 389); Verducci (1980, pp. 266-271).

Purpose.

To measure the maximal oxygen consumption of an examinee while riding a cycle ergometer.

Objectivity.

Not reported.

Reliability.

Not reported.

Validity.

.74 between the Astrand-Ryhming predicted maximal oxygen consumption and maximal oxygen consumption as measured by deVries.

Age and Sex.

Females and males, age 15 - adult.

Equipment.

A cycle ergometer, metronome, stopwatch, and stethoscope.

Space Requirements and Design.

A clear, level area approximately 3m (10') square with the cycle ergometer positioned in the center.

Directions.

The examinee positions the cycle ergometer's seat at a height so her/his leg is completely extended when the foot reaches the bottom of the pedaling cycle. The balls of the feet should be placed on the pedals. The metronome is set at a cadence of 100 beats per minute (bpm),'s which allows one beat for each downstroke and a constant 50 revolutions per minute (rpm). The workload selected depends on the fitness level, health, and age of the examinee. The examinee who is unconditioned should use 300 to 450 kilopounds per meter (KPM) for women and 300 to 600 KPM for men. For conditioned examinees, women should use 450 to 600 KPM and men 600 to 900 KPM. When the examinee is riding at 50 rpm, a workload of one KP = 300 KPM and for each .5 KP added, the workload is increased 150 KPM. The examinee pedals the cycle ergometer at a constant pace of 50 rpm for six minutes. During the last 20 seconds of each minute, the examinee's heart rate is monitored by the tester's placing a stethoscope below the pectoralis muscle or by palpitating the carotid pulse. The examinee's average heart rate for the fifth and sixth minutes are compared. If the two heart rates are not within five beats per minute of each other, the exercise is continued until a constant heart rate is maintained. If the examinee's heart rate is below 130 or above 150 beats per minute during the exercise, the workload should be increased or decreased, respectively.

Scoring.

The score is the mean heart rate of the fifth and sixth minutes, which is entered into a table, and a maximal oxygen uptake value in liters per minute is obtained. If the examinee is over 30 years of age, the maximal oxygen uptake value is multiplied by an age correction factor. The age corrected maximal oxygen uptake is then divided by the examinee's body weight (in kilograms) to arrive at a final score expressed as $ml/O^2/kg/min$.

Norms.

Corbin & Lindsey (1985, pp. 44-45) men and women; deVries (1971, pp. 91-92) men and women; Hoeger (1989, pp. 25-27) men and women.

REVIEW

LARRY W. TITLOW, Ph.D.

Professor of Physical Education
University of Central Arkansas
Conway, AR 72032

Cycling has long been considered a satisfactory means to assess cardiovascular fitness since the workload can be standardized, controlled, and monitored. The external workload can be determined and thus a graded and measured load can be used. While the reported validity of the test is not especially high, the test appears to measure the purported component satisfactorily. Test reliability is satisfactory but requires careful monitoring of the workload by the tester. An area of concern in using this test is how the heart rate is determined. If a calibrated electronic pulse monitor is unavailable, test reliability can be greatly affected by manual palpation accuracy. The same problem exists for test objectivity; it is dependent upon the ability to determine heart rate accurately. Examinee performance should not be affected by tester competence other than in determining heart rate. Examinees are capable of monitoring a personal test.

The test requires a calibrated cycle ergometer, commonly available in college and university human performance laboratories but not in public school settings. The cycle requires little space but must be equipped with a calibrated speedometer; otherwise, a metronome will be required to determine speed. The only other equipment needed is a timer. There should be no problem with space requirements or mobility of the equipment. The test requires little training, except for manual palpation accuracy for the

tester. Only one tester is required. One examinee can be tested in approximately 10 minutes. While not particularly feasible for large groups, it can be used for small groups (<30). The test is submaximal, but only one trial is allowed as there is a tendency for examinees to experience localized muscular fatigue of the legs. The protocol does not lend itself for use as a training method since it is too short to be satisfactory for cardiovascular endurance development. Length is probably what makes the protocol most desirable as a test and least desirable as a training tool.

Test validity is assumed for an adult population (>15 years) and an age correction factor is provided by Astrand. Workload can be adjusted so the test is suitable for all fitness levels. The test appears to discriminate among fitness levels as indicated by concurrent validity studies with other measures of cardiovascular endurance.

All cardiovascular endurance tests have inherent risks; this test is no exception. Examinees with a known history of heart or cardiovascular disease or who are over age 40 should be carefully examined by a physician before being allowed to proceed with testing. These examinees must be carefully monitored throughout the test and recovery for any signs or symptoms of unusual cardiac events.

Scoring the test is relatively easy as it requires only locating heart rate and workload on a table (or Astrand's nomogram) provided in the references. Most references provide information on maximal oxygen uptake in l/min. or ml/min.; one could compare this data to an appropriate norm table to obtain fitness level. Once an examinee learns how to obtain pulse during the test, self testing can be accomplished. This would not be recommended, however, as it is desirable to have a trained tester available in the event of difficulties.

SUMMARY

Major Strengths:

1. Requires little time or space to administer test.

2. Requires only a cycle ergometer and a timer.

3. Adaptable for all fitness levels, age (>15 years), and both sexes.

Major Weaknesses:

1. Only feasible for small groups (< 30).

2. Requires a reliable means of determining heart rate.

3. Provides an underestimate of oxygen uptake.

The Astrand-Ryhming Test is an acceptable test of cardiovascular endurance that could be used for research when better tests (i.e., maximal measurements) are unavailable. The test underestimates actual maximal oxygen uptake by 15 to 20 percent because of the lack of linearity between heart rate and oxygen uptake at near maximal levels of exertion. The error in prediction is larger among unconditioned, sedentary individuals, and smaller in highly conditioned athletes. The error is least when examinees achieve a heart rate of approximately 150 bpm. A prob-lem is to determine the workload that can be used to achieve this heart rate range. Terry et al. (*Journal of Sports Medicine and Physical Fitness,* 1977, 17:361-366) report a procedure to determine test workload. Ambient temperatures must also be considered when using this protocol since heat stress can invalidate the procedure.

The test's greatest use would be in testing small groups to determine fitness level quickly for exercise prescription. The same protocol could then be used to monitor changes brought about by training. When used for training evaluation, the errors in prediction are no worse than the errors encountered when measuring maximal effort.

Norms are provided for quick reference to fitness level.

EUROFIT BICYCLE ERGOMETER TEST (PWC170)

Reference.
Committee of Experts on Sports Research (1988). *European test of physical fitness.* Rome, Italy: Council of Europe, pp 16, 23, 30-40.

Additional Sources.
None.

Purpose.
To measure "...the ability to perform continuous physical activity where the principle limiting factor is the functional capacity of the entire cardiorespiratory system from lungs to muscles" (Committee, 1988, p. 23).

Objectivity.
Had to be high to meet their criteria, but an exact figure is not reported (Committee, 1988, p. 16).

Reliability.
Had to be high to meet their criteria, but an exact figure is not reported (Committee, 1988, p. 16).

Validity.
Had to be high to meet their criteria, but an exact figure is not reported (Committee, 1988, p. 16).

Age and Sex.
Females and males, age 6 - 18.

Equipment.
A cycle ergometer which can be used with children, a body weight scale, a stethoscope, and two stopwatches.

Space Requirements and Design.
A clear, level area approximately 3m (10') square with the cycle ergometer positioned in the center.

Directions.
The examinee's body weight is determined in the standard way, measured to the nearest 0.1 kg. The examinee then sits on the cycle with the ball of each foot on the pedals. The seat height is adjusted so that the examinee's knee is slightly bent when the pedal is at its lowest point. The handle bar is adjusted so that it permits the examinee to lean slightly forward while keeping the arms straight. The metronome is set at 120 beats per minute (bpm) in order to produce 60 revolutions per minute (rpm). The test requires the examinee to pedal continuously for not more than nine minutes. The workload is increased twice during the ride: at the end of three minutes and at the end of six minutes. The heart rate is counted by the tester's placing the stethoscope on the examinee's chest. The heart rate is taken three times for 15 second periods at the end of three minutes, six minutes, and nine minutes. Both the heart rate and workload for each of these work periods should be recorded. Ideally, the first workload should produce a heart rate of 90 to 120 bpm, and the third workload should produce a heart rate slightly less than 170 bpm. The manual provides detailed instructions on heart rate measurement (Committee, 1988, pp. 32-33) and workload increases (Committee, 1988 pp. 34-35).

Scoring.
The score, expressed in watts per kilogram, is determined by plugging into the following formula:

$$PWC170 = [(W3 - W2)/(HR3 - HR2) \times (170 - HR3) + W3]/BWt$$

Where HR2 and HR3 are the heart rates for the second and third workloads, W2 and W3 are the second and third workloads in Watts, and BWt is the examinee's body weight in kilograms.

Norms.
Not reported.

REVIEW

JAMES DECKER, Ph.D.

Assistant Professor
Health, Physical Education,
Recreation and Safety
East Carolina University
Greenville, NC 27858-4353

The Eurofit Bicycle Ergometer Test (PWC170) provides a submaximal assessment of cardiorespiratory endurance. No evidence of validity or reliability is provided for the Eurofit Test. Rather, the test constructors contend that since assessments of similar nature (i.e., physical working capacity tests utilizing a working heart rate of 170 bpm) have been used frequently in the literature, satisfactory validation of the test's procedures has been demonstrated. In essence, physical working capacity tests utilize the relationship between an examinee's working heart rate, workload, and oxygen consumption to assess cardiorespiratory endurance.

The Eurofit Bicycle Ergometer Test is designed to provide a satisfactory compromise between simple field assessments (e.g., walk/run tests) and elaborate laboratory assessments (e.g., maximal oxygen uptake tests). In this regard the Eurofit Bicycle Ergometer Test handsomely achieves its purpose. Limited space and equipment are required. Examinees being tested need only to pedal at a constant cadence of 60 rpm for a maximum of nine minutes. During this time the resistance (i.e., workload) of the cycle ergometer is increased progressively in order to achieve a working heart rate of approximately 170 bpm.

At least two testers are required to administer the Eurofit Bicycle Ergometer Test feasibly. Primary tester duties include: monitoring the examinee's heart rate at specific intervals, determining appropriate workload increases, adjusting the cycle's resistance, and recording data throughout the test. Due to the critical nature of the above described activities, testers should have some experience in laboratory procedures. For instance, at specified intervals testers must ascertain the elapsed time between 15 heart beats, consult a heart rate chart, consult another chart to determine the appropriate amount of workload increase and lastly, adjust the cycle ergometer resistance. In particular, the reliable heart rate measurement of examinees as they pedal the cycle requires considerable practice on a variety of examinees. Furthermore, each tester must be thoroughly trained in the testing protocol since hesitation in performing duties or incorrect adjustments in the workload will invalidate the test.

One of the primary advantages of the Eurofit Bicycle Ergometer Test is that it demonstrates how each examinee responds to various workloads. Appropriate exercise workloads can, therefore, be ascertained and activities prescribed. However, the major benefit of the test is its identification of the relative cardiorespiratory endurance of examinees based upon their physical working capacity.

SUMMARY

Major Strengths:

1. Relatively little facilities and equipment are required.

2. It can easily be administered in 10 to 15 minutes.

3. It does not require maximum exertion from the examinee.

Major Weaknesses:

1. As with any submaximal test, fitness levels achieved may be substantially in error (as much as ten percent).

2. Only one examinee at a time can be tested.

3. No norms are provided.

4. Testers must be experienced in both, laboratory procedures and the test protocol.

The Eurofit Bicycle Ergometer Test is an acceptable assessment of examinee's cardiorespiratory endurance. Although it is designed to use modest facilities and equipment, testers must be experienced in laboratory methods. This test is adequate for estimating cardiorespiratory endurance levels: however, for research purposes, a maximum oxygen uptake test is more appropriate.

MONTANA BICYCLE TEST

Reference.
Sharkey, B. J. (1984). *Physiology of fitness.* Champaign, IL: Human Kinetics, pp 264-265.

Additional Sources.
None.

Purpose.
To predict the aerobic fitness of an examinee.

Objectivity.
Not reported.

Reliability.
Not reported.

Validity.
"When conducted properly this test correlates highly with treadmill or bicycle ergometer tests of the maximal oxygen intake (aerobic fitness)" (Sharkey, 1984, p. 264).

Age and Sex.
Young males.

Equipment.
A 68.58cm (27") 10-speed bicycle, a stopwatch, and a method of determining wind velocity.

Space Requirements and Design.
A level, five mile (8.05 kilometers) out and back course or loop course.

Directions.
Prior to taking the test, the examinee's percentage of body fat is determined following standard procedures. On the day of testing, the wind velocity should be less than 10 mph (16.09 kilometers per hour). After adequate warm up and rest, the examinee assumes a stationary position on the bicycle at the starting line. Upon the command, "Ready, Go," the examinee rides the five mile course as fast as possible. Throughout the test, the chain must be kept on the 50 tooth chain wheel in front and the 18 tooth sprocket in back. The examinee must use the drop position on the handlebars. The stopwatch is started on the signal, "Ready, Go," and is stopped when the examinee crosses the finish line. This time is then converted to minutes and decimal fractions (e.g., 12.5 = 12 minutes and 30 seconds).

Scoring.
The score is determined by plugging the examinee's five mile time and the examinee's percent of body fat into a table (Sharkey, 1984, p. 265).

Norms.
Not reported.

REVIEW

CHARLES W. ASH, Ph.D.
Associate Professor
Physical Education
State University of New York at
Cortland
Cortland, NY 13045

The Montana Bicycle Test is designed to predict aerobic fitness. Although no validity correlation coefficient exists, the test constructor suggests that "when conducted properly this test correlates highly with treadmill or bicycle ergometer tests of the maximal oxygen intake (aerobic fitness)" (Sharkey, 1984, p. 264). Currently, the test has no coefficients for objectivity and reliability. The actual test procedure does not require the assistance of another individual. However, the tester must assess the percent of body fat of the examinee before the fitness table can be used.

The availability of a level out and back or loop course without grade elevation for 8.05 kilometers (5 miles) could be of concern depending upon local topography. The specific gear ratio (i.e., 50 tooth chain ring in front and an 18 tooth sprocket in the back) could be a problem because a 50 tooth chain ring is not common. Competitive cyclists typically use a 53 or 52 chain ring; whereas a novice would use a 52; possibly a 50 or a 48 chain ring size.

The test is easy to administer. It would require one tester, who would steady the examinee on the bicycle at the starting line and serve as the timer, and an assistant to help control traffic at the turn around point of an out and back course. Even though it would take 12 to 20 minutes to complete each test, a way to increase administrative efficiency would be to start examinees at 2 to 3 minute intervals.

The test does not provide any practice trials because of the rigorous nature of the test. However, examinees could practice independently to experience the test provided they are alerted to the precautions needed at the turn around point. This practice could also provide the added incentive for examinees to use these trials for cardiorespiratory conditioning purposes.

Currently, the test has been designed for males only with no specific age group identified.

The scoring procedure is objective for the bicycle time trial, and if the percent body fat determination is reliable, then these two values are applied to a table to predict the examinee's maximal oxygen consumption. This value must then be applied to a normative chart from other aerobic fitness tests (e.g., Astrand-Ryhming Test) to establish the aerobic fitness classification.

The Montana Bicycle Test does not lend itself to scientific research purposes because the data have not been subjected to scientific scrutiny/corroboration. However, the test constructor plans to update the test in the next edition of his textbook. When that occurs, this would fill a void for testing cyclists on their own bicycle using a time trial procedure.

No norms have been established for the test.

SUMMARY

Major Strength:

1. It is the only competitive road cycling test to predict maximal oxygen consumption.

Major Weaknesses:

1. A sufficiently large data base apparently has not been established for normalization.

2. The test must be performed in a specific gear. This may prohibit an examinee from using the desired gear to reach a specific pedalling frequency in which he has been accustomed.

The Montana Bicycle Test would be adequate for research purposes if the data base were expanded and validated more fully through scientific review. It has significant potential because of its uniqueness to competitive cycling. The test has limited application to teaching because of its specific application to individuals experienced in cycling.

PWC170 PHYSICAL WORKING CAPACITY TEST

References.
Sjostrand, T. (1947). Changes in the respiratory organs of workmen at an ore smelting works. *Acta Medica Scandinavia,* 196 Suppl: 687-699.

Wahlund, H. (1948). Determination of the physical working capacity. *Acta Medica Scandinavia,* Suppl: 215.

deVries, H. A. (1971). *Laboratory experiments in physiology of exercise.* Dubuque: Wm. C. Brown, pp 83-87.

Additional Sources.
Safrit (1986, p. 259); Safrit (1990, p. 389).

Purpose.
To measure the cardiorespiratory endurance of an examinee by predicting PWC170.

Objectivity.
Not reported.

Reliability.
Not reported.

Validity.
r = .88 between the PWC170 Test and maximal oxygen consumption as measured by deVries (1971, p. 84).

Age and Sex.
Females and males, elementary to adult age.

Equipment.
A cycle ergometer, metronome, stopwatch, and stethoscope.

Space Requirements and Design.
A clear, level area approximately 3m (10') square with the ergometer positioned in the center.

Directions.
The cycle ergometer's seat height should be set so the examinee's leg has a slight bend at the knee as the foot reaches the bottom of the pedaling cycle. The balls of the feet should be placed on the pedals. The metronome should be set at a cadence of 100 beats per minute (bpm) which allows 1 beat for each downstroke and a constant 50 revolutions per minute. While the examinee is pedaling, the heart rate is taken during the last 30 seconds of each minute. This heart rate is monitored with a stethoscope or by palpitation of the carotid pulse. With no resistance on the cycle ergometer, the examinee pedals until he/she can maintain rhythm with the metronome. The examinee continuously pedals for two consecutive six minute periods. The cycle ergometer's resistance is set (i.e., estimated, based on the examinee's fitness level) to produce a heart rate of 120 to 140 bpm for the first six minute period. During the second six minute period, the resistance should be increased and set (i.e., estimated, based on the examinee's response to the first workload) to produce a heart rate of 150 to 170 bpm. The heart rate is taken the last 30 seconds of every minute.

Scoring.
The score is calculated from the heart rate and resistance (i.e., workload) scores. These two scores are plotted on graph paper with heart rate on the vertical and workload on the horizontal. A straight line is drawn through these two points so that it intersects the horizontal line originating from 170 bpm. A perpendicular line is dropped from this intersection to give the estimated amount of workload needed to produce a heart rate of 170 bpm. The score is expressed in kilogram/meters per minute.

Norms.
Gauthier et al. (1983, pp. 6-8) boys and girls; Simons et al. (1990, p. 97) girls.

REVIEW

B. DON FRANKS, Ph.D.

Professor of Kinesiology
Louisiana State University
Baton Rouge, LA 70803

This PWC 170 Test, if carefully administered by trained testers, is a good indicator of cardiorespiratory endurance (CRE). It has a high validity coefficient (with maximal oxygen uptake) and can be administered in a reliable and objective manner. It is not as good as measuring maximal oxygen uptake directly. The longer time per stage means that the examinee will more likely have reached steady state by the end of the stage than by the end of the more common 2 to 3 minute stages, which will result in a better prediction. It is similar to other cycle ergometer submaximal test protocols in that it can be used at the beginning of a fitness program to estimate CRE. It can also be used to determine changes in CRE over time. This test differs in that it predicts the PWC at a heart rate of 170, whereas most tests predict maximal oxygen uptake.

This test can be used only in a fitness center that has the personnel and time to test examinees individually. It requires a cycle ergometer and a trained professional to administer the test. It does not require much space. The tester must be trained to use and calibrate the ergometer, set the appropriate resistance, and accurately measure heart rate during work. The PWD 170 differs from most of the graded exercise test protocols which set the workload and measure the physiological response to it (e.g., the ACSM Cycle Ergometer protocol, ACSM, 1986). This test is similar to the YMCA test (Golding et al., 1982) in that it uses different resistances based on the heart response, but the YMCA protocol provides directions concerning change of resistance based on the heart rate response to the previous workload. The PWC 170 requires the tester to be able to estimate the workload that will result in a heart rate within a certain range, thus requiring more skill by the tester. It would require about 20 minutes per examinee to administer as well as a few minutes to plot the results. It is a safe test (it could be used at the beginning of a fitness program: whereas, an endurance run should not be used until after a beginning conditioning program). This test can discriminate CRE among examinees and is appropriate for all ages, except those too young or too deconditioned to ride a cycle ergometer. It would not be acceptable for most research studies for which maximal oxygen uptake would be measured directly. It is less expensive than a treadmill and more expensive than a bench step test. The body weight is supported by the seat, which helps partial out the effect of weight, but also makes it a poorer predictor of performance where body weight is carried.

SUMMARY

Major Strengths:

1. The test is safe.

2. It is a valid test of cardiorespiratory endurance.

Major Weaknesses:

1. It is not the best test for research, yet it is too expensive (i.e., in terms of equipment, trained personnel, and time) to be used in many testing situations.

2. The prediction of the physical working capacity at a heart rate of 170 is not a commonly used value and is therefore more difficult to interpret than the predicted maximal oxygen uptake.

3. If the desire is simply to compare CRE before and after training, then one of the set work protocols with shorter stages would be better (get response to more levels of work in the same amount of testing time).

4. If the desire is to extrapolate from a submaximal test to heavier work, then this test should be modified to estimate maximal oxygen uptake rather than PWC at a heart rate of 170.

The test is acceptable for those situations for which a submaximal cycle ergometer test is desired, trained personnel are available, and time is allotted for individual testing.

REVIEW REFERENCES

American College of Sports Medicine (1986). *Guidelines for graded exercise testing and exercise prescription* (3rd ed.). Philadelphia: Lea & Febiger.

Golding, L.A. et al. (1982). *The Y's way to physical fitness*. Chicago: National Board of YMCA.

YMCA PHYSICAL WORKING CAPACITY TEST

Reference.
Golding, L. A. et al. (1989). *Y's way to physical fitness: The complete guide to fitness testing and instruction.* Champaign, IL: Human Kinetics, pp 89-106, 113-124.

Additional Sources.
Baumgartner & Jackson (1991, p. 313).

Purpose.
To measure an examinee's response to submaximal work and thus predict maximal working capacity and maximal oxygen consumption.

Objectivity.
Not reported.

Reliability.
Not reported.

Validity.
Not reported.

Age and Sex.
Females and males, age 18 - 65 + .

Equipment.
A cycle ergometer, body weight scale, a metronome, two stopwatches, and a stethoscope.

Space Requirements and Design.
A clear, level area approximately 3m (10') square with the cycle ergometer positioned in the center.

Directions.
Since some examinees are not familiar with cycling, a practice session should be held a few days before the test. On the day of the test, the examinee should abstain from physical exertion and from eating and smoking two hours prior to being tested. The examinee's body weight is determined in the standard way.

Once the tester has calibrated both the cycle ergometer and the metronome, the examinee assumes a seated position on the ergometer with the balls of her/his feet on the pedals. The seat height is adjusted so that the examinee's knee is straight when the pedal is at its lowest point. The metronome is set at 100 beats per minute (bpm) to produce 50 revolutions in one minute. The examinee then pedals without a load to become familiar with the pace. After one minute of practice, the ergometer is set with a .5 Kp workload (equivalent to 150 kpm/min) and the examinee pedals for three minutes. While using the stethoscope and a stopwatch, the tester counts the heart rate at the second and third minutes of pedaling. The difference between the two heart rate counts should not be greater than five bpm and if it is, the pedaling is continued an extra minute or more until two consecutive counts are within five beats of each other. In determining the heart rate, the tester measures the time for 30 beats by starting the stopwatch on a beat and stopping it on the 30th beat. This count is used to determine the beats per minute. Golding et al. (1989, p. 98) provide a heart rate conversion table.

After recording the first workload and heart rate, the tester increases the workload a second time. The examinee then pedals for three minutes or more until two consecutive heart rate counts are within five beats per minute. If the first workload did not produce a heart rate greater than 110 bpm, the workload is increased a third time following the same procedures as above. The examinee continues pedaling throughout the test even when the workload is being changed. Golding et al. (1989, p. 91) provide guidelines for administering the proper workloads in order to obtain the two desired heart rates between 110 bpm and 150 bpm.

Scoring.
The score is determined by plotting the two exercise heart rates which were between 110 bpm and 150 bpm and their respective workloads. A straight line is drawn connecting these two points and extended to the examinee's maximal heart rate (max HR = 220 - age). A perpendicular line is then drawn from the examinee's maximal heart rate to the baseline at which most of the examinee's maximal physical working capacity and maximal oxygen uptake are read. Golding et al. (1989, p. 100) provide a sampe form.

Norms.
Golding et al. (1989, pp. 113-118, 119-124) men and women.

REVIEW

STEVEN J. ALBRECHTSEN, Ph.D.

Director
Human Performance Laboratory
University of Wisconsin-Whitewater
Whitewater, WI 53190

The YMCA Physical Working Capacity Test is a popular submaximal test to estimate maximal oxygen consumption through the use of a cycle ergometer. Adequate information concerning the validity, reliability, and objectivity of the test has not been determined.

Submaximal cycle tests are particularly appropriate when there are contraindications for a maximal exercise test. These tests estimate maximal oxygen consumption based on the assumption of linear relationships between heart rate, workload, and oxygen consumption. However, these relationships become nonlinear after maximal heart rate has been reached but before maximal oxygen consumption has been achieved. In addition, estimating maximal heart rate on the basis of age is not reliable for many examinees. These problems introduce potential sources of error causing submaximal cycle tests to underestimate maximal oxygen consumption.

Reliability is frequently a problem with tests based on heart rates because of the variety of factors that can influence heart rates independently of exercise during these tests. Objectivity may be a problem with less experienced testers who frequently have difficulty obtaining accurate heart rates during exercise. The accuracy of heart rates determined by measuring the time for 30 heart beats decreases as heart rate increases. More accurate and objective heart rates may be obtained with 30 second pulse counts. Exercise cycles are increasingly available in a variety of settings. However, the majority of these exercise cycles do not qualify as cycle ergometers because they cannot be accurately calibrated and/or calibration cannot be easily verified. Achieving accurate workloads requires the use of an accurately calibrated metronome and also requires that the tester monitor the examinees for pedaling compliance throughout the test.

The Astrand-Ryhming Test (1954) is perhaps the best known submaximal cycle test and provides a "bench-mark" for evaluating similar tests. The Astrand-Ryhming Test may be classified as a single stage test during which a datum point is obtained and used with a constant intercept to determine the slope of the linear relationships between heart rate, workload and oxygen consumption. The YMCA Physical Working Capacity Test may be classified as a multi stage test which seeks to improve the determination of slope by measuring two workloads, instead of assuming a constant intercept. The slope determined from such a test should be more reliable when the two data points are as far apart as possible.

Unfortunately, two data points within the heart rate range of 110 to 150 bpm may be too close together to determine the slope of the linear relationships reliably. Furthermore, a larger range of heart rates is not possible, and an even narrower range of heart rates is physiologically indicated. Stroke volume increases and does not level off until approximately 45 percent of maximal oxygen consumption while anaerobic metabolism plays an increasing role above approximately 70 percent of maximal oxygen consumption. In recognition of these physiological considerations, Astrand and Rodahl (1986) recommend the use of heart rates between 120 and 150 bpm.

The Astrand-Ryhming Test requires only six or seven minutes and utilizes a nomogram or tables for data analysis. The YMCA Physical Working Capacity Test requires six to nine minutes or longer, and the data analysis involves a graphical procedure that does not take into account the leveling off of heart rate below maximal oxygen consumption or individual differences in maximal heart rate. The graphical analysis procedure is not difficult, but it is time consuming and provides a false sense of sophistication.

SUMMARY

Major Strengths:

1. Most examinees are familiar with exercise cycles which are becoming increasingly available.

2. The test is relatively easy to administer and does not involve maximal exercise.

Major Weaknesses:

1. Adequate information concerning the validity, reliability, and objectivity of the test has not been determined.

2. The test may require additional time and involves a time consuming graphical analysis procedure, but may not provide more reliable results than single stage tests.

The YMCA Physical Working Capacity Test is an acceptable test for teaching when the resources for more sophisticated tests are not available and/or when there are contraindications for a maximal exercise test. The YMCA Physical Working Capacity Test is an unacceptable test for research because the test involves the estimation and not the actual measurement of maximal oxygen consumption.

REVIEW REFERENCES

Astrand, P. O., & Ryhming, I. (1954). A nomogram for calculation of aerobic capacity (physical fitness) from pulse rate during submaximal work. *Journal of Applied Physiology,* 7:218-221.

Astrand, P. O., & Rodahl, K. (1986). *Textbook of work physiology*. New York: McGraw-Hill.

12-MINUTE CYCLING TEST

References.

Cooper, K. H. (1982). *The aerobics program for total well-being.* New York: M. Evans & Co., p 143.

Miller, D. K. (1988). *Measurement by the physical educator: Why and how.* Indianapolis: Benchmark Press, pp 148-149.

Additional Sources.

None.

Purpose.

To measure the cardiorespiratory endurance of an examinee through cycling.

Objectivity.

Not reported.

Reliability.

Not reported.

Validity.

Not reported.

Age and Sex.

Females and males, age 13 - 60.

Equipment.

A three speed bicycle, stopwatch, and tape measure.

Space Requirements and Design.

A flat, measured area or a measured distance on a street with little or no traffic that would enable the examinee to ride a bicycle safely. The course should be marked every 400m (440 yds).

Directions.

Before attempting the test, the examinee should become aware of how to cycle and pace for distance. The testing day should not have a wind of more than 10 miles per hour. Following a warm up, the examinee assumes a position at the starting line. On command, "Ready, Go," the examinee bicycles as far as possible within a 12 minute period. Following the 12 minute test, the examinee is asked to continue riding to cool down.

Scoring.

The score is the distance that the examinee bicycled within the 12 minute period measured in kilometers (miles).

Norms.

Barrow et al. (1989, p. 138) boys, girls, men, and women; Cooper (1982, p. 143) boys, girls, men and women; Kirkendall et al. (1980, p. 302) women;

Kirkendall et al. (1987, p. 176) boys, girls, men, and women; Miller (1988, p. 149) boys, girls, men, and women.

REVIEW

SCOTT E. FRAZIER, P.E.D.

Assistant Professor
Physical Education
University of Wisconsin-Stevens Point
Stevens Point, WI 54481

There are several measurement concerns with the 12-Minute Cycling Test as presented; these concerns relate to the lack of standardized equipment used when performing the test. According to the guidelines, the examinee may perform the test with any type, make, or model of bicycle as long as it is a three speed. Therein lies one major measurement problem. There are a wide range of bicycles that fit into that category. As any serious biker will attest, there are huge differences between bicycles costing a hundred dollars and those that sell for over a thousand dollars. There are aerodynamic, tire, and weight differences, in addition to countless other advantages in the expensive models. In the sport of bicycling, the equipment can have an impact on performance results. This important factor would certainly reduce the validity of the test.

The argument could be put forth that the test is at least reliable for a test-retest or pretest-posttest situation. However, many variables could change from one test period to the next, even for the same examinee and bicycle. Factors such as tire pressure, level of humidity, and amount of sunlight may influence the test results and decrease reliability. Scores may not be as precise as with standardized, calibrated laboratory ergometers. Perhaps this is the reason that reliability and validity figures are not included or are unknown for this particular test.

SUMMARY

Major Strengths:

1. The test is practical and easy to administer.

2. It is a very simple field test for determination of baseline fitness.

Major Weakness:

1. The lack of reported reliability and validity preclude usage of the test for research purposes.

The test is unacceptable for research, but may be acceptable for some teaching situations and assessment of individual fitness levels.

RUN AND/OR WALK TESTS OF CARDIORESPIRATORY ENDURANCE

CARLSON FATIGUE CURVE TEST

References.
Mathews, D. K. (1978). *Measurement in physical education*. Philadelphia: W. B. Saunders, pp 259-261.

Carlson, H. C. (1945). Fatigue curve test. *Research Quarterly* 16(3):169-175.

Additional Sources.
None.

Purpose.
To measure the cardiorespiratory endurance and power of an examinee through running in place.

Objectivity.
Not reported.

Reliability.
Not reported.

Validity.
Not reported.

Age and Sex.
Not reported.

Equipment.
A stopwatch, paper, and pencil.

Space Requirements and Design.
A clear, level area approximately 2m (6') square with the examinee in the center.

Directions.
The examinee sits on the floor and measures her/his pulse rate for 10 seconds. This pulse rate count is multiplied by six and recorded.

The examinee then assumes a standing position. On command, the examinee runs in place as fast as possible for a period of 10 seconds. At the end of 10 seconds of running, the examinee rests for 10 seconds. During the running phase, the feet must be raised only high enough to clear the floor. The number of times the right foot touches the floor must be noted by the examinee and recorded. At the end of 10 seconds of rest, the examinee, on command, runs in place another 10 seconds followed by 10 seconds of rest. The 10

seconds of running and 10 seconds of rest equals one inning. Immediately after 10 innings have been completed, the examinee sits on the floor and the pulse rate is taken. This pulse rate is then multiplied by six and recorded. The pulse rate should be measured again at 2, 4, and 6 minutes after the cessation of running. The count of all right foot contacts at the completion of 10 innings should also be summed and recorded.

Scoring.
The "production" score is determined by the sum of right foot contacts made during the 10 innings of running. A "condition" index is derived by plotting the pulse rate and evaluating the degree of recovery after running.

Norms.
Not reported.

REVIEW

PHYLLIS T. CROISANT, Ph.D.

Associate Professor
Physical Education
Eastern Illinois University
Charleston, IL 61920

Accuracy of the examinee's self count of right foot contacts is a concern affecting all scientific aspects of the Carlson Fatigue Curve Test. Twenty-five physical education students at Eastern Illinois University performed this test while simultaneously being videotaped. The mean difference in the self counted production score and the score counted from a slow motion replay of the videotape was 51.3 steps (range of 6 to 137), or mean difference of five foot contacts per inning. Experience in taking the test did not result in more accurate scores as the mean difference between self and video counts on a second day of testing was 54.8 steps (range of 1 to 171). Counts made by partners also showed large discrepancies from the video count, 46.8 and 64.2 steps on days one and two, respectively. The largest errors in self count occurred when the examinee performed over 40 right foot contacts per 10 second inning, with most examinees reporting undercounts. Examinees averaging fewer than 35 steps per inning tended to overcount.

Test-retest reliability of the Carlson Fatigue Curve Test was determined for 25 physical education students repeating the test at a 48 to 120 hour interval. The test-retest correlation of production scores taken from the videotape was 0.92. However, the test-retest correlation was only 0.51 for self counted production scores.

High intensity intermittent running of 10 seconds duration followed by 10 seconds rest has been shown to elicit high levels of oxygen uptake and cardiac output without significant elevation of blood lactate (Christensen et al., 1960). Phosphagen and oxygen stores in the working muscles are utilized during the work bout and replenished during the rest period, placing high demand upon the cardiorespiratory system without engaging anaerobic glycolysis. This process suggests construct validity of the Carlson Fatigue Curve Test. In the sample of 25 physical education students, the production score from videotape had a correlation of -0.54 with time for a mile run. There was a correlation of -0.72 between production score from videotape and maximal oxygen consumption for nine of the students. A negative correlation between the production score and VO_2max was not expected and was due to two members of the cross county team who had the highest maximal oxygen consumptions but the lowest production scores. With these scores removed, the correlation was essentially zero.

The Carlson Fatigue Curve Test requires little equipment or time and is extremely easy to use. One tester can administer the test to an entire class in less than 10 minutes. Carlson recommended that a series of tests should be administered daily for 10 days. A learning effect seems to be present as the mean production score increased by 19 steps from test one to test two in our sample. With continued daily use of the test, a training effect would be anticipated as the examinees are performing interval training. If accurate self counting were possible, the test could be motivational as examinees see daily improvement.

SUMMARY

Major Strengths:

1. It uses little equipment or time.

2. Many examinees may be tested simultaneously by one tester.

3. It is suitable for use as a conditioning drill.

Major Weaknesses:

1. Self scoring is inaccurate and inconsistent.

2. Validity as a test of cardiorespiratory endurance has not been established.

3. Norms are not available.

The Carlson Fatigue Curve Test as presented is inadequate as a test of cardiorespiratory endurance and power. The researcher will continue to use measurement of maximal oxygen consumption as a standard, while the practitioner is advised to consider one of the "walk run" or "step tests" in which scoring is less of a problem, validity has been established, and norms are available.

REVIEW REFERENCE

Christensen, E. H. et al. (1960). Intermittent and continuous running. *Acta Physiol. Scand.*, 50:269.

DISTANCE RUN/WALK TESTS

References.

Johnson, B. L., & Nelson, J. K. (1986). *Practical measurements for evaluation in physical education.* Edina, MN: Burgess, pp 154-158.

Safrit, M. J. et al. (1988). The validity generalization of distance run tests. *Canadian Journal of Sport Sciences,* 13(4):188-196.

Additional Sources.

Barrow et al. (1989, pp. 106, 109, 118, 130-133); Baumgartner & Jackson (1982, pp. 250-251); Baumgartner & Jackson (1987, pp. 283, 288-289, 303-304); Baumgartner & Jackson (1991, pp. 265, 270-276, 286);

Bosco & Gustafson (1983, pp. 138-140); Clarke & Clarke (1987, pp. 150-151, 160); Hastad & Lacy (1989, pp. 180-186, 230, 233, 236-237); Jensen & Hirst (1980, pp. 108-110); Johnson & Nelson (1986, pp. 154-158); Kirkendall et al. (1980, pp. 272, 274, 297);

Kirkendall et al. (1987, pp. 153, 155-156, 166-167, 174-177, 401); Miller (1988, pp. 145-148); Safrit (1981, pp. 222-228, 242-243); Safrit (1986, pp. 230-233, 283-285, 443-444); Safrit (1990, pp. 244-245, 353-357, 416-418); Verducci (1980, pp. 273-276, 280, 286-288).

Purpose.

To measure the cardiorespiratory endurance of an examinee via running either a specified distance in a measured amount of time or for a specified time for a measured amount of distance.

Objectivity.

Not reported.

Reliability.

r = .94 by Doolittle and Bigbee (1968) for the 12 minute run cited in Johnson and Nelson (1986, p. 154).

600 Yard Run-Walk Test: r = .92 by Willgoose and Askew (1961) for junior high school boys and girls cited in Johnson and Nelson (1986, p. 156).

Validity.

r = .64 to .90 for the 12 minute run when the criterion used was maximum oxygen intake cited in Johnson and Nelson (1986, p. 154).

600 Yard Run-Walk Test: r = .96 (third grade boys), r = .88 (fifth grade boys), and r = .76 (seventh grade boys) were obtained by Biasiotto and Cotten (1972) cited in Johnson and Nelson (1986, p. 156).

Age and Sex.

Nine and Twelve-Minute Run-Walk Tests: Females and males, junior high school through college.

Six Minute Run-Walk Test: Females, junior high school through college.

1.5 Mile Run: Females and males, age 13 and older.

1 Mile Run: Females and males, age 10 - 12.

600 Yard Run-Walk Test: Females and males, age 6 -12.

800 Meters (Canadian Association, 1980, p. 34): Females and males, age 6 - 9.

1600 Meters (Canadian Association, 1980, p. 34): Females and males, age 10 - 12.

2400 Meters (Canadain Association, 1980, p. 34): Females and males, age 13 - 17.

Equipment.

A whistle, a stopwatch, and plastic cones to designate the distance intervals.

Space Requirements and Design.

A 400 meter/440 yard track or a smooth, level, open area with a measured distance (e.g., 50 yard square or a rectangle 40 x 100 yards) marked off. Increments of 10 yards or more must be marked off. The distance of each increment is determined by the size of the area used for the run/walk.

Directions.

Timed Runs for Distance (Twelve, Nine, and Six Minute Run/Walk Tests):

To facilitate these tests, the examinees are organized with a partner. The examinees then go to the designated starting point and on command, "Ready, Go," they begin. Once started, the examinees attempt to run and/or walk as many laps around the course as possible in the allotted time. The examinee's partner keeps count of the number of laps completed, and upon hearing the "stop" whistle, the partner goes to the spot on the course where the examinee finished. The distance covered is determined by multiplying the number of laps by the length of each lap and adding the number of yards past the starting line during the last lap. This distance is recorded.

Distance Runs for Time (1.5 mile, 1 mile, 600 yards and 800, 1600 and 2400 meters Run/Walk Tests):

To facilitate these tests, the examinees are organized with a partner. The examinees go to the designated starting point, and on command, "Ready, Go," they begin. At the end of the required run/walk distance, the timer reads aloud the times as the examinees pass the finish line. Partners of examinees should remember the proper time and turn it in to be recorded.

Scoring.

Timed Runs for Distance (Twelve, Nine, and Six Minute Run/Walk Tests):

The score is the distance covered, in yards or meters, during the allotted time.

Distance Runs for Time (1.5 Mile, 1 Mile, and 600 yards and 800, 1600, and 2400 meter Run/Walk Tests):

The score is the time required to complete the specified distance.

Norms.

Alabama (1988, pp. 13-15, 26-27) boys and girls for mile; American Alliance (1975, pp. 31-33, 39-41, 48, 53, 58-60) boys, girls, men, and women for 600 yards, mile, 1.5 mile, 9 minute and 12 minute;

American Alliance (1980, pp. 23-28) boys and girls for mile, 1.5 mile, 9 minute, and 12 minute; American Alliance (1985, pp. 11-15, 20-21) men and women for mile and 9 minute; American Alliance (1988, pp. 28-29) boys and girls for mile; American Alliance (1990, pp. 10-11, 39) boys and girls for .5 mile, mile, 1.5 mile, 9 minute and 12 minute;

Arizona (1983, pp. 3-28) boys and girls for mile; Barrow et al. (1989, pp. 105, 110, 124-126, 130, 134-135) boys, girls, men and women for 600

yards, mile, 1.5 mile, 9 minute, 12 minute, and steady state run; Baumgartner & Jackson (1982, pp. 252-254) boys and girls for mile, 1.5 mile, 9 minute, and 12 minute;

Baumgartner & Jackson (1987, pp. 284-286, 290-291) boys and girls for 600 yards, mile, 1.5 mile, 9 minute, 12 minute and steady state run; Baumgartner & Jackson (1991, pp. 263, 266-267, 274-276, 287-289) boys and girls for 600 yards, mile, 1.5 mile, 9 minute, 12 minute, and steady state run;

Canadian Association (1980, pp. 37-60) boys and girls for 800m, 1600m and 2400m; Chrysler/AAU (1990, p. 6) boys and girls for 440 yards, 880 yards, 1320 yards and mile; Clarke & Clarke (1987, p. 162) boys and girls for mile; Corbin & Lindsey (1983, p. 36) boys, girls, men, and women for 12 minute;

Corbin & Lindsey (1985, p. 43) boys, girls, men, and women for 12 minute; Evans (1973, p. 386) rugby players for 600 yards; Fitness Institute (1981, no page numbers) boys, girls, men, and women for 1.5 mile; Fleishman (1964A, p. 60) boys and girls for 600 yards; Franks (1989, pp. 42-47) boys and girls for mile;

Getchell (1983, pp. 52-53, 56) men and women for 1.5 mile and 2 mile; Governor's Commission (no date) boys and girls; Greenberg & Pargman (1989, p. 68) men and women for 1.5 mile; Harrison & Bradbeer (1982, pp. 24-25) boy and girl athletes for 12 minute;

Hastad & Lacy (1989, pp. 182-184, 187, 284) boys and girls for mile, 1.5 mile, 9 minute and 12 minute; Hawaii (1989, pp. 19-20) boys and girls for 300 yards; Haydon (1986, pp. 56-57) boys and girls for mile and 1.5 mile; Hoeger (1989, pp. 21, 27) men and women for 1.5 mile; Jackson & Ross (1986, p. 29) sex and age not stated for 1.5 mile and 12 minute;

Jensen & Hirst (1980, p. 109) men and women for 12 minute; Johnson & Nelson (1986, pp. 155, 157-158, 203-205, 207) boys, girls, men, women, and army for 300 yards, 600 yards, mile, 1.5 mile, 9 minute and 12 minute; Kirkendall et al. (1980, pp. 280-283, 288-291, 301, 305) boys, girls, men, and women for 400 yards, 600 yards, mile, 1.5 mile, 9 minute, and 12 minute; Kirkendall et al. (1987, pp. 160-161, 170-171, 175, 406-407) boys, girls, men, women, and special populations for 400 yards, 600 yards, mile, 1.5 mile, 9 minute, and 12 minute; Lindsey et al. (1989, p. 9) men and women for 1.5 mile;

Maryland (1986, pp. 21-22) boys and girls for mile and 9 minute; McCaughan (1975, p. 16) boys for 880 yards; Miller (1988, pp. 146-147, 233-234) boys, girls, men and women for 600 yards, mile, 1.5 mile, 9 minute, and 12 minute; National Marine (no date, p. 16) boys and girls for 600 yards;

Prentice & Bucher (1988, pp. 97, 102) men and women for 1.5 mile and 12 minute; President's Council (1987, pp. 3-6) USSR boys and girls for 1500m, 2000m and 3000m; President's Council (1988, pp. 2, 7) boys and girls for mile; President's Council (1989, p. 8) boys and girls for mile;

Pyke (1986, p. 8) boys and girls for 1.6km; Ross et al. (1985, p. 64) boys and girls for mile; Ross et al. (1987, p. 70) boys and girls for .5 mile and mile; Rhode Island (1989, pp. 24-26) boys and girls for mile; Safrit (1981, p. 225) men and women for 1.5 mile and 12 minute;

Safrit (1986, pp. 232-233, 285, Appendix A-35) boys and girls for 600 yards, mile, and 9 minute; Safrit (1990, pp. 342, 345, 347, 352, 356-357, 416, Appendix A-36) boys and girls for 600 yards, .5 mile, and 20 minute steady state jog; Shannon (1989, p. 45) high school football players for 440 yards;

South Carolina (1983, pp. 15, 30-38) boys, girls, men, and women for mile and 9 minute; Stokes et al. (1986, p. 170) men and women for 1.5 mile and 12 minute; Virginia (1988, pp. 18, 22) boys and girls for mile.

REVIEW

J. JESSE DEMELLO, Ed.D.

Associate Professor
Health and Physical Education
Louisiana State University in
Shreveport
Shreveport, LA 71115

Astrand and Rodahl (1970) consider cardiorespiratory fitness (Aerobic Capacity) to be the most valid index of physical fitness. Cardiorespiratory capacity (CRC) has been directly correlated to the ability of an individual to participate successfully in physical activity requiring a sustained effort (i.e., activity lasting more than five minutes of constant work). Therefore, it is imperative that there be a valid, consistent, and objective instrument that measures CRC feasibly.

Distance Run/walk Tests are the most commonly used instruments when estimating CRC in field conditions. When concurrently validated to laboratory measurements of maximal oxygen consumption, distance runs have been shown to have moderate to high (-0.66 to -0.90) validity. However, it should be noted that distance runs shorter than one mile and/or less than nine minutes duration may not be valid measures of cardiorespiratory function (Jackson & Coleman, 1976). Additionally, one needs to recognize that distance runs measure more than one physiological variable (Cureton, 1982) because distance run performance is affected by body composition, running efficiency, motivation, and pace.

Distance Run/Walk Tests are usually highly reliable. Reliability coefficients of 0.75 to 0.94 have been obtained. However, it should be noted that most reliability studies have been conducted utilizing adult and adolescent examinees.

The reviewer was unable to find any estimation of objectivity for these tests. However, due to the fact that the scores on these tests are based on concrete observation, it is anticipated that these tests will have a high degree of objectivity.

From a practical standpoint, these tests are very feasible if a field or a large indoor facility is available. The only equipment needed is a stopwatch. The tests are easy to administer if the class and/or group is paired as recommended. The distance runs for time are recommended instead of timed runs for distance because these tests require less preparation time. Distance runs for time also decrease the amount of possible measurement error by requiring fewer tasks of the testers, thus possibly increasing the validity and reliability of the measurement.

As to the number of trials, the instructions do not address the issue specifically (i.e., the instructions leave us with the impression that one trial is adequate). However, most measurement specialists recommend two trials. Either have a practice run of equal distance or time to be followed with a subsequent test run (three or more days later) or administer the test twice and use the mean time for the two tests as the criterion score. This method does double the time required; however, it improves the validity and reliability of the scores significantly.

The tests could be incorporated into a drill to promote CRC conditioning. The tests are fairly safe to administer and because of their objective nature they could be used for self evaluation purposes.

From the standpoint of appropriateness, these tests could be administered to any examinee who is between 6 and 35 years of age and free from any apparent disease or condition which may rule out safe participation. Any test requiring less than nine minutes duration and/or less than one mile in length are not recommended due to possible validity questions. This validity question, of course, brings to mind the possible inappropriateness of these tests for the six to nine year old age group. This has been the topic of much discussion within the profession and will probably continue to be a controversial topic in the future. However, from a measurement standpoint it makes no sense whatsoever to use an instrument which lacks validity.

The test does not have suitable precision for research purposes unless it is used with large populations and in conjunction with other related measures of fitness, such as body composition and estimates of regular physical activity.

Up to date norms are available for age and gender. Norms can be found in most measurement and evaluation textbooks, and, of course, they can be also be obtained from AAHPERD and/or the President's Council on Physical Fitness.

SUMMARY

Major Strengths:

1. The tests do not require much equipment.

2. The tests can be easily administered.

3. The tests are very mass testable.

Major Weaknesses:

1. The difficulty of administering the longer tests to the six to nine year old age group.

2. The poor validity of the tests requiring less than nine minutes and/or less than one mile distance.

Overall, these tests are acceptable for teaching, coaching, and research if: (1) we limit the tests to the longer distances, (2) we use the tests when evaluating large populations, and (3) we evaluate results taking into consideration other related fitness parameters such as body composition and physical activity history. Nonetheless, these tests are of value because they evaluate a unique physical ability that is not measured in most other tests of human physical performance, that is the ability of an examinee to sustain a certain level of energy expenditure for an extended period of time.

REVIEW REFERENCES

Astrand, P., & Rodahl, K. (1970). *Textbook of work physiology.* New York: McGraw-Hill.

Cureton, K. J. (1982). Distance running performance tests in children - what do they mean? *Journal of Physical Education, Recreation and Dance,* 53:64-66, October.

Jackson, A. E., & Coleman, A. E. (1976). Validation of distance run tests for elementary school children. *Research Quarterly,* 47(1):86-94.

ENDURANCE SHUTTLE RUN TEST

Reference.
Committee of Experts on Sports Research (1988). *Eurofit: Handbook for the eurofit tests of physical fitness*. Rome, Italy, pp 16, 25-29.

Additional Sources.
None.

Purpose.
To measure the cardiorespiratory endurance of an examinee through the use of a maximal progressive shuttle run.

Objectivity.
Had to be high to meet their criteria, but an exact figure is not stated (Committee, 1988, p. 16).

Reliability.
Had to be high to meet their criteria, but an exact figure is not stated (Committee, 1988, p. 16).

Validity.
Had to be high to meet their criteria, but an exact figure is not stated (Committee, 1988, p. 16).

Age and Sex.
Females and males, age 6 - 18.

Equipment.
A prerecorded audio tape of the test protocol, a tape recorder, a tape measure, and marking tape.

Space Requirements and Design.
A clear, level area approximately 3m x 30m (10' x 90') with two parallel lines marked 20m (65.6') apart in the middle of the 30m length.

Directions.
The examinee stands behind one line and upon the signal given on the prerecorded tape, begins the test at a walking pace. The examinee moves toward the other line, touches the line with one foot, reverses direction, and continues moving back and forth between the two lines. The speed at which the examinee moves is controlled by the tape, giving off buzzing sounds at regular intervals. The examinee must pace herself/himself so as to be at or within one to two meters of the correct line when the prerecorded tape gives off the signal. During the first phase of the test, the speed is slow, but the pace increases slowly and steadily with each passing minute. The objective

is that the examinee follow the proper pace for as long as possible. The test is terminated when the examinee can no longer maintain the proper pace, and the number of the last minute completed, announced over the prerecorded tape, is noted. The length of the test thus varies with the condition of the examinee; that is, the more fit the examinee, the more minutes the test is continued.

Scoring.
The score is the number of the last minute the examinee maintained the proper pace.

Norms.
Not reported.

REVIEW

MATTHEW T. MAHAR, Ed.D.

Assistant Professor
Physical Education
Springfield College
Springfield, MA 01109

The Endurance Shuttle Run was developed as part of Eurofit, a physical fitness assessment battery, by the Committee of Experts on Sports Research. The purpose of the Endurance Shuttle Run is to estimate aerobic power of school aged children (6 to 18 years).

The Endurance Shuttle Run was developed as a field test to enable assessment of several examinees in a relatively short time. The test constructors reported that the Endurance Shuttle Run replaced the 6-Minute Run test as the field test of cardiorespiratory fitness because the Endurance Shuttle Run demonstrated high validity and reliability estimates.

The Endurance Shuttle Run and the entire Eurofit test battery is published in a handbook. The handbook outlines the general requirements for inclusion of a test in the battery and presents adequate descriptions of all tests. The space requirements of the Endurance Shuttle Run are minimal, requiring only a flat surface 20 meters in length. Several examinees can be measured simultaneously if the test course is sufficiently wide. The handbook suggested that the test could be performed either outdoors or indoors. Most of the required equipment is typically available in schools; however, a prerecorded tape of the protocol must be acquired to indicate proper procedures (e.g., pace and step number).

The most fit examinees will endure for longer periods of time. Speed of movement begins at a slow pace (8 kph or 4.96 mph) and increases each minute of the protocol. Examinees follow the set pace so as to be at one end of the 20 meters when the tape sounds. Examinees continue until they can no longer keep pace with the tape. The highly fit examinees who complete the entire protocol will exercise for 23 minutes and end at a pace of 18.5 kph (11.47 mph). The lack of published norms makes it difficult to determine whether this test adequately discriminates among examinees with high cardiorespiratory fitness levels.

The Endurance Shuttle Run may take more time to administer than other comparable cardiorespiratory field tests, such as the 1-Mile or 9-Minute Run. In a physical education class situation, examinees who do not continue for the entire protocol (i.e., less fit examinees) must be supervised while the highly fit examinees continue. In addition, many of the examinees will end the test in failure (i.e., inability to continue), which result is not true of several other cardiorespiratory field tests. The psychological impact of such testing on examinees is unknown.

As with other maximal aerobic fitness tests, examinees must be motivated to perform at their maximal capacity to obtain a valid measure of cardiorespiratory fitness. Scoring procedures are objective as examinees must note their last completed step from the tape. However, examinees are unable to use the Endurance Shuttle Run for self evaluation unless a copy of the prerecorded tape is available.

The Eurofit handbook states that the tests (including the Endurance Shuttle Run) are not to be practiced as drills to increase aerobic capacity. Thus, the effect of practice on Endurance Shuttle Run test performance is unknown. It is possible that examinees need to learn the pace of the prerecorded tape, but this apparently is not of great concern to the test constructors.

One of the weaker aspects of the test is that no norms are available. It is stated that each country which participates will be responsible for establishing its own norms.

No reliability or validity estimates are provided in the Eurofit handbook. The handbook stated that reliability and objectivity measures had to be high for inclusion of a test in the battery, but did not give an indication of the magnitude of the coefficient required or of the number of examinees used to estimate the test's consistency.

Additionally, it was stated that test criteria included evidence of construct and concurrent validity. However, specific procedures for validating the Endurance Shuttle Run were not reported. It would be helpful to know if the Endurance Shuttle Run results were significantly correlated to measured maximal oxygen consumption values as an estimate of concurrent validity. Other maximal field tests of cardiorespiratory fitness (e.g., 12-Minute Run and 1.5-Mile Run) have been validated in this manner.

Profile charts are recommended to help interpret Endurance Shuttle Run scores to examinees. Profile charts are to be based on national sex and age group norms. A profile chart is constructed on a scale ranging from 0 to 20, with a score of 10 at the 50th percentile. Individual scores are then plotted on these charts to provide an overall picture of the examinee compared to her/his peers. No specific information is provided on how to translate Endurance Shuttle Run scores into specific training recommendations.

SUMMARY

Major Strengths:

1. Minimal space requirements.
2. Feasibility for mass testing.
3. Objective scoring procedures.

Major Weaknesses:

1. Specific validity estimates are not presented.
2. Specific reliability estimates are not presented.
3. The test may take more time to administer than other comparable tests.
4. The test lacks published norms.

Overall, the Endurance Shuttle Run seems to be measuring the appropriate construct of aerobic fitness. However, this reviewer cannot recommend its use in a physical education class setting because of the lack of published norms or criteria to be met and the absence of documented reliability and validity estimates in the handbook. Other maximal field tests of aerobic fitness seem more appropriate for use at this time.

FAIRBANKS SUBMAXIMAL TEST

References.
Fairbanks, J. G. (1978). Submaximal walking test: Prediction of max VO^2 and physical fitness in adult males. Unpublished dissertation, Brigham Young University.

Jensen, C. R., & Hirst, C. C. (1980). *Measurement in physical education and athletics*. New York: MacMillan, pp 112-113.

Additional Sources.
None.

Purpose.
To predict maximum oxygen consumption of an examinee based on heart rate after exercise.

Objectivity.
r = .95 between self measured recovery pulse and telemetry measured recovery pulse.

Reliability.
Not reported.

Validity.
r = .69 recovery pulse and VO^2max, r = .96 between telemetry measured exercise pulse and telemetry measured recovery pulse.

Age and Sex.
Males, age 24 - 42.

Equipment.
A paper, a pencil, two plastic cones, and a stopwatch.

Space Requirements and Design.
A clear, level area approximately 35m (110') long with the two cones marked off 30.48m (100') apart.

Directions.
The examinee rests 10 minutes before the test and then counts the pulse at the wrist for one minute. After recording the pulse count and when ready, the examinee starts the stopwatch and begins walking the 30.48m (100') distance, turning around the cone at each end. The examinee should use a normal, brisk walking pace to cover the 100 feet in 15 to 16 seconds (between 4.26 and 4.55 mph). After five minutes of walking at a consistent pace, the examinee stops walking, stands motionless, and takes his pulse during the

first 10 seconds of recovery from the exercise. If the examinee fails to locate his pulse during the first two seconds of recovery, the whole test must be repeated.

Scoring.
To determine maximum oxygen consumption, the examinee's scores are plugged into the following formula.

$$\text{Max } VO^2 \text{ (ml/kg/min)} = 111.6 - 0.06198 \text{ (Weight)} - 0.4564 \text{ (Recovery pulse)} - 0.0867 \text{ (Resting pulse)}.$$

Body weight is expressed in pounds, and both the resting pulse and the recovery pulse are expressed in beats per minute. The answer will be the predicted number of millimeters of oxygen the examinee uses per kilogram of body weight per minute at maximum work.

Norms.
Fairbanks (1978, p. 53) men; Jensen & Hirst (1980, p. 113) same standards as Fairbanks.

NOTE: It is highly recommended that examinees practice counting their exercise recovery pulse several times before taking the test since they must repeat the test if they do not initiate the count within the first two seconds of recovery.

REVIEW

SUSAN M. MOEN, Ph.D.

Assistant Professor
Physical Education
Dallas Baptist University
Dallas, TX 75211

The purpose of the Fairbanks Submaximal Test is to estimate aerobic fitness and to predict maximal oxygen consumption using recovery heart rate following five minutes of walking at a specified pace. True validity is not given because there is no mention of the correlation between the results of a VO^2max test in which respiratory gases were collected and predicted VO^2max using the formula derived by the test constructor. Similar tests shown to be relatively valid include the Queens College Step Test (McArdle et al., 1972), whose validity coefficient is -0.75 between recovery pulse rate and VO^2max and a shuttle run test (Ramsbottom et al, 1988) with a coefficient of 0.92. The unknown validity as well as reliability of the Fairbanks Submaximal Test might be enhanced by the use of walking rather than running; this avoids the problems of lack of motivation, effective pacing, and running efficiency that are often inherent in running tests. Also, a lower heart rate would be expected compared with that resulting from a running or step test, making it easier for examinees to count their pulse rates accurately.

Apparently, reliability was not determined. Reliability is a particularly important criterion when using heart rate to estimate fitness because many factors can influence it, such as nervousness, time of day, and digestion as well as ability to count the pulse rate accurately. Because pulse rate is taken by the examinee, the test constructor used the relationship between self measured recovery pulse and telemetry measured recovery pulse to evaluate the objectivity of the test. A high positive correlation is desirable. The test does not require active participation of another individual who could affect the performance of the examinee.

The practical aspects of this test are excellent. Little space and no special facilities are needed. Only one tester would be required, and minimal practice would be necessary for the tester to learn the required walking pace of the examinees. Further, several examinees could be tested at the same time, and the test takes five minutes to administer. Only one trial is given. It seems necessary, therefore, for the examinees to practice walking the specified pace and locating their pulse quickly and counting it before the official test is given. Because of the short duration of the test and the minimal effort required of fit individuals, the test would not be useful for conditioning. The test appears appropriate for the intended age range, and it seems it could discriminate among a wide range of fitness levels. The Queens College Step Test imposes

too low a maximal value for women causing it to be invalid for those who are highly fit. Safety aspects of the Fairbanks Test are excellent. The test can be used easily for self evaluation provided examinees are skilled in quickly locating and then accurately counting their own pulse rate. Because VO^2max predicted from a submaximal heart rate is generally only within 10 to 20 percent of a individual's actual value, the test could not be used for research purposes even if validity and reliability were known. Once these coefficients are determined, the test might be suitable for fitness classes and self evaluation. Only ranges of VO^2max norms are given for the test. The test was developed only on adult males and, therefore, cannot be extrapolated to females.

SUMMARY

Major Strengths:

1. The test is inexpensive, easy to administer, and can be given to many examinees in a very short time.

2. The test can be administered in many different settings requiring little space and no special facilities.

3. The test mode, walking, is one in which skill, pacing, and motivation are unlikely to affect test results.

4. The test is extremely safe for all examinees.

Major Weaknesses:

1. The test has not been properly validated, and test reliability is unknown.

2. The test is applicable only to males aged 24 to 42 years, eliminating its use for most school aged males and all females.

The test is currently unacceptable because validity and reliability are unknown. If, however, these coefficients were determined, the test might be excellent for teaching and self evaluation, although not for research purposes.

ROCKPORT WALK TEST

References.

Kline, G. M. et al. (1987). Estimation of VO^{2}max from a one-mile track walk, gender, age and body weight. *Medicine and Science in Sports and Exercise,* 19:253-259.

Coleman, R. J. et al. (1987). Validation of 1-mile walk test for estimating VO^2 in 20-29 year olds. *Medicine and Science in Sports and Exercise,* 19(2):Sup 29.

O'Hanley, S. et al. (1987). Validation of a one mile walk test in 70-79 olds. *Medicine and Science in Sports and Exercise,* 19(2):Sup 28.

Rockport (1989). *The Rockport guide to fitness walking.* Marlboro, MA.

Ward, A. et al. (1987). Estimation of VO^{2}max in overweight females. *Medicine and Science in Sports and Exercise,* 19(2):Sup 29.

Additional Sources.

Baumgartner & Jackson (1991, pp. 315-316); Safrit (1990, pp. 279-280).

Purpose.

To estimate maximum oxygen consumption of an examinee by using a submaximum one mile walk.

Objectivity.

Not reported.

Reliability.

r = .93 for heart rate and r = .98 for walking time using the test-retest method.

Validity.

r = .92 between estimated VO^{2}max and measured VO^{2}max using a treadmill protocol.

Age and Sex.

Females and males, age 30 - 69.

Equipment.

A stopwatch.

Space Requirements and Design.

A 400 meter or 440 yard track or a measured, smooth, level one mile surface.

Directions.

The examinee is encouraged to take several practice walks on the track days prior to the test in order to reduce any learning effect and to establish a steady walking pace. On test day, after 5 to 10 minutes of stretching, the examinee assumes a standing position behind the starting line and on the command, "Ready, Go," begins walking the one mile as fast as possible. The tester starts the stopwatch on, "Go," and stops it when the examinee's chest breaks the plane of the finish line. The time is recorded to the nearest hundredth of a minute.

Scoring.

Multiple regression analysis was used to develop the following equation to predict VO^{2}max.

VO^{2}max = 132.853 - (0.0769 x W) - (0.3877 x A) + (6.315 x G) - (3.2649 x T) - (.1565 x HR)

where:

W = body weight in pounds

A = age in years

G = gender with 1 = males and 2 = females

T = time required to walk mile measured to nearest 0.01 minute

HR = heart rate for last two minutes of mile walk

Norms.

Rockport (1989, no page numbers) men and women.

NOTE 1: The above multiple regression equation has since been validated for 20 to 29 year olds by Coleman et al. (1987), for 70 to 79 year olds by O'Hanley et al. (1987) and for overweight women by Ward et al. (1987).

NOTE 2: The norms in the *Rockport Guide* are based on the examinee's time required to walk the mile and the examinee's heart rate measured for 15 seconds immediately after cessation of walking and then multiplied by four.

REVIEW

TERESA SHARP, M.Ed.

Research Assistant
Clinical Nutrition Unit
Vanderbilt University Medical Center
Nashville, TN 37232-8285
and

SHARON SHIELDS, Ph.D.

Associate Professor
Teaching and Learning
Peabody College of Vanderbilt
University
Nashville, TN 37232-8285

The Rockport Walk Test has been validated in the literature. Reliability has been reported at $r = .93$ for heart rate and $r = .98$ for walking time using the test-retest method. Validity is reported as $r = .92$ between estimated VO^2max and measured VO^2max using a treadmill protocol. The test is definitely reproducible by various testers thus substantiating its objectivity. The test does not require the active participation of another individual which makes the scoring more objective. However, the tester is put into a role of being a motivator to the examinee to elicit optimal performance on the test.

Facility and equipment requirements are minimal thus making the test extremely practical for any setting. No equipment problems should exist. Test administration is easily performed and very little training is required. The test should take no longer than 15 to 30 minutes to administer depending on the age and fitness level of the examinee. However, several examinees may participate in one trial thus facilitating large group testing. One trial is recommended in administering the test; however, the recommended practice walks will reduce any learning effect. The test can be used as a drill to promote learning and conditioning. The test is appropriate for the age, gender, and skill level of the examinees for whom the test was designed. The test, administered under the re-quired conditions, should pose no undue orthopedic or cardiovascular risk to the examinees. The test scoring is objective and can be easily utilized by an examinee for self evaluation. Based on validity and reliability scores, the test is suitable for field based research endeavors. Norms are available and up to date. The test, however, has not been validated for populations between the ages of 30 to 70 years. The test has been validated for populations 20 to 29 years old and 70 to 79 years old and in overweight women.

SUMMARY

Major Strengths:

1. A valid and reliable test.
2. Easily administered.
3. Can be used for self evaluation.
4. Application for all age groups.
5. Norms are available.

Major Weaknesses:

1. The results of all age groups have not been validated.

2. Has some dependency on examinee motivation.

3. Health screening information needs to be acquired before test administration to evaluate the examinee's ability to withstand the test.

The test is acceptable as an assessment of cardiovascular fitness. This test is very appropriate for use as a field based measure due to the minimal equipment requirements. The test also lends itself as an easy self evaluation tool; however, examinee motivation may bias the test results. Testers should be aware of the lack of validity for age groups between 30 and 70 years of age.

SUBMAXIMAL WALK TEST

Reference.
Jackson, A. S., & Ross, R. M. (1986). *Understanding exercise for health and fitness*. Houston: MacJ-R Publishing, pp 22, 24-27.

Additional Sources.
None.

Purpose.
To estimate VO^{2}max of an examinee through the use of a safe physical activity - walking.

Objectivity.
Not reported.

Reliability.
Not reported.

Validity.
Not reported.

Age and Sex.
Not reported, but suitable for females and males, age 14 - adult.

Equipment.
A stopwatch.

Space Requirements and Design.
A 400 meter (440 yard) track or a clear, level area where such a distance can be measured and marked.

Directions.
Prior to taking the test, the examinee should practice counting her/his pulse at the wrist. The pulse should be taken for 15 seconds and multiplied by four to give the beats per minute (bpm). After gaining proficiency in taking the pulse, the examinee should then practice walking at a steady pace that will produce a heart rate of 120 to 150 bpm. Once the examinee becomes skilled at walking the proper pace, the test can be administered. On the command, "Ready, Go," the examinee walks the 400m (440 yards) at a constant pace that produces a heart rate of 120 to 150 bpm. The tester starts the stopwatch on the command, "Go," and stops it when the examinee's chest crosses the finish line. Immediately after crossing the finish line, the examinee takes her/his pulse count for 15 seconds and multiplies it by four to give bpm.

Scoring.
The examinee converts the walking performance into miles per hour (mph) with the following formula:

Walking Speed (mph) = (D/T) x 60:

Where D = distance walked in decimal form (i.e., .25 miles) and T = the time it took to walk the distance in decimal form (e.g., 4 minutes and 30 seconds would be 4.50).

The maximum oxygen uptake score is calculated from the following formula:

VO^{2}max = Walking Factor - Heart Rate Factor - Age Factor.

All three factors in the above formula are determined by plugging the examinee's data into a table (Jackson and Ross, 1986, p. 26).

Norms.
Jackson & Ross (1986, p. 22) men and women.

REVIEW

DAVID E. CUNDIFF, Ph.D.

Professor
Health and Physical Education
Campbellsville College
Campbellsville, KY 42718

The purpose of the Submaximal Walk Test is to estimate VO^{2}max through the use of a safe physical activity - walking. The test constructors state that the test was developed at the University of Houston. The fact that no reference is given indicates that the research data used to construct the test was not published. Therefore, no data are available on the test's objectivity, reliability or validity. No appropriate age range is given although a norm table has age divisions starting at age 20 and continuing through age 69.

The test requires a precisely marked (400 meter or 440 yard) track or clear, level area. Many communities do not have tracks and if they do, they are not always accessible to the public. No mention is made of the possible effect of varying temperatures on heart rate. Since the estimated VO^2 is based on the pace and heart rate response, some range of temperature for test administration should be given. For example, a four minute, 440 yard walk in 90 degree heat might elicit heart rate of 150 beats per minute (bpm) and the same pace in 60 degree weather might elicit a heart rate of 130 bpm. The equipment required should not present a problem to most people.

The test directions indicate that practice on taking heart rate is needed but gives no indication how one might know when he/she are measuring it accurately (e.g., having someone else take her/his pulse under the same conditions). Taking the pulse for 15 seconds might be acceptable, if started within 5 seconds of exercise termination, but the directions state a delay up to 15 seconds would be acceptable. If this delay occurred, the 15 second count would end at 30 seconds post exercise. Currently heart rates are recorded for either 6 or 10 seconds and started within 5 seconds of exercise termination to minimize the possibility of heart rate slowing down before recording is completed. No information is provided as to how long it would take an inexperienced examinee to practice pace, take heart rate accurately, walk test, and perform the calculations to determine VO_2max and fitness category. Information is not provided about whether the test discriminates fitness levels accurately at 25 years of age as well as 65 years of age. Directions state that the test is safe but no precautions are mentioned. This omission is particularly troublesome in the area in which it is emphasized that the walking speed should be fast enough to elicit a heart rate response between 120 and 150 beats per minute. Some individuals on heart medications may not be able to increase their heart rate this high without potential or serious medical consequences. Leg length may make a difference in the heart rate response to the same speed and should be considered.

SUMMARY

Major Strengths:

1. The Submaximal Walk Test would be an excellent method to teach and practice heart rate pacing and post exercise recording of heart rate in apparently healthy individuals.

2. Little equipment and just a flat walking surface are required to administer the test.

Major Weaknesses:

1. No information is provided or a reference cited on the scientific aspects of the test (i.e., reliability, validity, or objectivity).

2. No guidelines are given on precautions related to age or health status.

3. No guidelines are given for environmental conditions (e.g., temperature).

4. The test lacks precise instructions for post exercise heart rate recording (e.g., start counting pulse within five seconds of test termination).

5. Norms and directions are not be available to the general public.

The Submaximal Walk Test is not be an acceptable test for determining VO_2max for research purposes. The test would be useful in teaching heart rate pacing and post exercise heart rate counting.

UNIVERSITY OF MONTREAL TRACK TEST (UM-TT)

Reference.
Leger, L., & Boucher, R. (1980). An indirect continuous running multistage field test: The universite de montreal track test. *Canadian Journal of Applied Sport Sciences*, 5(1):77-84.

Additional Sources.
None.

Purpose.
To provide a maximal progressive multistage running test which can be used to estimate an exanubee's VO^{2}max and to provide a less strenuous alternative to the 12 minute run.

Objectivity.
Not reported.

Reliability.
r = .97 by test-retest method.

Validity.
r = .96 between UM-TT predicted VO^{2}max and VO^{2}max measured directly using a running multistage treadmill test.

Age and Sex.
Males, age 20 - 40 years.

Equipment.
Four plastic cones, a prerecorded audio tape with the test's directions and sound signals on it for pacing purposes, a tape recorder, and a tape measure.

Space Requirements and Design.
A 166.7m (182 yds) or 200m (218 yds) indoor track with inclined curves and a cone placed on the inside edge of the track at every quarter section of the track (i.e., 41.68m or 50m between cones).

Directions.
The examinee takes a standing position behind the starting line. Upon the signal emitted by the prerecorded tape, the examinee begins moving at a speed of five Mets or six km.h-1. The examinee is paced by sounds being emitted from the prerecorded tape. The examinee moves at the given pace for each stage of two minutes duration. The speed at each stage is increased one Met over the previous stage. The examinee tries to complete as many stages as possible. The time is announced every 30 seconds to help the examinee decide whether or not to complete the stage. The test is terminated when the examinee falls at least 9.15m (30') behind the proper pace after the sound signal is emitted or the examinee feels incapable of completing the stage.

Scoring.
The score is the number of stages completed, which is then used to estimate VO^{2}max (see Leger & Boucher, 1980, Table 1, p. 81).

Norms.
Leger & Boucher (1980, p. 77) men and women.

REVIEW

HAROLD B. FALLS, Ph.D.

Professor of Biomedical Sciences
Southwest Missouri State University
Springfield, MO 65804

The UM-TT test score correlates well with directly measured VO^{2}max in males ages 20 to 40. The relationship (r = 0.96) is excellent and indicated the test is valid for use in estimating VO^{2}max. It should be noted that the original study did not include a validation sample for females. Reliability with females, however, was investigated and found to be lower than in males (r = 0.88 versus 0.97). The lower value in females implies that validity would also be somewhat lower. Nonetheless, the test would probably have acceptable validity when used with females. In a later study, Leger & Lambert (1982) validated a 20 meter shuttle run version of the UM-TT using VO^{2}max as the criterion. Although the validity coefficient for the shuttle run test was lower when compared with the UM-TT (r = 0.84 versus 0.96), it is acceptable, and the study did include a sufficient number of females. Further, the correlation between results on the shuttle run and UM-TT in a group of 35 females and 35 males was r = 0.92. In addition, Leger & Lambert (1982) found no significant difference in the slopes of regression lines for the VO^{2}max vs 20m shuttle run relationship in females and males with the tests conducted on both high and low friction surfaces.

The reliability of the test is quite good for both females and males. Objectivity has not been determined. However, if the instructions for administering the test are followed, there should be no problem with objectivity. Further, even when examinees are tested in groups as a time saving measure, the performance of one examinee should have minimal effect on that of another.

The original version of the test requires a 166.7 or 200 meter indoor track with banked turns. However, this facility requirement could be easily modified with no likely effect on the validity or reliability. The test could be administered on any indoor or outdoor circular course of 166.7 or 200 meters, or any multiple of these. The original reference includes a table giving split times for the two course distances.

Examinees could be tested in pairs as is commonly done with most distance run tests. One examinee of the pair is tested while the other records the distance covered. In the UM-TT, the scoring member would also observe to assure the examinee was keeping pace with the cones on the course.

Tape recording the instructions and a signal for pacing would be convenient, but does not appear an absolute necessity. The tester could call these verbally during the test. It would take about 20 minutes to test the average examinee on this test. However, as many as 30 to 40 examinees could be tested in that same amount of time. The UM-TT is a one trial test. One trial may not be sufficient to assure adequate reliability unless the examinees are practiced in running. As with any running test, the examinees should practice until they are thoroughly familiar with the procedures and pacing. Performing the test itself as a learning and/or conditioning activity is acceptable and desirable.

The latter stages of the test are maximal. Therefore, precautions normally taken with any maximal cardiovascular activity should be observed. Since the test merely yields an estimate of VO^2max, it is not acceptable as a research instrument where absolute measures of VO^2max are desirable. It could be useful, however, if only relative measures are acceptable.

Leger and his colleagues have tested several thousand students at the University of Montreal. They probably could supply norms for that population. In addition, a table in the original reference can be used to yield a direct estimate of VO^2max. Norms for VO^2max are available from several sources.

SUMMARY

Major Strengths:

1. It has acceptable validity for adult males and probably acceptable validity for adult females.

2. The reliability is acceptable in both females and males.

3. The test is easy to administer and requires a minimum of special facilities, equipment, expertise, and assistance from others.

4. Only the last stages of the test are maximal. The first few stages are submaximal. This procedure could be a safety feature for examinees over 30 years of age. It is also likely to aid motivation.

5. The test has a strong conceptual foundation. It is based on an excellent analysis of the energy and oxygen consumption requirements and mechanical efficiency for various speeds of running.

Major Weakness:

1. The test has one possible weakness if administered on a short non banked course with very fit examinees who can complete more than 10 or 11 stages of the test. These examinees may reach speeds during the last stages of the test which may make it difficult for them to negotiate the turns on the course.

This test is adequate for research and/or teaching for which it is not critical that an absolute estimate of VO^2max be obtained. It yields a reasonably accurate estimate of VO^2max that can be used for classifying groups on cardiovascular fitness or assessing the status of training responses in athletes.

REVIEW REFERENCE

Leger, L., & Lambert, J. (1982). A maximal multistage 20-m shuttle run test to predict VO^2max. *European Journal of Applied Physiology,* 49:1-12.

3-MILE WALKING TEST (NO RUNNING)

References.
Cooper, K. H. (1982). *The aerobics program for total well-being.* New York: M. Evans & Co., p 142.

Miller, D. K. (1988). *Measurement by the physical educator: Why and how.* Indianapolis: Benchmark Press, p 148.

Additional Sources.
None.

Purpose.
To measure the cardiorespiratory endurance of an examinee through walking.

Objectivity.
Not reported.

Reliability.
Not reported.

Validity.
Not reported.

Age and Sex.
Females and males, age 13 - 60.

Equipment.
A stopwatch.

Space Requirements and Design.
A 440 yard track or a measured, flat area that would enable the examinee to walk three miles.

Directions.
The examinee should be allowed to warm up prior to the walking test. On the command, "Ready, Go," the examinee attempts to walk three miles as fast as possible. The examinee cannot run during the test.

Scoring.
The score is the time in minutes and seconds required to walk three miles.

Norms.
Alabama (1988, pp. 50-51) boys and girls for 2 miles; Barrow et al. (1989, p. 136) boys, girls, men and women; Cooper (1982, p. 142) boys, girls, men and women; Kirkendall et al. (1980, p. 302) women; Miller (1988, p. 149) boys, girls, men and women; President's Council (1988, p. 6) boys and girls for 2 miles.

REVIEW

RUSSELL H. LORD, Ed.D.
Professor of Educational Foundations
Eastern Montana College
Billings, MT 59101-0298

Since the stated purpose of the 3-Mile Walking Test is to assess cardiorespiratory endurance through walking and examinees attempt to walk three miles as quickly as possible, there seems small need to establish traditional psychometric validity data for the test. Indeed, such supportive data are not provided. Traditional indicators of reliability are also omitted, along with any mention of the objectivity of the test.

While the omission of such technical data seems to be, and probably is, less critical to the 3-Mile Walking Test than to most tests, such omission still poses problems. To what extent do day to day performances vary for examinees who must work at or near their maximum to perform this test? Any fluctuations would obviously affect the reliability of the test. In contrast, what about the large number of females and males, ages 13 to 60, for whom walking three miles imposes minimal demand? How accurately does this test assess their cardiorespiratory endurance?

Despite omissions of important psychometric data, it is hard to imagine their absence posing all that serious a problem in this test. Several reasons operate to moderate the omissions: (1) the stated purpose is clearly matched to the task presented, (2) the assessment avoids, for the most part, claims that the test is measuring constructs very far removed from the task itself, (3) objectivity could only be compromised through techniques, and (4) day to day consistency in walking three miles would seem to be enhanced by the ceiling effect of not being allowed to run. The test is not proclaimed as an assessment of something that must be inferred indirectly and with considerable care from the physical measurement obtained. Instead the test is claimed to measure the physiological component upon which the task is directly based. Some problems might arise from confusing endurance with maximal effort, or over the definition of what is meant by "cannot run," but such problems should be manageable. It seems unlikely that many testers or examinees would apply vastly different criteria in determining what was meant by walking but not running. Only for examinees having certain physical disabilities would validity seem to become an issue, and the related issues of objectivity and reliability would seem to become problematic only when measurement is grossly mishandled.

A major advantage of the 3-Mile Walking Test is its limited demands for (1) facilities and space, (2) special equipment, (3) leadership skills, and (4) time. Every practicing educator should already possess all of the knowledge required to follow the directions for administration and scoring; and have access to all of the facilities and equipment needed to administer the 3-Mile Walking Test. While dangers introduced by this or any test are always possible, they are certainly minimal in this test.

Individuals wishing to administer and score the test for themselves in an ongoing process of self evaluation could certainly do so. The norms with which to compare themselves are sufficiently recent for use, and provide reference points for boys, girls, men, and women. The 3-Mile Walking Test certainly seems appropriate for research purposes, but its assessment of cardiorespiratory endurance must suffer from a ceiling effect.

SUMMARY

Major Strengths:

1. The test's basis in the work of Cooper and the familiarity of many potential users with aerobics.

2. Its easy administration and scoring.

3. Its high degree of safety.

4. The current norms for both genders across the intended age range.

Major Weaknesses:

1. The omission of reliability, validity, and objectivity data.

2. Questions as to the impact of the ceiling effect on its assessment of cardiorespiratory endurance.

Overall, the 3-Mile Walking Test is certainly an acceptable test, suitable and safe for use by a wide range of individuals who do not need extensive knowledge or skills to administer and score it appropriately. Validity data should establish the extent to which scores on the 3-Mile Walking Test agree or disagree with other established measures of cardiorespiratory endurance. Such data across diverse populations of varying levels of cardiorespiratory fitness could confirm the extent to which the test is or is not an excellent test having several appropriate uses for which other tests are either too hazardous, require too much specialized equipment, or encounter other limitations.

20M SHUTTLE RUN TEST

References.

Leger, L. et al. (1984). Capacite aerobic des Quebecois de 6 a 17 ans - Test navette de 20 metres avec paliers de 1 minute. *Canadian Journal of Applied Sport Sciences,* 9(2):64-68.

Leger, L., & Gadoury, C. (1989). Validity of the 20m shuttle run test with 1 min stages to predict VO^2max in adults. *Canadian Journal of Sports Sciences,* 14(1):21-26.

Leger, L., & Lambert, J. (1982). A maximal multistage 20m shuttle run test to predict VO^2max. *European Journal of Applied Physiology,* 49:1-12.

Van Mechelen, W. et al. (1986). Validation of two running tests as estimates of maximal aerobic power in children. *European Journal of Applied Physiology,* 55:503-506.

Additional Sources.

None.

Purpose.

To estimate the maximum aerobic power of an examinee.

Objectivity.

Not reported.

Reliability.

$r = .95$ using one minute stages and test-retest method (Leger & Lambert, 1982, p. 11); $r = .98$ using two minute stages and test-retest method (Leger & Lambert, 1982, p. 1).

Validity.

$r = .92$ using two minute stages compared with another continuous multistage running test (Leger & Lambert, 1982, p. 1); $r = .76$ with VO^2max for a combined group of boys and girls age 12 - 14 (Van Mechelen et al., 1986, p. 503); $r = .89$ to $r = .93$ using one minute stages and adults (Leger & Gadoury, 1989, p. 25).

Age and Sex.

Females and males, age 6 - adult.

Equipment.

A prerecorded tape with the test's directions and pacing sounds on it, tape recorder, marking tape, tape measure, and a stopwatch.

Space Requirements and Design.

A clear, level area approximately 3m x 25m (10' x 75') with two parallel lines, approximately 2m (6') long, marked off 20m (65.6') apart in the center of the 25m length.

Directions.

With the examinee standing ready behind one line, the tester turns on the tape recorder. When the prerecorded tape gives the signal, the examinee moves to the other line, reverses direction and returns to the starting line. The examinee continues to move back and forth behind the two lines at a rate of 7.5 km/h -1 for two minutes (NOTE: One minute exercise stages have generally replaced the original two minute exercise stages. Leger and Lambert (1982) reported a $r = .97$ between the one minute and two minute protocols.) The prerecorded tape helps the examinee maintain the proper pace. The pace is increased 0.5 km/h -1 each two minute period. The tester announces the time every 30 seconds of each two minute stage to help the examinee decide whether to attempt to complete that stage. The test is terminated when the examinee feels he/she is unable to continue or when the examinee falls at least three meters off the pace when the 20 meter signal sounds. The examinee tries to complete as many stages as possible.

Scoring.

The score is the number of stages completed which is then used to estimate VO^2max (see Leger & Lambert, 1982, Table 2, p. 5).

Norms.

Leger et al. (1984, pp. 65, 67) boys and girls using one minute exercise periods instead of two minute periods.

REVIEW

JAMES E. GRAVES, Ph.D.

Assistant Scientist
Department of Medicine
University of Florida
Gainesville, FL 32610
and

LYNN B. PANTON, M.S.

Department of Exercise and Sport
Sciences
University of Florida
Gainesville, FL 32610

Traditionally the Shuttle Run has been used to evaluate speed and agility. In 1982, Leger and Lambert (1982) developed a maximal multi stage shuttle run to predict the maximal aerobic power (VO_2max) of adults. The original protocol consisted of two minute stages which resulted in relatively long tests for many examinees. A protocol consisting of one minute stages has been reported to save administrative time and facilitate examinee motivation (particularly with school children). Validity coefficients for the test using one minute stages are slightly higher than those reported for the two minute stage test. Thus, the one minute protocol has generally replaced the two minute protocol.

Reliability of the 20M Shuttle Run is high for both children ($r = 0.89$; Leger, 1988) and adults ($r = 0.95$; Leger & Lambert, 1982; Leger et al., 1988). The validity of the test has been extensively studied (Leger & Lambert, 1982; Leger et al., 1984; Van Mechelen et al., 1986; Paliczka et al., 1987; Leger et al., 1988; Ramsbottom et al., 1988; Leger & Gadoury, 1989) and is acceptable for predicting VO_2max. Standard errors of prediction (range = 3.4 to 4.7 ml x kg-1 x min-1) are generally less than 10 percent of reported mean values for adults (Paliczka et al., 1987; Leger et al., 1988; Leger et al., 1989) and children (Van Mechelen et al., 1986) although Leger et al. (1988) reported a standard error of prediction of 12.1 percent (5.9 ml x kg-1 x min-1) for children 8 to 19 years of age. Predicted VO_2max values from the 20M Shuttle Run Test (one minute stages) correlated well with 10K ($r = 0.93$; Paliczka et al., 1987) and 5K ($r = 0.96$; Ramsbottom et al., 1988) race times for adults.

The accuracy of the 20M Shuttle Run is comparable to or slightly better than that of other field tests for predicting VO_2max. However, laboratory controlled maximal tests using performance time on a treadmill usually provide the most accurate prediction of VO_2max (SEE =

2.5 to 4.0 ml x kg-1 x min-1) (Pollock & Wilmore 1990, p. 284). For research purposes, a direct measure of VO_2max is required.

The 20M Shuttle Run can be used on men and women ranging in age from 6 years through adult and norms exist for children up to 17 years of age. In children (up to 18 years), age has a significant influence on the relationship between the number of test stages completed and VO_2max (Leger et al., 1988) and must be considered for accurate prediction. Although objectivity has not been reported, the use of a prerecorded tape to direct the pace of the test makes it unlikely that different testers would affect the results. It may be important, however, to provide verbal encouragement during the test to obtain the best results.

The test is easy to administer and requires minimal space and equipment. It is well suited for mass testing but, obviously, space requirements will increase when testing large groups. The test can be administered indoors on a variety of surfaces and thus the test is not influenced by weather conditions. Due to the maximal nature of the test, it is important to screen examinees for risk factors and contraindications to exercise prior to testing.

SUMMARY

Major Strengths:

1. Reliability and validity of the test is well established.

2. The test is easy to administer and well suited for testing large groups.

3. Space requirements and cost of equipment are minimal.

Major Weaknesses:

1. Due to the maximal nature of the test, examinees must be screened for risk factors and contraindications prior to testing.

2. The test yields an estimate of VO_2max that is associated with a moderate amount of variability and cannot be used for research purposes.

3. There may be groups of individuals (e.g., uncoordinated children or highly fit adults) for whom the test is not valid.

The 20M Shuttle Run Test is an adequate test for predicting VO_2max in children and adults. The test is easy to administer, inexpensive, requires little space, and is well suited for group testing. Due to the maximal nature of the test, examinees must be screened prior to testing for risk factors and contraindications. Because the test yields a prediction of VO^2max, it is not appropriate for research purposes.

REVIEW REFERENCES

Leger, L. et al. (1988). The multistage 20 metre shuttle run test for aerobic fitness. *Journal of Sports Sciences,* 6:93-101.

Leger, L. et al. (1984). Capacite aerobic des Quebecois de 6 a 17 ans - test navette de 20 metres avec paliers de 1 minute. *Canadian Journal of Applied Sport Sciences,* 9(2):64-68.

Leger, L, & Gadoury, C. (1989). Validity of the 20M shuttle run test with one minute stages to predict VO^2max in adults. *Canadian Journal of Sports Sciences,* 14(1):21-26.

Leger, L., & Lambert, J. (1982). A maximal multistage 20m shuttle run test to predict VO^2max. *European Journal of Applied Physiology,* 49:1-12.

Paliczka, V. J. et al. (1987). A multistage shuttle run as a predictor of running performance and maximal oxygen uptake in adults. *British Journal of Sports Medicine,* 21(4):163-165.

Pollock, M. L., & Wilmore, J. H. (1990). *Exercise in health and disease* (2nd ed.). Philadelphia: W. B. Saunders Company.

Ramsbottom, R. et al. (1988). A progressive shuttle run test to estimate maximal oxygen uptake. *British Journal of Sports Medicine,* 22(4):141-144.

Van Mechelen, W. et al. (1986). Validation of two running tests as estimates of maximal aerobic power in children. *European Journal of Applied Physiology,* 55:503-506.

STEP TESTS OF CARDIORESPIRATORY ENDURANCE

CANADIAN AEROBIC FITNESS TEST*

*Formerly known as the Canadian Home Fitness Test: Advanced Version.

Reference.

Canadian Standardized Test of Fitness (CSTF), 3rd ed. (1986). Ottawa, Ontario, Canada: Fitness and Amateur Sport Canada, pp 10-11, 17, 28-29, 34-35.

Additional Sources.

None.

Purpose.

To measure the efficiency of an examinee's circulatory and respiratory systems to supply the working muscles with the needed oxygen.

Objectivity.

Not reported.

Reliability.

Not reported.

Validity.

Not reported.

Age and Sex.

Females and males, age 15 - 69.

Equipment.

A stethoscope, sphygmomanometer, stopwatch, and a double step bench with each step 20.3cm (8") high and with handrails on each side are needed. Details for the construction of the bench are provided in CSTF (1986, p. 17). A tape recorder and an audio cassette tape with the proper cadence on it are also needed.

Space Requirements and Design.

A clear, level area approximately 3m (10') square with the bench in the center.

Directions.

Before beginning the test, the examinee's resting blood pressure and resting heart rate are determined following standard procedures. The blood pressure cuff is also worn throughout the test. The examinee takes a standing position in front of the bench and begins a three minute warm up period of stepping at a cadence of 65 to 70 percent of the average aerobic power expected of an individual 10 years older. The cas-

sette tape contains the stepping cadence and time signals. A table (CSTF, 1986, p. 10) is used to determine the stepping cadence based upon the examinee's age and sex. A six count stepping cadence is used as follows: (1) the right foot is placed on the first bench step, (2) the left foot is placed on the second bench step, (3) the right foot is placed next to the left on the second bench step, (4) the left foot is lowered to the first bench step, (5) the right foot is lowered to ground level, and (6) the left foot is lowered to ground level next to the right foot. The examinee must follow this cadence throughout the test as well as place both feet completely on the top bench step, fully extend the knees and stand erect each time. Examinees should be told that they may stop stepping anytime they feel discomfort. The tester should stop the test if the examinee "begins to stagger, complains of dizziness, extreme leg pain, nausea, chest pain, or shows facial pallor."

When the cassette gives the three minute signal, the examinee stops stepping and remains standing motionless while her/his heart rate is measured. The stethoscope is placed over the examinee's sternum or the second intercostal space on the left side of the sternum. The heart rate count is started with the termination of the signal, "COUNT" (do not count a heart beat that occurs during the word COUNT) and terminated with the first sound of the signal, "STOP." This 10 second heart rate count is used to determine if a second three minute session of stepping is to be initiated. If this count is equal to or exceeds the ceiling post exercise heart rate found in a table (CSTF, 1986, p. 11), the test is terminated. If the count does not equal or exceed the ceiling heart rate, the second stepping session is initiated. The same procedures are used to determine if a final, third stepping session is to be initiated. Examinees in the 60 to 69 age group are to terminate the test after the second session of stepping regardless of how well they performed.

After completing the last three minute session of stepping, the examinee sits down. The tester takes the examinee's post exercise blood pressure between 0:30 and 1:00 minute and between 2:30 and 3:00 minutes after cessation of stepping. The tester then takes a 15 second heart rate count between 3:00 and 3:30 minutes after cessation of stepping. These post exercise measures are taken primarily as a safety precaution to be sure the examinee's heart rate has dropped below 100 and her/his blood pressure below 150mm Hg systolic and below 100mm Hg diastolic.

Scoring.

The score is the 10 second heart rate count and the final stepping stage completed.

Norms.

Canadian Standardized (1986, p. 35) boys, girls, men and women.

NOTE: The results of the step test can also be used to predict maximal aerobic power (CSTF, 1986, p. 15). Standards and percentiles are provided for predicted maximal aerobic power on p. 34 of the reference.

REVIEW

ELIZABETH J. SCHUMAKER, D.P.E.

Associate Professor
Physical Education
Stetson University
DeLand, FL 32720

The Canadian Standardized Test of Fitness closely parallels important variables of submaximal stress testing used in a laboratory setting. It measures cardiac function during exercise as the workload is increased. As in similar tests, heart rate is used to predict oxygen uptake. This is not as accurate as measuring with a spirometer but the reliability of this test may be enhanced by the fact that the tester measures the examinee's heart rate as opposed to each examinee monitoring her/his own heart rate. This factor should allow for greater accuracy in monitoring heart rate. The other factor related to the monitoring of heart rate, which should increase the reliability of this test when compared to others, is the use of the stethoscope to listen to the heart rate instead of palpation of the carotid artery.

There are several precautionary procedures which reduce the risk factor of the test. The monitoring of heart rate and blood pressure, the inclusion of handrails on the two step bench and an adequate warm up for the test make this test more attractive for use with an older population. However, precaution still should be taken for examinees over the age of 35 and they should be screened carefully and tested with a physician present or with their physician's permission.

The absence of reliability and validity coefficients is a critical issue. This problem should be addressed by the test constructors. These coefficients are important if one would like to use the test, for example, in a field study for which a more sophisticated means of testing is not available. It is difficult to consider this test when comparing it to similar tests which have been tested for reliability and validity.

Unlike other step tests which are fairly simple to administer, this test required several hours of practice for the testers before they became proficient and consistent. The training sessions required additional volunteers to provide adequate training. However, the training sessions provided a good learning experience for the testers as well as the volunteers but as a general cardiorespiratory endurance test for large numbers of examinees, such as a school or college physical education class, this test would be too time consuming. However, for a campus wellness program for which there is a need for cardiorespiratory endurance testing, once the reliability and validity are established, this test could be a very good alternative.

SUMMARY
Major Strengths:
1. Appropriate for a wide age range.
2. Provides good precautionary measures.
3. More closely parallels laboratory measures of cardiorespiratory endurance than other step tests.
4. Has potential for use in field research.

Major Weaknesses:
1. Lacks reliability and validity coefficients.
2. Requires careful training of testers.
3. Time consuming.

4. Requires more equipment than comparative step tests.

When comparing the Canadian Aerobic Fitness Test to both laboratory cardioresporatory endurance tests and other step tests, it would appear to be valid and reliable providing testers have been trained properly.

A very critical issue is the absence of objectivity, reliability and validity coefficients. If this data were provided, the test, in all likelihood, could be used for both research and fitness assessment. There also needs to be a stronger statement regarding the use of this test for populations over 35, especially high risk individuals.

CANADIAN HOME FITNESS TEST

Reference.
Bailey, D. A. et al. (1976). Validation of a self administered home test of cardiorespiratory fitness. *Canadian Journal of Applied Sport Sciences,* 1:67-78.

Additional Sources.
None.

Purpose.
To provide a simple measure of cardiorespiratory endurance which can easily be administered in the home.

Objectivity.
Not reported.

Reliability.
r = .79 by test-retest method.

Validity.
Coefficients range from r = .40 to r = .76 for different age groups and two sexes with a cycle ergometer test.

Age and Sex.
Females and males, age 15 - 70.

Equipment.
A bilevel bench with the first step 20.32cm (8") high and the second step 40.64cm (16") high with a hand rail support on one end, an audio tape with the test's directions and lively music prerecorded, and a tape recorder. A staircase with eight inch high steps is intended to be substituted for the bench.

Space Requirements and Design.
A clear, level area approximately 3m (10') square with the bench in the center.

Directions.
With the examinee standing facing the bench, the tester starts the tape recorder. After the tape gives a warning signal and the, "Ready, Go," signal, the examinee begins stepping for three minutes at a rate designed for a individual 10 years older than the examinee. Five seconds after the three minutes of stepping, the prerecorded voice gives the signal to start counting the pulse at the wrist and 10 seconds later a second signal is given to stop counting. If the 10 second pulse exceeds the predetermined level (see Table 3, p. 70 of the above reference), the test is terminated. If the pulse is less than the predetermined level, a second three minutes of stepping is initiated 15 seconds after the completion of the pulse count. During the second bout of exercise, the examinee steps at a rate designed for her/his age group. At the completion of this second bout of exercise, the pulse is taken five seconds after the cessation of stepping. If this 10 second pulse count exceeds the predetermined value, the test is terminated. If the pulse is less than the predetermined level, a third three minutes of stepping is initiated 15 seconds after the completion of the pulse count. During this third bout of exercise, the examinee steps at a rate designed for a individual 10 years younger than the examinee. The pulse count is taken in the same manner described above after this third and final bout of exercise. The 60 plus year old age group does not take this third bout of exercise.

Scoring.
The score is the 10 second pulse count and the duration of stepping.

Norms.
Bailey et al. (1976, p. 73) boys, girls, men and women; Canadian Minister (1979, p. 21) men and women; Stephens et al. (1986, p. 15) men and women.

REVIEW

JAMES KLINZING, Ph.D.
Associate Professor
Health, Physical Education and
Recreation
Cleveland State University
Cleveland, OH 44115

The purpose of this step test is to provide a convenient method for the typical individual to estimate her/his current level of cardiorespiratory endurance. The test utilizes two eight inch steps of a stairway. A sample of 1,544 Canadians from the city of Saskatoon were administered the test in order to establish its scientific feasibility. A cycle ergometer test was administered to 1,292 of these people in order to determine the validity of the Home Fitness Test. Validity correlations ranged from a poor level of .40 to an acceptable level of .76 for different age groups and the two sexes. The reliability as determined by the test-retest method was .79, which is satisfactory for the intended home use of this test. The objectivity of the test was not determined, but cannot be considered to be satisfactory since large discrepancies between palpated pulse counts and recorded heart rates were noted. Since this test is designed for self administration, accurate pulse counting needs to be assured for meaningful results.

This test is a practical method by which the typical individual can determine her/his level of cardiorespiratory endurance. Two eight inch steps are readily available on a stairway in most homes. The test can be completed in less than 11 minutes. The music containing the instructions and stepping cadences can be obtained from the Fitness and Amateur Sport Branch, Health and Welfare, Ottawa, Ontario, Canada K1A 0X6. A metronome could also be used to set the cadence. Without either of these items the proper cadence would be difficult to achieve.

A major concern of the above study is that the examinees did not accurately count pulse rates at the end of each stepping period. Limited practice and noisy conditions contributed to the problem. People using this test should practice taking resting and exercise pulse rates several times on different days and use the final test results for evaluation of cardiorespiratory endurance. Regular participation in stepping could serve as a training technique, if boredom can be overcome.

The instruction kit contains a medical survey to be completed prior to taking the test and describes symptoms which indicate the need to stop the test. This process enhances the suitability of the test for the target population of females and males 15 to 69 years. No serious or lasting medical problems of any type occurred during the development of the test.

This test is suitable for its intended purpose of providing a quick estimate of cardiorespiratory endurance in the home. Because of the submaximal nature of the test and the use of heart rate as the measurement criterion, it is unsuitable for research purposes. Other more accurate measures are available for research in the area of physical fitness. Norms are provided for both sexes and all age groups.

SUMMARY

Major Strengths:

1. The test can be self administered in a comfortable home setting.

2. The test can be given in less than 11 minutes.

3. Norms are provided for both sexes and all age groups, 15 to 69 years.

Major Weaknesses:

1. Adequate pulse counting practice is needed to achieve accurate results.

2. Special equipment, the test music or a metronome, may not be readily available for all interested in taking the test.

3. A limited possibility of a medical emergency could result, especially if an examinee fails to complete the pretest medical survey or ignores symptoms during the test.

If used properly, this is an acceptable test for the self administered evaluation of cardiorespiratory endurance. With practice almost all examinees should be able to count their pulse accurately. If an individual were to commence a training program, the test provides a convenient method of monitoring the training effect. Stepping cadence needs to be paced with the music developed for the test or with a metronome. Many people will not bother to get either and therefore will not use the test in their homes.

CARDIOVASCULAR EFFICIENCY FOR GIRLS AND WOMEN (SKUBIC & HODGKINS) TEST

References.

Skubic, V., & Hodgkins, J. (1963). Cardiovascular efficiency test for girls and women. *Research Quarterly*, 34(14): 191-198.

Hodgkins, J., & Skubic, V. (1963). Cardiovascular efficiency scores for college women in the united states. *Research Quarterly*, 34(4):454-461.

Skubic, V., & Hodgkins, J. (1964). Cardiovascular efficiency test scores for junior and senior high school girls in the United States. *Research Quarterly*, 35(2):184-192.

Johnson, B. L., & Nelson, J. K. (1986). *Practical measurements for evaluation in physical education*. Edina, MN: Burgess, pp 164-166.

Additional Sources.

Bosco & Gustafson (1983, p. 134); Clarke & Clarke (1987, pp. 139-140); Kirkendall et al. (1980, pp. 304-305); Miller (1988, p. 152).

Purpose.

To measure the cardiovascular endurance of girls and women through bench stepping.

Objectivity.

Not reported.

Reliability.

r = .82 (Skubic & Hodgkins 1963).

Validity.

r = .79 with 5 minute step test (Skubic & Hodgkins, 1963).

Age and Sex.

Junior high school, senior high school, and college age females.

Equipment.

A bench 46cm (18") high, a stopwatch, and a metronome or an audio tape with the cadence prerecorded. A tape recorder is also needed if a prerecorded tape is used.

Space Requirements and Design.

A clear, level area approximately 3m (10') square with the bench and the examinee in the center.

Directions.

The directions for the test are the same as for the Harvard Step Test with the exception of the use of an 46cm (18") high bench, 24 steps/minute cadence, and a maximum exercise time of three minutes. Only one pulse count is taken at the carotid artery during the one to one and one-half minute period after the cessation of stepping. If the examinee stops before the three minutes, the same directions are applied as in the Harvard Step Test.

Scoring.

The following formula is used to derive the score.

Cardiovascular Efficiency Score = Number of Seconds completed x 100/Recovery pulse x 5.6.

Norms.

Hodgkins & Skubic (1963, pp. 187, 456-461) girls and women; Johnson & Nelson (1986, p. 166) girls and women; Kirkendall et al. (1980, p. 305) girls and women; Miller (1988, p. 152) girls and women; O'Connor & Cureton (1945, p. 314) girls.

REVIEW

LARRY D. ISAACS, Ph.D.

Professor
Health, Physical Education and Recreation
Human Performance Laboratory
College of Education and Human Services
Wright State University
Dayton, OH 45435

This test of cardiovascular efficiency for girls and women uses recovery heart rate as the criterion measure. In general, the test assumes that the more highly conditioned (cardiovascular) an individual is, the faster the exercise heart rate will return to a resting level.

The validity of any test which uses post exercise heart rate is dependent upon a number of factors. First, the accuracy in which heart rate is determined is a critical factor. Second, because of the nature of the stepping task, many examinees may undergo local muscular fatigue before experiencing any significant central cardiovascular effect. Third, researchers have found that the correlations between a heart rate recovery step test and maximal oxygen uptake are higher when heart rate is determined five seconds following exercise and lower when heart rate is determined one minute after exercise. The present test is an example of the less desirable latter case. Test-retest reliability is acceptable (r = .82).

The test does not specifically require the active participation of other individuals. However, most authorities recommend that the examinee be paired with another individual for the purpose of helping determine the post exercise heart rate.

Practical aspects regarding test administration are appealing. More specifically, the test can be administered to large groups in very little time, little in the way of equipment is required and what equipment is required is inexpensive, and the test is easy to administer and requires no special leadership skills.

The test is suitable for the intended age levels. Furthermore, the test constructors have reported that the test does discriminate among females designated as trained, active, and sedentary.

One potentially dangerous aspect of the test includes tripping on the step bench - somewhat similar to falling up a stair. This unsafe aspect of the test is most likely to occur toward the latter stages of the test when the examinee may experience local muscular fatigue. As a safeguard, the tester may wish to incorporate a spotter who would stand in front of the examinee during test administration. This could be the same individual assigned to help the examinee determine post exercise heart rate.

As mentioned previously, scoring objectivity is critically important. The research seems to support the notion that objectivity coefficients are larger when pulse counting is performed by adults as compared to junior high school students. Therefore, it is absolutely essential that

examinees, as well as other test participants (if used), be trained and practice pulse counting on several occasions prior to test administration. Special attention should be paid to explaining how to take a pulse count at the carotid artery, noting that too much pressure on the carotid artery can alter heart rate. With training, it is possible for examinees to score themselves and use the test for self evaluation.

This test was well researched and a national sample was used to establish norms for junior high girls, senior high girls, and college age women. Unfortunately, the norms are presented according to these three categories and not according to age. This can be misleading because a close examination of the original research reveals that the test constructors used girls between 9 and 14 years of age to represent the junior high age group, girls between 15 and 19 years of age to represent the senior high age group, and no age ranges were reported for the college age group. In today's educational system, children between 9 and 11 years of age will be in elementary school, not junior high school. No doubt, this somewhat confusing point is a result of the test's age. The test and its accompanying norms were reported in 1963 and 1964. As such, these norms are possibly outdated.

SUMMARY

Major Strengths:

1. Inexpensive.

2. Requires little equipment.

3. Can test large numbers in a small amount of time.

Major Weaknesses:

1. Validity is contingent upon a very accurate pulse measurement.

2. Local muscular fatigue may occur before a cardiovascular effect is encountered.

3. Norms are outdated and illogically presented.

This test is unacceptable for research and/or teaching purposes for primarily two reasons. First, the test norms are outdated and second, since the development of this test, more up to date and task specific cardiovascular tests are available.

COTTEN GROUP CARDIOVASCULAR STEP TEST
(MODIFIED OHIO STATE STEP TEST)

References.

Cotten, D. J. (1971). A modified step test for group cardiovascular testing. *Research Quarterly*, 42(1):91-95.

Kirkendall, D. R. et al. (1987). *Measurement and evaluation for physical educators.* Champaign: Human Kinetics, pp 179-181.

Additional Sources.

Johnson & Nelson (1986, pp. 156, 158-160); Kirkendall et al. (1980, pp. 306-307).

Purpose.

To measure the cardiorespiratory endurance of a group of examinees accurately and efficiently.

Objectivity.

Not reported.

Reliability.

r = .95 for college men and r = .75 for high school boys (Cotten, 1971, pp. 93-94).

Validity.

r = .84 between step test and time it required the heart rate to reach 180 bpm on the Balke Treadmill Test.

Age and Sex.

College age males.

Equipment.

A bleacher step 43cm (17") high, test instructions and cadences prerecorded on an audio tape, and tape recorder.

Space Requirements and Design.

A clear, level area approximately 2m (6') square for each of the examinees in the group being tested.

Directions.

Prior to being tested, the group of examinees is paired off and a 15 minute rest period provided. During the rest period, the pairs should practice taking each other's pulse. Upon completion of the rest period, a demonstration of a complete inning (i.e., 30 seconds of stepping followed by 20 seconds of rest) should be presented.

Following the demonstration, the examinee assumes a standing position in front of the bench. The tape recorder is then started and provides the following instructions: On the command, "Go," the examinee begins stepping to the cadence of 24 steps per minute for a period of 30 seconds. On the command, "Stop," there is a cessation of stepping and after a period of 5 seconds there is a command, "Count," during which the pulse rate of the examinee is taken by the examinee's partner for a period of 10 seconds. At the end of the 10 second pulse count, a command, "Prepare to exercise," is given, followed by the command, "Go," thus beginning a new inning.

The test continues for a period of 18 innings or until the examinee's pulse rate has reached 25 beats/10 seconds (i.e., 150 beats/minute). The test is divided into three phases, with each phase consisting of six innings. The three phases follow each other in a continuous pattern and their cadence are as follows:

Phase 1 = 24 steps/minute;

Phase 2 = 30 steps/minute; and

Phase 3 = 36 steps/minute.

The examinees should be reminded of the increase in the cadence prior to innings 7 and 13.

Scoring.

The score is the inning number in which the pulse rate reaches 25 beats/10 seconds (i.e., 150 beats/minute). If all 18 innings are completed, a score of 19 is awarded.

Norms.

Not reported.

REVIEW

BEN R. LONDEREE, Ed.D.
Associate Professor
Health and Physical Education
University of Missouri-Columbia
Columbia, MO 65211

The Cotten Group Cardiovascular Step Test is a modified version of the Ohio State Step Test (Kurucz, et al., 1969). In the original version examinees used a handrail and the work rate was increased by a combination of changes in bench height and cadence. The modifications make the test more administratively feasible in a gymnasium.

The scientific criteria are satisfactory. The validity of .84 was lower than the .94 value reported for the original version (Kurucz, et al., 1969). Cotten (1971) speculated that the modifications caused the reduced validity. Reliability was excellent (.94) for college men but rather poor for high school boys (.75). Cotten (1971) indicated that numerous, obvious counting errors were responsible for the latter low value. The results also suggested that more instruction and practice might be necessary for younger groups. Mathews and Fox (1973) reported a modified version of the Ohio State Step Test for use with elementary school boys (lower step heights) and reported a validity of .90 and a reliability of .96. However, this modified version, like its predecessor, was not suitable for mass testing. Cotten did not provide norms; only 34 examinees were tested. The test constructor rationalized that bleacher heights vary among gymnasiums so that local norms should be used.

Even though the Cotten modifications improved the administrative feasibility of the step test, significant instruction and practice appear to be required for valid and reliable results. Perhaps instruction and brief practice on one more previous occasion would solve this problem. The 15 minute rest and practice prior to the test appear to be a long time for students in an activity class to remain inactive. In addition, one trial of the test requires 15 minutes plus startup and finishing time. If the test is given to one-half of the class at a time, the total administration time would require at least 50 minutes. A distance run probably would be easier to administer; however, pacing and motivation are common problems associated with mass distance run tests. Bleachers are available in many gymnasiums. Stable locker room type benches

probably could be substituted when bleachers are not available. Almost all schools have a tape recorder. Since most inexpensive and moderately priced tape recorders have a pulley drive, versus a gear drive, the tester should verify with a stopwatch that the tape recorder runs consistently at the proper speed.

A problem common to all step tests is failure of examinees to perform the correct amount of work. First, examinees may have trouble maintaining the cadence. Second, examinees may fail to attain a fully erect posture when mounting the step. In either case, the examinee will do less work than expected and will achieve an erroneously high score. The tester must monitor these problems carefully and correct them quickly.

The scoring system has an upper limit of 19. During test validation with 34 male college physical education major students only one student achieved a score of 19 on the step test and a corresponding Balke Treadmill Test score of 30 minutes (an excellent score). The next best step test score was 17. Therefore, it is unlikely that the upper score will pose as an artificial ceiling unless used with trained endurance athletes. Conversely, one member of the validation group lasted only 3 minutes on the step test and 12 minutes on the treadmill test. It would appear that a false floor does exist for the step test when used with poorly conditioned, younger, or female examinees. Use of a lower bench height would alleviate this problem but would require a different set of norms.

SUMMARY
Major Strengths:
1. Valid test of circulorespiratory endurance when administered under controlled conditions.

2. Highly reliable with male college physical education students who were given adequate instruction.

3. Equipment usually is available so the test requires no extra expenditures.

Major Weaknesses:
1. Test requires considerable instruction and practice to obtain valid and reliable results.

2. The tester must monitor cadence and proper form closely to obtain valid results.

3. Test requires 50 minutes to administer to a class.

4. The test has an artificial floor for poorly conditioned, younger, or female examinees.

REVIEW REFERENCES

Kurucz, R. L., et al. (1969). Construction of a submaximal cardiovascular step test. *Research Quarterly,* 40(1):115-122.

Mathews, D. K., & Laubach, L. L. (1973). *Measurement in physical education,* Philadelphia: Saunders, p. 257.

F-EMU STEP TEST (MODIFIED OHIO STATE STEP TEST)

Reference.
Witten, C. (1973). Construction of a submaximal cardiovascular step test for college females. *Research Quarterly,* 44(1):46-50.

Additional Source.
Safrit (1981, pp. 220-221).

Purpose.
To measure the cardiorespiratory endurance of an examinee through a submaximal step test.

Objectivity.
r = .95 between examinees' pulse count and electrocardiograph recordings.

Reliability.
r = .90 by test-retest.

Validity.
r = .85 between Balke Treadmill Test and step test scores.

Age and Sex.
College age females.

Equipment.
A tri-level bench with heights of 36cm (14"), 43cm (17"), and 51cm (20"), metronome, and a stopwatch.

Space Requirements and Design.
A square clear, level area approximately 3m (10') with the bench and the examinee in the center.

Directions.
The test is composed of 20 innings which are divided into four workloads with each workload consisting of 5 innings. Each inning consists of 30 seconds of stepping followed by 20 seconds of rest. The four workloads are divided as follows:

Phase 1 Innings 1 to 5, 24 steps/minute on the 36cm (14") bench;

Phase 2 Innings 6 to 10, 30 steps/minute on the 36cm (14") bench;

Phase 3 Innings 11 to 15, 30 steps/minute on the 43cm (17") bench;

Phase 4 Innings 16 to 20, 30 steps/minute on the 51cm (20") bench.

The examinee begins the test on the command, "Go," and continues stepping for a period of 30 seconds. On the command, "Stop," the examinee rests for 5 seconds and then on the command, "Count," the pulse rate is taken for 10 seconds. At the end of the 10 second pulse count, the command, "Stop and prepare to exercise," is given. After five seconds of rest, the command, "Go," is given to signify the start of another inning. The above procedure continues until all 20 innings are completed or until the examinee's pulse rate reaches at least 28 beats/10 seconds (168 beats/minute).

Scoring.
The score is the inning during which the examinee's pulse rate reaches at least 28 beats/10 seconds.

Norms.
Witten (1973, pp. 48-49) women.

REVIEW

JAMES A. RICHARDSON, Ed.D.

Assistant Professor
Exercise Science and Wellness
The University of South Dakota
Vermillion, SD 57069

With the basic assumption that "heart rate is one of the basic measures of the efficiency of the heart as a machine," then this test, as a diagnostic tool, is weak.

The consistency of this test lies in the reduction of the error margin that exists in direct relation to the number of hands on experiences that the tester has with the test and its application in the laboratory and in the field. The differences between the application of the test in the laboratory and in the field can be significant. The conditions of the test as administered in the laboratory can be strictly controlled by the tester from the standpoint of equipment (i.e., metronome, stopwatch, benches, and work space) and environment (i.e., air temperature, humidity, and lighting). In the field, the difference in the equipment may influence the test's results - i.e., the metronome (is it mechanical or electronic?), the stopwatch (is it mechanical or electronic?), the bench (is the workmanship such that the various levels are plum and level?), or the work space (is the work space level, and consistent in surface resistance to the stepping?).

The experience of the tester is critical to the success of gaining the results that could be achieved in the laboratory. The test is objective, unless the tester fails to follow the protocol exactly. This test, as with most human involved evaluations, is not very forgiving. In other words - it is not user friendly.

The active participation of the tester is essential from the standpoint of controlling the examinee in the consistency of stepping, the placing of the entire foot on the top of the level in use, the straightening of the knees when the foot is on the top of the bench, and the straightening of the torso when the cycle is completed. The leadership and experience factors involved in this test can be significant in relation to the potential for confusion, missed timing, starts and stops, consistency of stepping, and regularity of stepping.

The space requirements limit the number of people that can be tested at one time. Therefore, space is a significant limitation when testing large numbers, or mass testing. The equipment required may place a financial burden on schools, and/or laboratories that have limited funds.

The number of bouts that the examinee is required to complete to make definitive decisions concerning the examinee causes this test to have problems on the whole.

It would be counterproductive to use this test as a training tool in quest of cardiovascular conditioning. The use of this test as a tool to train testers would be somewhat advantageous in test organization if the population in question is parallel to that of the original work. The test is suitable for its intended age and sex group.

The test constructor does not discuss any of the danger signs related to sudden and critical intervention. Some of these signs are: inability to keep the tempo of the metronome in the stepping; deep panting; flushness of the face; sudden cold sweating; and significant changes of air temperature, air quality (molds, mildew, etc.), and humidity level of the room or space provided.

In terms of heart rate, the scoring is objective. Only when the population for which this test was prepared is utilized is the test suitable for research purposes. This condition is also a limitation of the test.

SUMMARY

Major Strength:

1. The test can be completed by an examinee without the assistance of another individual. This is based on the premise that the examinee can take her own pulse, set a metronome, and read a clock.

Major Weaknesses:

1. The scope of the age of the examinees is limited.

2. The scope of the sex of the examinees is limited.

3. The examinee must participate in multiple bouts to achieve the desired heart rate.

4. The examinee must participate in multiple levels in search of the desired heart rate.

5. The examinee must be able to take her own pulse.

6. The examinee must be able to set a metronome.

The F-EMU Step Test is inadequate for research. Since there are no norms upon which to base decisions, it is not possible to compare the results with those of another group. The limitation of the available statistics causes this test to be less than useful in a research setting.

GALLAGHER & BROUHA TEST FOR HIGH SCHOOL BOYS
(MODIFICATION OF HARVARD STEP TEST)

References.

Gallagher, J. R., & Brouha, L. (1943). A simple method of testing the physical fitness of boys. *Research Quarterly,* 14(1):23-30.

Clarke, H. H., & Clarke, D. H. (1987). *Application of measurement to health and physical education.* Englewood Cliffs: Prentice Hall, pp 141-142.

Additional Sources.

Bosco & Gustafson (1983, p. 133); Kirkendall et al. (1980, p. 304); Miller (1988, p. 152).

Purpose.

To measure an examinee's fitness level for physical work and the ability to recover.

Objectivity.

Not reported.

Reliability.

Not reported.

Validity.

Not reported.

Age and Sex.

Males, age 12 - 18.

Equipment.

Benches 46cm (18") and a 51cm (20") high, a ruler, a stopwatch, and a metronome or an audio tape with the cadence prerecorded.

Space Requirements and Design.

A clear, level area approximately 3m (10') square with the benches and the examinee in the center.

Directions.

The body surface area of the examinee must be determined before administering the test. The DuBois Body Surface Chart Nomograph (see Gallagher & Brouha, 1943, p. 29; Clarke & Clarke, 1987, p. 142) is used. A ruler is laid on the nomograph connecting the examinee's body height with the examinee's body weight. The point at which the ruler crosses the middle column represents the body surface area of the examinee.

Examinees with a body surface area of less than 1.85 square meters use the 46cm (18") bench while those with a 1.85 body surface of 1.85 square meters or more use the 51cm (20") bench. The cadence is 30 steps/minute for a maximum time of four minutes. The remainder of the directions are the same as those of the Harvard Step Test.

Scoring.

Same as for the Harvard Step Test.

Norms.

Bosco & Gustafson (1983, p. 133) boys; Clarke & Clarke (1987, p. 141) boys; Gallagher & Brouha (1943, p. 28) boys; Kirkendall et al. (1980, p. 304) boys; Miller (1988, p. 152) boys.

REVIEW

PAUL G. VOGEL, Ph.D.

Associate Professor
Physical Education
Michigan State University
East Lansing, MI 48824

This test was designed to measure the ability of 12 to 18 year old males to perform hard work. The scores are based upon the principle that an individual's level of physical fitness can be estimated by the rate at which the heart slows after it has responded to a standard bout of exhausting work. The test is based on the body's ability to handle relatively short, high intensity work and equates the obtained scores to physical fitness.

The test is described by its constructors as a measure of physical fitness. Although high scores on this test no doubt are related to a type of fitness (aerobic capacity and muscular strength and endurance of muscles located in the thigh and hips), it is inappropriate to equate performance on the test with physical fitness. Physical fitness, as the term is currently used, embodies much more than can be inferred from a test which primarily measures aerobic capacity and muscular strength and endurance of the hip and leg extensors.

No evidence of the reliability of the test is provided. However, the testing procedure and scoring are well described. The test appears to have good potential to produce reliable scores within and across testers. Also, no evidence of the test's validity is provided. Accordingly, this test cannot be recommended for research purposes.

Although the test could be used for research purposes subsequent to documenting its reliability and validity, there is no compelling reason to do so. Other laboratory measures based on oxygen uptake are available that have demonstrated strong reliability and validity (Bruce et al., 1974; Cooper, 1977). Neither can the test be strongly recommended for use in program evaluation or applied research studies. Again, other measures are available that have documented psychometric qualities, [although the acceptability of their psychometric characteristics have been questioned (Safrit, in press)] are more commonly used, have more recent norms and/or criterion referenced standards, and provide an educational component (AAHPERD, *Health*, 1980; AAHPERD, *Technical*, 1985; AAHPERD, *Physical*, 1988; *Fitnessgram*, 1987).

To the test constructors' credit, the test was developed for a clearly defined population and consideration was given to minimizing the effect of body size on test results (though no documentation or rationale for the cut off point used to divide large and small boys or for 18" and 20" benches was given). Also, the test involves commonly used musculature and no special skill. Administratively, the test is of short duration and is feasible for mass testing. The major deterrent to its administration would be obtaining the benches. Otherwise, only a stopwatch and metronome and/or recorded cadence are required. Pulse counters can be easily obtained by training students or interested others.

The test procedure could be used as an activity to develop aerobic fitness and muscular strength and endurance of the hip and leg extensors for individuals and/or groups. It could also be used as a self testing activity for those who wish to: (1) determine their aerobic status, (2) determine if their fitness program is resulting in desirable changes, and/or (3) determine how they compare to boys tested during the early part of the century.

SUMMARY

Major Strengths:

1. A well described testing and scoring procedure.

2. Relative ease of administration.

3. Suitability for mass or individual testing.

4. Possible use as a structured activity to develop aerobic capacity in conjunction with muscular strength and endurance of the leg and hip extensors.

5. Commonly attainable equipment.

6. Provision for examinees of different sizes.

Major Weaknesses:

1. Undocumented reliability, objectivity and validity.

2. Outdated norms and arbitrary cut off scores labeling relative fitness levels.

3. Norms for boys only.

4. The implication that it measures physical fitness when it addresses only a narrow component of physical fitness.

In summary, this test offers little to recommend its use. The weaknesses of this test far outweigh its strengths. Accordingly, it is not recommended for use in research or evaluation settings.

REVIEW REFERENCES

AAHPERD (1980). *Health related physical fitness test manual.* Reston, VA: American Alliance for Health, Physical Education, Recreation and Dance.

AAHPERD (1985). *Technical manual.* Reston, VA: American Alliance for Health, Physical Education, Recreation and Dance.

AAHPERD (1988). *The AAHPERD physical best program.* Reston, VA: American Alliance for Health, Physical Education, Recreation and Dance.

Bruce, R. A. et al. (1973). Maximal oxygen intake and nomographic assessment of functional aerobic impairment in cardiovascular disease. *American Heart Journal,* 85:546-562.

Cooper, K. A. (1977). *The aerobics way.* New York: M. Evans.

Fitnessgram user's manual (1987). Dallas: Institute for Aerobics Research.

Gallagher, J. R., & Brouha, L. (1943). A simple method of testing the physical fitness of boys. *Research Quarterly,* 14:23-30.

Safrit, M. Methods of measurement for physical fitness in children and youth. In *The Measurement of Physical Fitness in Children, Youth, Adults and Older Adults.* Washington, DC: National Institute of Health (in press).

GALLAGHER & BROUHA TEST FOR HIGH SCHOOL GIRLS
(MODIFICATION OF HARVARD STEP TEST) TEST

References.

Brouha, L., & Gallagher, J. R. (1943). A functional fitness test for high school girls. *Journal of Health and Physical Education,* 14(10):517, 550.

Clarke, H. H., & Clarke, D. H. (1987). *Application of measurement to health and physical education.* Englewood Cliffs: Prentice Hall, p 140-141.

Additional Source.

Clarke & Clarke (1987, pp. 140-141).

Purpose.

To measure the examinee's fitness level for physical work and the ability to recover from it.

Objectivity.

Not reported.

Reliability.

Not reported.

Validity.

Not reported.

Age and Sex.

High school age females.

Equipment.

A bench 41cm (16") high, a stopwatch, and a metronome or an audio tape with the cadence prerecorded.

Space Requirements and Design.

A clear, level area approximately 3m (10') square with the bench and the examinee in the center.

Directions.

The techniques and directions are the same as for the Harvard Step Test except that the bench is 41cm (16") high and the maximum exercise time is four minutes.

Scoring.

The score is derived by the long form formula presented in the Harvard Step Test.

Norms.

Clarke & Clarke (1987, p. 141) girls.

REVIEW
CHERYL NORTON, Ed.D.

Associate Professor
Human Performance
Metropolitan State College
Denver, CO 80204

The step test as proposed by Gallagher and Brouha is a commonly used method of assessing cardiovascular functioning in response to physical work. It does not, however, measure this capacity as accurately as an evaluation of maximal oxygen uptake. Because the test discriminates between trained and untrained individuals, it can be used to screen individuals for appropriate fitness activities, show improvement in condition with training, and as an educational device, to understand better cardiovascular functioning with exercise.

The strength of the test lies in its ease of administration. Not only can groups be tested at one time, but equipment and space needs are minimal and inexpensive. Because the test requires little time (approximately 7.5 minutes/examinee) and is conducted indoors, weather and scheduling are typically not a problem. The test does require an assistant to work with each examinee; however, partners can be trained to do this task. If the test is used for research purposes, specially trained testers should be used to insure consistency of measures.

It should be noted that there are factors associated with this test that can produce variability in the results. Because the examinee must raise her weight onto a bench, the relative leg strength to body weight ratio is assessed as well as cardiovascular efficiency. Typically for high school females, not only is the leg strength poor but the body weight lifted has a high percentage of fat content. Thus, it is possible that the limiting test factor for an examinee is not the ability to bring oxygen into the body but the relative strength capacity of the leg muscles. Consequently, it must be kept in mind that this test is measuring work capacity. As such, other factors may also influence the outcome of the test such as room temperature, time of day, previous exercise before the test, altitude, humidity, current state of health, and, most importantly, the examinee's motivation. Consequently, test scores could vary on a day to day basis. In addition, it is easy for the examinee to "cheat" on this test (i.e., do less work than the test requires). Not coming to a full erect position on the bench or failing to follow the cadence results in an under-achievement of work.

Another problem which must be taken into consideration when using this test is the inability to standardize the relative workload each examinee does. Because the bench is a fixed height, and the examinees have different leg lengths and standing heights, the work done to raise the body this fixed distance provides for variability in the biomechanical task of stepping. As a result it is possible to place considerable strain on the knee joint. This consideration, coupled with a varying cardiovascular condition of examinees, suggests that for some examinee, this test will require a maximal effort. Other examinees may find only a submaximal effort is needed. Consequently, short, poorly conditioned and/or overfat examinees will find this test very stressful.

Probably the most limiting feature of the test is the lack of normative data. While the scoring of the test is simple, objective, and reasonable for high school students, without norms the only use for the test is a pre and post training comparison or the provisions of a relative class ranking.

SUMMARY

In summary, the test is of value as a screening/educational tool to provide examinees with a practical experience regarding physiological assessment of work. The test discriminates between examinees who have highly or poorly developed cardiovascular systems; however, other factors such as the leg strength/body weight ratio and bench size effect the ability of the examinee to perform the test. The convenience and lack of expense associated with the test make it a good tool for class situations.

The Gallagher & Grouha Test is an acceptable test for teaching purposes with very limited research application unless the focus of the research was to provide normative data for the test.

HARVARD STEP TEST

References.

Brouha, L. (1943). The step test: A simple method of measuring physical fitness for muscular work in young men. *Research Quarterly,* 14(1):31-36.

Carver, R. P., & Winsmann, F. R. (1970). Study of measurement and experimental design problems associated with the step test. *Journal of Sports Medicine and Physical Fitness*, 10(2):104-113.

Karpovich, P. V. (1965). *Physiology of muscular activity.* Philadelphia: W. B. Saunders, pp 240-243.

Safrit, M. J. (1981). *Evaluation in physical education.* Englewood Cliffs: Prentice Hall, pp 216-218.

Additional Sources.

Baumgartner & Jackson (1982, pp. 276-277); Bosco & Gustafson (1983, pp. 131-133); Clarke & Clarke (1987, pp. 137-139); Jensen & Hirst (1980, pp. 110-112); Johnson & Nelson (1986, pp. 163-164);

Kirkendall et al. (1980, pp. 303-306); Kirkendall et al. (1987, pp. 177-179); Miller (1988, pp. 150-151); Mood (1980, pp. 279-280); Safrit (1986, pp. 250-253); Safrit (1990, pp. 384-385); Verducci (1980, pp. 271-273).

Purpose.

To measure an examinee's fitness level for physical work and the ability to recover.

Objectivity.

Not reported.

Reliability.

Not reported in Brouha (1943), but r = .65 and r = .77 for college men and r = .65 for eighth grade boys were reported by Meyers (1969) cited in Safrit (1981, p. 217).

Validity.

Not reported in Brouha (1943), but r = .41 was obtained by Hettinger (1961) using VO^2max as the criterion cited in Safrit (1981, p. 217).

Age and Sex.

College age males.

Equipment.

A bench 51cm (20") high, stopwatch, and a metronome or an audio tape with the cadence prerecorded.

Space Requirements and Design.

A clear, level area approximately 3m (10') square with the bench and the examinee in the center.

Directions.

On command, the examinee begins stepping at a cadence of 30 steps/minute. The examinee should stand erect when both feet are on the bench or on the floor. The stepping is continued for a period of five minutes or until the examinee becomes too exhausted to continue. If the examinee stops stepping prior to the five minutes, the amount of time completed is recorded. At the cessation of the stepping, the examinee sits and remains still.

The following forms are provided to measure the pulse rate:

A. Original Long Form - Sitting pulse rate taken 1 to 1.5, 2 to 2.5, and 3 to 3.5 minutes following the stepping.

B. Short Form - Sitting pulse rate is taken 1 to 1.5 minutes following the stepping.

Scoring.

The Physical Efficiency Index (PEI) is computed using either of the following two methods:

A. Original Long Form

PEI = Duration of stepping in seconds x 100/2 x sum of three pulse counts in recovery.

B. Short Form

PEI = Duration of stepping in seconds x 100/5.5 x pulse count for 1 to 1.5 minutes after exercise.

Norms.

Brouha (1943, p. 32) boy athletes; Clarke & Clarke (1987, p. 138) men; Jensen & Hirst (1980, pp. 112-113) ages and sex not specified; Johnson & Nelson (1986, p. 166) men; Karpovich (1965, pp. 240-242) boy athletes; Kirkendall et al. (1980,

p. 303) men; Kirkendall et al. (1987, p. 178) men; Miller (1988, p. 151) men; Safrit (1986, p. 252) men.

REVIEW

JAMES R. MORROW, JR., Ph.D.

Professor
Health and Human Performance
University of Houston
Houston, TX 77204-5331

The Harvard Step Test, perhaps the original cardiorespiratory endurance test that could be used in mass fitness testing, is essentially a "recovery heart rate test" based on the principle of rapid heart rate recovery following exercise in fit individuals. The test can be used in large groups and can be self administered to determine current fitness level as well as changes in fitness. Originally developed for college age men, the test has been modified for use with women and younger children. Unfortunately, while the test does provide an efficient means with which to test large groups, requiring little equipment and little time, there are limitations to its use.

Reported reliabilities are adequate to high. However, objectivity and validity issues result in limitations in its acceptability. The test is based on the principle that the heart rate recovers more quickly toward the resting value following exercise in fit individuals than in those less fit. Thus, accurate heart rates must be recorded following the exercise bout. A benefit to the test is that it causes the examinee to assess heart rate and may encourage the examinee to use heart rate as an indication of exercise intensity and monitoring during training. The test is five minutes in length, though scores can be determined if the examinee must discontinue the test early. The time, cadence, and stepping height make the test reasonably strenuous and thus contraindicated for some individuals (e.g., elderly and unfit).

Accurate measure of recovery heart rate is essential. Whether the original or short version is administered, heart rate must be determined one minute following cessation of the stepping. At the measurement time, it may be difficult for younger children to feel the pulse accurately and

record the value, thus invalidating the measurement. Accuracy in heart rate measurement can be obtained with training prior to administering the test. Heart rate measurements have been shown to be objective and valid when individuals are trained in obtaining heart rate. However, little evidence exists for this essential accuracy in younger populations which may use various modifications of the test.

The test has demonstrated moderate discriminate and convergent (concurrent) validity. It does not correlate well with measures of strength and psychomotor performance. However, moderate correlations have been found between the results and oxygen consumption, treadmill time, and distance running performance. Construct validity has been provided by testing various groups known to differ in fitness levels. Additional construct validity is provided by changes in test performance for individuals who increase or decrease training behaviors.

Various modifications in time, cadence, and stepping height have been made in attempts to make the test more appropriate for specific groups (see various other step tests reviewed in this volume). The time for completion has been reduced to alleviate the strenuous nature of the test. Adjustments in the stepping height have been made to adjust for leg length differences. Unfortunately, an examinee's body weight could be significantly related to test performance. Two examinees with the same leg length, with considerably different weights, could complete the entire test. However, the heavier examinee will have accomplished considerably more work.

While the test is acceptable for use in self monitoring and large group testing, it is typically inappropriate for research purposes (though similar step tests have been used for wide scale public health surveys). Practice testing sessions for cadence and heart rate recording should be utilized. Classification indices for various groups are presented by Miller (1988).

REVIEW REFERENCE

Miller, D. K. (1988). *Measurement by the physical educator: Why and how.* Indianapolis: Benchmark Press.

KASCH PULSE RECOVERY TEST

Reference.
Barrow, H. M., & McGee, R. (1979). *A practical approach to measurement in physical education.* Philadelphia: Lea & Febiger, pp 196-199.

Additional Sources.
Bosco & Gustafson (1983, p. 136); Hastad & Lacy (1989, pp. 189-192).

Purpose.
To measure the ability of an examinee's heart and circulatory system to adjust to and recuperate from hard work.

Objectivity.
Not reported.

Reliability.
Not reported.

Validity.
r = -.53 when compared with a maximal oxygen uptake cycle ergometer test cited in Barrow and McGee (1979, p. 196).

Age and Sex.
Females and males of all age.

Equipment.
A bench 31cm (12") high, stopwatch, and metronome.

Space Requirements and Design.
A clear, level area approximately 3m (10') square with the bench and the examinee in the center.

Directions.
The examinee should rest a minimum of five minutes prior to the test and should not have smoked for one hour or eaten for two hours prior to the test. After the appropriate rest, the examinee assumes a standing position in front of the bench and on command, begins stepping at a cadence of 24 steps/minute. The examinee should stand erect when both feet are on the bench or on the floor. The stepping is continued for a period of three minutes unless the examinee becomes overly exhausted and has to stop. The lead foot may be changed when stepping up on the bench, but not more than three times. Immediately following the three minutes of stepping,

the examinee sits down and locates her/his pulse. The pulse count is initiated 10 seconds after the cessation of the stepping and is taken for one minute.

Scoring.
The score is the examinee's pulse rate taken for one minute.

Norms.
Barrow & McGee (1979, p. 199) boys, girls, men and women; Hastad & Lacy (1989, p. 192) boys, girls, men and women.

REVIEW

SAMUEL CASE, Ph.D.

Professor of Physical Education
Western Maryland College
Westminster, MD 21157

The Kasch Pulse Recovery Test was designed as a submaximal exercise tolerance test for use with a population of post rheumatic patients. The original test was designed using a sample of 27 post rheumatic boys aged 8 to 13 years. Since that time, the test has been included in measurement books as a test to be used with individuals of all ages and of either sex.

The validity coefficients are not given in the primary source (Kasch, 1961). However, since that time, a validity coefficient of -.53 has been obtained by comparing the results of the test with maximal oxygen uptake as measured on a cycle ergometer. This is an unsatisfactory validity coefficient. Reliability and objectivity coefficients are not given, but according to the primary source a test-retest design was used in the construction of the test to insure reliability. However, the test constructor cautions that in addition to recovery pulse rate, ventilation rates and oxygen consumption are also essential in making an adequate assessment.

The requirements for administering the test are reasonable. Nothing extraordinary is required in terms of equipment, facilities, or space. Furthermore, if the examinees are taught to take the pulse accurately, one tester could easily test an entire class very efficiently.

This test is not suitable for drill or conditioning purposes. Bench stepping is boring and has little, if any, carry over value. Because of the low exercise intensity, that is stepping on a 12 inch platform at a rate of 24 times a minute, this test may not discriminate between the fit and the highly fit.

If the pulse rate is accurately counted and recorded, the test is easily scored, and it can be self administered. Norms are available for both sexes. Although the norms for males aged 6 to 60 were attained scientifically, the norms for women were arbitrarily assigned. This factor compromises the credibility of the test.

SUMMARY

Major Strengths:

1. The requirements in terms of equipment and space are neither extensive nor expensive.

2. The skills needed to accomplish and administer the test are not excessive.

Major Weaknesses:

1. The low published validity coefficient.

2. Scientifically designed norms are not available for females.

This test met an important need when it was originally developed. However, since that time much progress has been made in the design of fitness tests for both individuals in the laboratory and for groups in a class setting, and today, better designed and more accurate tests are available for both situations. Therefore, this test is unacceptable for research purposes or for use in the normal classroom situation.

REVIEW REFERENCE

Kasch, F. W. (1961). A comparison of the exercise tolerance of post rheumatic and normal boys. *Journal of the Association for Physical and Mental Rehabilitation,* 15:35-40.

KENT STATE UNIVERSITY STEP TEST

Reference.

Harvey, V. P., & Scott, G. D. (1970). The validity and reliability of a one minute step test for college women. *Journal of Sports Medicine and Physical Fitness,* 10(3):185-192.

Additional Sources.

None.

Purpose.

To measure the cardiorespiratory endurance of an examinee through bench stepping.

Objectivity.

r = .91 and r = .96 between examinees' pulse count and that taken simultaneously with stethoscope.

Reliability.

r = .73 for test-retest method.

Validity.

r = .71 compared with the Skubic-Hodgkins Test.

Age and Sex.

College age females.

Equipment.

A bench 46cm (18") high, metronome, and stopwatch.

Space Requirements and Design.

A clear, level area approximately 3m (10') square with the bench and the examinee in the center.

Directions.

On command, the examinee begins stepping at a cadence of 30 steps/minute for a period of one minute.

One minute after the cessation of stepping, the pulse rate is taken for 30 seconds.

Scoring.

The score is the pulse rate taken 1 to 1.5 minutes after the cessation of stepping.

Norms.

Not reported.

REVIEW

DONNA J. TERBIZAN, Ph.D.

Assistant Professor
Health, Physical Education and Recreation
North Dakota State University
Fargo, ND 58105

The Kent State University Step Test may be acceptable for measuring cardiorespiratory endurance, but there are other tests that would meet this objective in better fashion. A test that takes only 1 minute to complete may not be as good a measure of cardiorespiratory endurance as another test of 12 minutes duration. If this test was constructed because administrative time was a factor, and with a reported reliability of 0.73, it seems to be as good as a longer test, but this reviewer would probably utilize a different test for this fitness aspect.

In practicality, this test may be functional. It does not take an inordinate amount of time, it is fairly valid and reliable, and it requires little equipment. It may be considered dangerous by some because of the height of the step bench and its effect on the knee joint of the examinees. Without norms it, cannot be determined if this test is suitable for the general public, although this reviewer believes that it can be if norms were provided. The Kent State University Step Test is not suitable for research purposes, because of its duration and danger aspects. There are better tests available for research.

SUMMARY

The major strength of this step test is its duration. If one were to be concerned with a large number of examinees in a testing situation, it may be acceptable. On the other hand, if the test is to be used for job advancement (e.g., military or police), the validity and reliability of this test is high enough to warrant its use.

The Kent State University Step Test is also weak in the area of duration. One may question whether a one minute test is a good measure of cardiovascular fitness, even with a reliability of 0.73. This test may also be considered by some as unsafe with the bench height being too high for some females, especially the shorter individuals. This test is not suitable for research purposes due to the noted weaknesses. Overall, the Kent State Test is an acceptable test for teaching with cautions, relative to bench height and duration of the test and an unacceptable for research purposes, relative to the duration of the test.

LSU STEP TEST

References.
Johnson, B. L., & Nelson, J. K. (1986). *Practical measurements for evaluation in physical education*. Edina, MN: Burgess, pp 160-163.

Nelson, J. K. (1976). Fitness testing as an educational process. In Broekhoff (ed.). *Physical Education, Sports and Sciences*. Eugene, OR: Microform Publications.

Additional Sources.
Clarke & Clarke (1987, p. 143); Hastad & Lacy (1989, pp. 186, 188-190).

Purpose.
To measure the cardiorespiratory endurance of an examinee through submaximal bench stepping and to provide a graphic illustration of pulse rate adjustments to exercise and recovery.

Objectivity.
Not reported.

Reliability.
Test-retest reliability coefficients for five pulse counts have been reported as follows: before exercise (.86), 5 seconds after exercise (.88), 1 minute after exercise (.85), 2 minutes after exercise (.87), and 3 minutes after exercise (.80).

Validity.
Construct validity has been established.

Age and Sex.
Females and males, grades 9 to 12 and adults.

Equipment.
Benches, chairs, or bleachers 43-46cm (17-18") high, graph paper, metronome, and stopwatch.

Space Requirements and Design.
A clear, level area approximately 3m (10') square with the bench and the examinee in the center.

Directions.
Before the test begins, the examinee should practice taking her/his own pulse rate several times using the radial artery. Three consecutive 10 second counts should be taken until the pulse rate has stabilized and the tester is satisfied that the examinee is competent in the pulse counting procedures.

The examinee stands in front of the bench and on the command, "Ready, Go," begins stepping at a cadence of 24 steps per minute for females and 30 steps per minute for males. The cadence should be established with the use of a metronome by multiplying the desired steps per minute by four. This way each step of "up, up, down, down" is synchronized with a click of the metronome. After two minutes of stepping, the commands, "Stop, sit down, find your pulse" are given, and after five seconds has elapsed, a ten second pulse rate is taken and recorded. Three 10 second recovery pulse rates are taken at one minute, two minutes, and three minutes after cessation of stepping.

Scoring.
The five 10 second pulse counts are recorded on the score sheet, the 10 second counts are then multiplied by six in order to express the scores in beats per minute. The beats per minute scores are then plotted on graph paper to provide an illustration of the pulse rate adjustment to exercise.

Norms.
Johnson & Nelson (1986, p. 162) men and women.

REVIEW

JAMES B. GALE, Ph.D.
Professor
Physical Education and Health
Sciences
Sonoma State University
Rohnert Park, CA 94928

The LSU Step Test has been designed to evaluate responses of the cardiovascular system to exercise. It is based on differences in recovery rates of individuals of different levels of cardiovascular training and VO_2max. It has been assumed that trained subjects who perform a single, absolute workload will have lower exercise and recovery heart rates (HR) than those who are less trained and/or that subjects who have higher VO_2max's will have lower exercise and recovery HR than those who have lower VO_2max's. The test constructors have used the term "cardiovascular endurance" where others might have used aerobic power (VO^{2}max). The ability to sustain a long duration activity (endurance) depends upon aerobic power and both quantity and quality of training.

This test requires little equipment or space and was designed to be self administered (i.e., the examinees take their own HR). Thus, it may be administered simultaneously to a large number of examinees in a brief period. Because it is not possible to measure one's own HR accurately during exercise, recovery HR may be measured as an indicator of the HR during exercise (first HR at five seconds post exercise) and as a moderate indicator of "fitness" related to the slope of the recovery HR response.

A pulse measured immediately after exercise is an accurate indicator of exercise HR and the HR response to an equal exercise intensity may indicate relative VO^{2}max or level of training. A problem with this test is that the bench stepping may not be of equal intensity for all examinees. Differences in the elevation of the center of gravity may be due to variations in body dimensions and biomechanics, including bending forward at the waist while stepping up.

More accurate estimates of VO^{2}max include the submaximal bicycle tests (e.g., Astrand-Ryhming or YMCA), the 12 or 15 minute runs (Cooper or Balke), and step tests which measure HR during exercise. Validation of this particular test was not made with either measured or estimated VO^{2}max, and therefore, it is not to be considered a valid test of aerobic power. However, this test was used to assess changes in cardiovascular fitness following a 15 week training program, and this may be the best application for this particular protocol. The test, elicited HR's below estimated maximums in both college age men and women and would, therefore, be considered safe to administer to this or similar populations. It may evoke supramaximal responses in older examinees and would be contraindicated.

Used as an educational tool, examinees may be able to observe changes in their own HR responses following training. If environmental conditions are well controlled (especially differences in temperature and clothing), the HR responses immediately post exercise, as well as during recovery, should become attenuated after a period of endurance training.

SUMMARY

In summary, the LSU Step Test is acceptable only for educational purposes. It allows for testing of a large number of examinees in physical conditioning programs. The results of this test could be used to introduce concepts of cardiovascular response to exercise and the effects of training on these cardiovascular responses.

MANAHAN-GUTIN ONE-MINUTE STEP TEST

References.

Manahan, J. E., & Gutin, B. (1971). The one minute step test as a measure of 600 yard run performance. *Research Quarterly,* 42(2):173-177.

Meyers, C. R. (1974). *Measurement in physical education.* New York: Ronald Press, pp 337-338.

Additional Sources.

None.

Purpose.

To measure the cardiorespiratory endurance of an examinee through bench stepping.

Objectivity.

Not reported.

Reliability.

r = .95.

Validity.

r = .82 between step test and 600 yard run/walk scores.

Age and Sex.

Ninth grade age females.

Equipment.

A bench 46cm (18") high and a stopwatch.

Space Requirements and Design.

A clear, level area approximately 3m (10') square with the bench and the examinee in the center.

Directions.

The examinee assumes a standing position with her right foot on the bench. For safety reasons, the examinee holds an assistant's hand during the entire test. On command, the examinee straightens the right leg and then returns to the starting position. The left foot does not come in contact with the bench. This sequence is repeated for a period of one minute. The examinee is permitted to change the lead foot if necessary.

Scoring.

The score is the number of times the examinee returns her left foot to the floor in one minute.

Norms.

Not reported.

REVIEW

WALTER R. THOMPSON, Ph.D.

Director
Laboratory of Applied Physiology
School of Human Performance and
Recreation
The University of Southern Mississippi
Hattiesburg, MS 39406-5142

The Manahan-Gutin One Minute Step Test has several advantages over more sophisticated evaluation instruments. First identified in the literature by Brouha in 1942, the step test was later revised by Brouha and Gallagher (1943). Since that time several other variations have appeared in the literature. The Manahan-Gutin One-Minute Step Test is yet another variation of this simple testing instrument.

The step test is the most inexpensive device to measure cardiorespiratory work (Barrow et al., 1989; Hastad & Lacy, 1989). It is also one of the more simple tests to administer with little inter observer variability. The Manahan-Gutin One-Minute Step Test requires the examinee to step up on a 46cm (18") bench as many times as possible in one minute. The observer simply counts the number of steps completed and not the heart rate immediately after exercise. Although no objectivity data are reported, it can be assumed to be very high.

The original purpose of the Manahan-Gutin One-Minute Step Test was to determine if it was an appropriate replacement for the 600 yard run (Manahan & Gutin, 1971). After several trials, the test constructors found the test to carry good validity. The test constructors claimed the use of this step test is four times more accurate than tests using post exercise heart rate. The test also carries good test-retest reliability. The increased reliability, according to the test constructors, of this test over the four count step test is the elimination of the "jump down" which is not permitted. One foot must remain in contact with the bench at all times.

The test does not require the active participation of another individual except to count steps. However, the test constructors suggest another individual may hold the hand of the examinee. Although this may be considered trivial, some assistance may be rendered if the hand is held high and the examinee exerts force against the hand assisting in the step up or step down. Therefore, careful instruction should be given to the examinee and the assistant that aid is not to be offered at any time. The test does not require the active assistance of another individual who could affect performance.

Previous step tests that require cadence or heart rate measurements have been determined to be difficult to administer, often not valid and seldom reliable. The test constructors have suggested that stepping as many times as possible in a specified period of time is similar to running. Therefore, equipment, space, and training personnel will cause no problem in the administration of this test. Since this test requires a partner, the only limitation for large group testing is the space requirements on a bench. The test takes only one minute to administer. Only one trial is recommended, which may not be an adequate representation of fitness.

The original test utilized ninth grade girls (n = 40) as examinees. While scoring for this test is objective with reasonable validity and reliability, no normative data are available. The examinees (although all were in the ninth grade) ranged in age from 160 to 188 months, a difference of 28 months. Body weight ranged from 87 to 176 pounds (89 pounds separating the lightest to the heaviest). There was a 9.3 inches difference between the shortest (59.5 inches) and the tallest girl (68.8 inches). A lack of homogeneity was a factor in the original publication of this test. No further refinement of the test is available nor are normative data for this or any other age group. This test has limited use for research purposes.

SUMMARY

Major Strengths:

1. This test (not unlike all step tests) has an advantage over other evaluation instruments in its relative simple construct.

2. It is inexpensive and dependent only upon the accuracy of a one minute clock and the counting ability of an observer.

3. The Manahan-Gutin One-Minute Step Test has "reasonable" validity and reliability compared to the 600 yard run. As such, it may be a good alternative if a facility is not available or weather forces indoor use.

Major Weaknesses:

1. Since no normative data exist for this test, its application is quite limited.

2. The examinee is expected to use the right leg only (although if it tires the examinee may switch legs), therefore not considering leg dominance.

The Manahan-Gutin One-Minute Step Test is not adequate for research and/or teaching because of the lack of normative data. This test has only been validated for ninth grade girls. The original publication indicated that the examinees had a wide range of height, weight, and age. Therefore, homogeneity is a problem. To become an acceptable test for research and/or teaching, large scale testing should be accomplished with subsequent norms developed and published.

REVIEW REFERENCES

Barrow, H. M. et al. (1989). *Practical measurement in physical education and sport*. Philadelphia: Lea & Febiger.

Brouha, L. (1942). The step test: A simple method of measuring physical fitness for muscular work in young men. *Research Quarterly*, 14:31-36.

Brouha, L., & Gallagher, J. R. (1943). A functional fitness test for high school girls. *Journal of Health and Physical Education*, 14(10):517.

Hastad, D. N., & Lacy, A. C. (1989). *Measurement and evaluation in contemporary physical education*. Scottsdale, AZ: Gorsuch and Scarisbrick.

Manahan J. E., & Gutin, B. (1971). The one minute step test as a measure of 600 yard run performance. *Research Quarterly*, 42(2):173-177.

NARSS MODIFIED HARVARD STEP TEST

References.

Carver, R. P., & Winsmann, F. R. (1970). Study of measurement and experimental design problems associated with the step test. *Journal of Sports Medicine and Physical Fitness,* 10(2):104-113.

Meyers, C. R. (1974). *Measurement in physical education.* New York: Ronald Press, pp 334-336.

Additional Sources.

None.

Purpose.

To measure the general capacity of an examinee to adapt to and recover from hard work.

Objectivity.

Not reported.

Reliability.

Not reported.

Validity.

Not reported.

Age and Sex.

Not reported, but editor assumes it is same as Harvard Step Test - college age males.

Equipment.

A bench 51cm (20") high with an adjustable horizontal bar at the back edge of the bench, metronome, tape recorder, and stopwatch.

Space Requirements and Design.

A clear, level area approximately 3m (10') square with the bench and the examinee in the center.

Directions.

The New and Rapid Stepping Score (NARSS) is a modified version of the Harvard Step Test (HST) which was developed to overcome the inadequacies of the HST. The major inadequacy the NARSS attempts to overcome is that the scores from the original HST of those who do not step the full five minutes are primarily the result of the duration of stepping while the scores of those that complete the full five minutes depend wholly on the heart rate response. A pretest resting pulse rate should be counted to screen out people with rates over 100 beats per minute,

since high initial rates invalidate the score. To effect standardization of the testing technique, it is recommended that the horizontal bar apparatus be gripped with both hands and adjusted so the forearms are horizontal when standing on the bench. The metronome is used with the tape recorder to make an accurate recording of 30 steps per minute as follows: up, up, down, one; up, up, down, two; up, up, down, three; etc. No crouching or bouncing is permitted while stepping. Examinees that lag more than one step behind cadence while stepping are stopped and assumed to be at the exhaustion point. The pulse count is taken during the interval 1 to 1.5 minutes after the start of the test (i.e., stepping). Other than these modifications, the same procedures that are used for the HST are followed.

Scoring.

The score is derived from using the rapid form of scoring the HST plus a correction factor which is supposed to estimate a five minute score regardless of the length of stepping.

NARSS Score = (duration in seconds x 100) / [(5.5 x pulse count) + .22 (300 - duration in seconds)].

Norms.

Not reported.

REVIEW

E. R. BUSKIRK, Ph.D.

Professor of Applied Physiology
The Pennsylvania State University
University Park, PA 16802

The test is a measure of endurance for those who exercise to their capacity, but for less than five minutes. Because the heart rate or pulse count is recorded between 1.0 and 1.5 minutes of stepping, a "steady state" heart rate is not obtained, but the recorded rate is proportional to the examinee's response to the intensity of the activity. For those who exercise for five minutes, the test depends totally on the pulse rate. Data on test reliability are not currently available in sufficient quantity to establish such values for different segments of the population that vary in age, gender, etc. There is no reason to suspect that reliable data could not be obtained through careful adherence to the test protocol when the test is administered to relatively homogeneous groups. The test should be objective even though administered by different testers if the test protocol is carefully followed. The test requires the participation of no more than one tester.

Facility and space requirements are minimal but the environmental conditions should be in the thermal comfort range for the intensity of the proposed stepping (i.e., 65-75 degrees with relatively low humidity). Only light weight clothing and shoes should be worn. The equipment required consists of the bench positioned on a non slip surface and a metronome. The bench should be sturdy enough to accommodate heavy examinees without moving. Radial pulse counting is adequate but electronic counting would be preferable. The test is easy to administer, but training of the tester is necessary so that the proper stepping cadence is achieved and maintained and the pulse count is made in a consistent way with proper entry and exit pulse counts. Maintenance of an upright body position is also important. The test should take no more than 10 minutes to administer to naive examinees. Some practice is necessary to establish the proper stepping sequence and cadence. Although not recommended, more valid and reliable data would undoubtedly be obtained if the test were repeated by each examinee following a 15 to 30 minute rest. The test could be used to produce some physical conditioning by repeated testing several times a week for several weeks, but other methods of physical conditioning would be more practical. The test has been utilized primarily by young men. The bench height would have to be lowered for children, the obese, most women, the elderly, etc. The only dangerous aspects perceived would be slipping on the bench or floor surface and falling with injury to the head or some other body part. Among those with car-

diovascular risk factors, the test could precipitate a myocardial event. Scoring is objective, although slightly complicated to perform without the assistance of a calculator. The test is of marginal suitability for laboratory research and is more suited to field research and presumably when relatively large numbers of examinees need to be tested and limited facilities and other resources are available. Adequate norms for different age groups, genders, etc., are not available.

SUMMARY

Major Strength:

1. The test is easy to administer and requires a minimum of equipment.

Major Weaknesses:

1. Dependence on a rather subjective endpoint with respect to duration of the test for those who step for less than five minutes. A slight miscue in cadence may take place for a variety of reasons. If the examinee exercises for five minutes, the test is exclusively dependent on the pulse count.

2. The radial pulse may be difficult to palpate in some examinees in view of the fact that they are moving and their arm will not remain in one position.

3. The assumed slope of the relationship between stepping duration in seconds and the HST score (0.22) may not apply to all examinees.

The test is acceptable for field research and for classroom demonstrations. Gross differences in physical condition with respect to stepping can be ascertained. The results will, in general, agree with other assessments of cardiorespiratory capacity, but careful adherence to the test protocol is essential. Benches of different heights are necessary to accommodate examinees who differ in age, gender, height, body fatness, etc. Behaviors during testing such as lagging or crouching will affect the score.

OHIO STATE UNIVERSITY STEP TEST

References.

Kurucz, R. L. (1967). Construction of the Ohio state university cardiovascular fitness test. Unpublished doctoral dissertation, Ohio State University.

Kurucz, R. L. et al. (1969).Construction of a submaximal cardiovascular step test. *Research Quarterly*, 40(1):115-122.

Mathews, D. K. (1978). *Measurement in physical education*. Philadelphia: W. B. Saunders, pp 275-277.

Additional Sources.

Baumgartner & Jackson (1982, pp. 274-276); Bosco & Gustafson (1983, pp. 137-138); Clarke & Clarke (1987, pp. 143-145); Jensen & Hirst (1980, pp. 113-114); Johnson & Nelson (1986, pp. 156, 158-160); Safrit (1981, pp. 218-220); Safrit (1986, pp. 253-254); Safrit (1990, pp. 384-385).

Purpose.

To measure the cardiorespiratory endurance of an examinee through a submaximal step test.

Objectivity.

Not reported.

Reliability.

r = .94 in a test-retest study.

Validity.

r = .94 when compared with the Balke Treadmill Test.

Age and Sex.

Males, age 18 and over.

Equipment.

A split level bench which is 38cm (15") high on one level and 51cm (20") high on the other level. A depth of 41cm (16") and a width of 46cm (18") for each level is desired. Two firmly mounted vertical bars with holes are placed at the back edge of the split level bench. A horizontal bar is placed through the two vertical bars. A metronome and a stopwatch are also required.

Space Requirements and Design.

A clear, level area approximately 3m (10') square with the bench and the examinee in the center.

Directions.

The examinee stands in front of the 38cm (15") high section of the bench. The examinee grasps the horizontal bar with both hands at approximately head height. On command, the examinee steps up and down for 30 seconds in cadence with the metronome, which is set at 96 beats per minute, producing 24 steps per minute. On the command, "Stop," the examinee sits down and finds his pulse rate. After sitting for 5 seconds, the command, "Count," is given and after 15 seconds the commands, "Stop," and "Prepare to exercise," are given. In other words, the pulse rate is taken for 10 seconds between the 5 and 15 second commands. After 5 more seconds have elapsed and on command, the examinee begins stepping again for another period of 30 seconds. During each stepping period, the examinee should assume an erect standing position when on the floor or bench.

Phase One

The test continues until the pulse rate has reached 25 or more (150 beats per minute) or six innings have been completed. An inning consists of 30 seconds of stepping followed by 20 seconds of rest in which 10 seconds are used to obtain the pulse rate.

Phase Two

This part of the test consists of the same procedures as mentioned above with the exception that the metronome is set at 120 beats per minute to produce 30 steps per minute. The second phase consists of six innings.

Phase Three

This phase follows the same directions as phase two with the exception that the examinee uses the 51cm (20") high level section of the bench. The third phase consists of six innings. The total number of innings in the test is 18, provided the examinee's pulse rate did not reach 25 or more prior to the inning 18.

Scoring.

The score is the inning in which the examinee's pulse rate reaches 25 or more beats in 10 seconds (150 beats per minute). If the examinee completes all of the 18 innings without the pulse rate reaching 25 or more beats in 10 seconds, a score of 19 is recorded.

Norms.

Bosco & Gustafson (1983, p. 138) men; Mathews (1978, p. 277) men.

REVIEW

CRAIG J. CISAR, Ph.D.

Associate Professor
Human Performance
San Jose State University
San Jose, CA 95192-0054

The Ohio State University Step Test does appear to have face validity in terms of measuring the physical component of cardiorespiratory endurance. In addition, the concurrent validity of the step test has been established by comparing its results with that of the Balke Treadmill Test (r = .94). The step test has also been reported to have a high test-retest reliability (r = .94) and, hence, only one trial of the test is needed to obtain valid results. The test would appear to be potentially an objective test if testers follow the detailed instructions outlined in the test protocol. Further, the objectivity of the test is enhanced by the fact that the measurements taken (i.e., heart rate responses to various workloads) are quantitative physiological responses rather than subjective, qualitative perceptions. An additional factor which enhances the reliability and validity of the step test is that the active participation of another individual is not required, hence; an examinee's performance is independently measured.

The Ohio State University Step Test has minimal facility and equipment requirements. Further, the step test is relatively easy to administer requiring only one tester. In fact, the test could be self administered. However, the examinee should be very familiar with the test protocol prior to beginning the test as strict adherence to the time intervals, heart rate monitoring, and changes in workloads which are critical in order to obtain reliable and valid results. The test may take up to 15 minutes to administer depending on the fitness level of the examinee being tested because of the progressive increments in workloads used in the test. Although this would tend to enhance the reliability and validity of the step test as a measure of cardiorespiratory endurance, it may make the test an impractical method for mass assessment of cardiorespiratory endurance. This latter point is accentuated by the fact that it is difficult to test more than one examinee at a time due to the equipment requirements and the decisions which need to be made on a timely basis during the test. Thus in terms of time to administer the test, the step test would appear to be best suited for individual cardiorespiratory endurance assessment rather than group fitness assessment. In addition, since the step test is not particularly practical for group fitness assessment, the test has limited application in terms of promoting learning and/or conditioning.

Since the test was developed on males aged 19 to 56 years, the test appears to be an effective discriminator of cardiorespiratory endurance in young to middle aged adult males, but would not be appropriate for assessing females or males younger than 19 years or older than 56 years.

The potential risks involved in using the test include dyskinesia and cardiac abnormalities. The use of the hand bar minimizes the dyskinetic related risks without altering the results. However, the risk of cardiac abnormalities tends to increase in older examinees who are required to work at a higher percent of maximal heart rate. For example, the required test termination heart rate of 150 b/min would be approximately 75 percent of maximal heart rate in a 20 year old, but 88 percent of maximal heart rate in a 50 year old.

Thus, it would seem reasonable to limit the maximum age of the examinee performing the test (without physician supervision) to the age of 35 years or less. The norms that exist for the test are limited, as they are separated into three broad age groups for males and they are described in terms of mean and standard deviation of the innings completed rather than in predicted maximal oxygen uptake which is considered to be the best single indicator of cardiorespiratory endurance. Finally, the step test is not of suitable precision for research, since other factors (e.g., caffeine, smoking, lack of sleep, and environmental heat stress) may affect heart rate response during the test. Also, local muscle fatigue may affect the results of the step test. Generally, determination of cardiorespiratory endurance in research requires direct assessment of maximal oxygen uptake rate via expired gas analysis.

SUMMARY

Major Strengths:

1. The test has high validity.

2. The test has high test-retest reliability and, hence, only one trial of the test is required.

3. The test has high objectivity and assesses an examinee's performance independently.

4. The test is relatively easy to administer requiring minimal facilities and equipment.

5. The test is appropriate for individual field assessment of cardiorespiratory endurance.

Major Weaknesses:

1. The test is not appropriate for group field assessment of cardiorespiratory endurance or for the promotion of learning and conditioning.

2. The test is limited to males aged 19 to 56 years; although, from a safety perspective the maximum age which should be tested is probably 35 years in order to limit the risks of cardiac abnormalities.

3. The test has limited useful normative data.

4. The test is not of suitable precision for research purposes.

In conclusion, the Ohio State University Step Test is an acceptable field test for assessing cardiorespiratory endurance in young adult males, but is inadequate for research purposes as well as the promotion of learning and conditioning.

OHIO STATE UNIVERSITY STEP TEST (CALLAN MODIFICATION)

References.

Callan, D. E. (1968). A submaximal cardiovascular fitness test for fourth, fifth and sixth grade boys. Unpublished doctoral dissertation, Ohio State University.

Mathews, D. K. (1978). *Measurement in physical education.* Philadelphia: W. B. Saunders, p 278.

Additional Sources.

Clarke & Clarke (1987, p. 145); Safrit (1981, pp. 221-222).

Purpose.

To measure the cardiorespiratory endurance of an examinee through submaximal bench stepping.

Objectivity.

$r = .96$ was derived by the test-retest method (Mathews, 1978, p. 257).

Reliability.

$r = .96$ was obtained by the test-retest method (Clarke, 1976, p. 166).

Validity.

$r = .90$ when correlated with a modified treadmill test and $r = .96$ between the work done in lifting the body during the bench stepping and the energy expended.

Age and Sex.

Fourth, fifth, and sixth grade males.

Equipment.

The same as for the Ohio State University Step Test with the exception that the bench depth is 34cm (13.5") and the two bench levels are 38cm (15") and 46cm (18") high. A stopwatch and metronome are also required.

Space Requirements and Design.

A clear, level area approximately 3m (10') square with the bench and examinee in the center.

Directions.

The length and number of innings, number of phases, cadence and the general directions follow those of the Ohio State University Step Test. The exceptions are that the: (1) tester obtains the pulse rate through the use of a stethoscope; (2)

maximum pulse rate for 10 seconds is 29 beats (174 beats/minute); (3) bench height on the third phase is 46cm (18"); and (4) the hand bar is adjusted to eye level.

Scoring.

The same as for the Ohio State University Step Test except the last inning of exercise is determined by a maximum pulse rate of 29 beats for 10 seconds (174 beats/minute).

Norms.

Mathews (1978, p. 278) boys and girls.

REVIEW

SYNE ALTENA, Ed.D.
Professor of Physical Education
Dordt College
Sioux Center, IA 51250

The Ohio State University Step Test as modified by Callan for grades four through six is a valid test of cardiorespiratory endurance. The test is reliable and objective. It does not require a second individual which could affect the results of the test.

The test poses several practical problems when administered to a group. The first problem concerns the requirement of a stethoscope to measure heart rate. It is very difficult to hear the heart rate when the test is administered to several examinees at the same time in a noisy gymnasium. The test requires a quiet area if the stethoscope is to be used. It is unlikely that a school would have the necessary stethoscopes available to test several examinees simultaneously. It is recommended that the carotid pulse be used.

The second problem deals with bench heights. The benches must be constructed because normal locker room benches and gymnasium bleachers do not match the required bench heights of the test. The benches must be constructed in one piece because there is no time to switch from one bench to another when the examinee is required to change bench heights.

The third problem with the test is the degree of expertise required on the part of the tester. Elementary school students would have a difficult time testing each other with any degree of reliability and objectivity.

The test does not require an excessive amount of time and is appropriate for the grade levels intended. The test seems to discriminate among its intended users but would not be suitable for a drill to promote conditioning because there is too much rest between innings. The test would be suitable for research purposes. The mean of the test seemed to be rather high compared to the mean of the examinees who were tested for this review.

SUMMARY

Major Strengths:

1. It is a vigorous test which discriminates cardiorespiratory endurance.

2. It is appropriate for males in the fourth, fifth, and sixth grades.

3. It is suitable for research purposes.

Major Weaknesses:

1. It requires the silence of a laboratory setting so one can hear through the stethoscope.

2. The bench heights are not practical and must be constructed.

3. Examinees cannot administer this test to one another.

4. A great deal of equipment would be needed to test a large group.

The Ohio State University Step Test, as modified by Callan, would be an acceptable test when used for research purposes. However, it does not seem to be practical for a teacher to administer this test on a regular basis.

QUEENS COLLEGE STEP TEST

References.

McArdle, W. D., et al. (1972). Reliability and interrelationships between maximal oxygen intake, physical work capacity, and step test scores in college women. *Medicine and Science in Sports,* 4(4):182-186.

McArdle, W. D., et al. (1973). Percentile norms for a valid step test in college women. *Research Quarterly,* 44(4):498-500.

Johnson, B. L., & Nelson, J. K. (1986). *Practical measurements for evaluation in physical education.* Edina, MN: Burgess, pp 160-161.

Kirkendall, D. R., et al. (1987). *Measurement and evaluation for physical educators.* Champaign, IL: Human Kinetics, pp 177, 182-183.

Additional Sources.

Baumgartner & Jackson (1982, pp. 277-278); Clarke & Clarke (1987, p. 140); Miller (1988, p. 150); Safrit (1986, pp. 255-256); Safrit (1990, pp. 385-386).

Purpose.

To measure and group a large number of females and males in terms of cardiorespiratory fitness.

Objectivity.

Not reported.

Reliability.

$r = .92$.

Validity.

$r = -.75$ with VO^2max.

Age and Sex.

College age females and males.

Equipment.

A stepping bench or bleachers 41 to 43cm (16-17") high, a metronome or tape recorder, and a stopwatch.

Space Requirements and Design.

A clear, level area approximately 3m (10') square with the bench and the examinee in the center.

Directions.

The metronome is set at 88 beats per minute to provide a cadence of 22 steps per minute for females and at 96 beats per minute to provide a cadence of 24 steps per minute for males. The examinee is then given a 15 second practice period at the required cadence. Upon completion of the practice session and on command, the examinee steps up and down on the bench for a period of three minutes. Five seconds after cessation of stepping, the standing pulse rate should be taken for 15 seconds and recorded.

Scoring.

The score is derived by multiplying the 15 second pulse rate by four, thereby obtaining the number of beats per minute.

Regression equations for predicting oxygen consumption for men and women were developed as follows:

Men:

$VO^2max = 111.33 - (0.42 \times$ step test pulse rate in beats per minute$)$.

Women:

$VO^2max = 65.81 - (0.1847 \times$ step test pulse rate in beats per minute$)$.

Where the step test pulse rate is the 15 second recovery heart rate, it should be multiplied by four.

Norms.

Baumgartner & Jackson (1982, p. 278) men and women; Johnson & Nelson (1986, p. 161) women; Kirkendall et al. (1987, p. 183) men and women; McArdle et al. (1973, p. 500) women; Miller (1988, p. 150) men and women; Safrit (1986, p. 255) men and women; Safrit (1990, p. 386) men and women.

REVIEW

JOSEPH J. GRUBER, Ph.D.
Professor of Physical Education
University of Kentucky
Lexington, KY 40506-0219

The purpose of this test is to measure cardiorespiratory endurance through bench stepping. The test was originally developed and validated on college women ages 17 to 24. The test has subsequently been extended to include college age males. The criterion of cardiorespiratory endurance accepted by physiologists is maximum oxygen consumption per kilogram of body weight. Since no respiratory gasses are collected and analyzed during the step test, the Queens College Test is an indirect estimate of maximum oxygen consumption. Equations for predicting VO2max have been developed for both college aged females and males. With a validity coefficient of -.75 and an $r^2 = .56$, approximately 56 percent of the variability in maximum oxygen consumption can be explained by the recovery heart rate from the bench step test. This statistic plus a standard error of prediction of 2.9ml places this test, quality wise, in the same category as other submaximal indirect field tests designed to predict maximum oxygen uptake. The test-retest reliability of .92 studied over a one week period in a school gymnasium is highly acceptable. Adherence to strict standardized directions for administration and scoring the Queens College Step Test will enhance the usage validity of the test score. There is no reported objectivity information in the literature. The test does not require the active participation of another individual that could affect the score of the examinee.

This test is easy to administer and score on an individual or a group basis. The test does not require elaborate equipment. It can be administered using gymnasium bleachers as long as the step height requirement is met. This reviewer has administered the test to a class of 25 students in 15 minutes. One-half of the class was tested first; the second half counted the pulse along with her/his partner to secure objectivity. Examinees must learn how to count their pulse on cue with accuracy. In addition, more valid data is secured if the examinees practice the test at least once a day before any testing is done for decision making. This test can be self administered repeatedly at school or at home as examinees monitor progress in a fitness pro-

gram. Short, heavy examinees may have difficulty maintaining the cadence for three minutes. There is no danger to examinees so long as they are in good health and have no orthopaedic or balance problems. Validity of testing is enhanced by having all test directions and cadence played to the class on a tape recorder. Predicted maximum oxygen consumption and recovery heart rate norms are available only for college age men and women. This test does not have sufficient precision to be used in a research study since it is an indirect measure of oxygen consumption. In addition, the three minute exercise session is far too brief to challenge the oxygen transport system with high validity.

SUMMARY

Major Strengths:

1. The test is an easy, inexpensive field test of endurance that can be administered on an individual or group basis in a short period of time.

2. The test's main strength is its application to college age men and women who desire to monitor their progress in a physical fitness program.

3. The test can be used in a school, health club, or clinic or by an individual who is on her/his own fitness program.

Major Weaknesses:

1. It is an indirect measure of cardiorespiratory endurance.

2. The exercise bout is too short if the objective is to predict oxygen consumption in highly fit individuals.

The test is acceptable and recommended for teaching in fitness classes because it is inexpensive in terms of time, money, equipment and personnel. The test is not recommended for use as a criterion measure in a research study for which oxygen consumption must be accurately measured with a minimum of error.

SHARKEY STEP TEST

Reference.
Sharkey, B. J. (1984). *Physiology of fitness.* Champaign, IL: Human Kinetics, pp 255-263.

Additional Sources.
None.

Purpose.
To predict the aerobic fitness of an examinee through a submaximal stepping exercise.

Objectivity.
Not reported.

Reliability.
Not reported.

Validity.
Not reported.

Age and Sex.
Females and males.

Equipment.
A bench 40cm (15.75") high for men and 33cm (13") high for women, a body weight scale, a metronome set at 90 beats per minute, and a stopwatch.

Space Requirements and Design.
A clear, level area approximately 3m (10') square with the bench in the center. Room temperature should be 65 to 75 degrees Fahrenheit.

Directions.
The examinee's body weight is determined following standard procedure. The examinee then assumes a standing position in front of the bench and upon the command, "Ready, Go," begins stepping. The examinee steps in cadence with the metronome (i.e., 22.5 steps per minute) for five minutes. As soon as the five minutes of stepping are completed, the examinee sits down on the bench and locates her/his pulse. The pulse count is taken for 15 seconds, beginning 15 seconds after cessation of stepping and ending 30 seconds after cessation of stepping.

Scoring.
A fitness score is determined by plugging the examinee's body weight and 15 second pulse count into a table (Sharkey, 1984, p. 258 for men; p. 259 for women). This fitness score and the examinee's age are then entered into another table (Sharkey, 1984, pp. 260-261) which gives the final age adjusted score.

Norms.
Sharkey (1984, p. 262) boys, girls, men and women.

REVIEW

BARBARA E. AINSWORTH, Ph.D.

Assistant Professor
Physical Education,
Exercise and Sport Science
University of North Carolina at
Chapel Hill
Chapel Hill, NC 27599-8700

The Sharkey Step Test is a modification of the Harvard Step Test and was developed to determine cardiovascular fitness (CV) of employees of the U.S. Forest Service. The test involves bench stepping in a rhythmic pattern to a metronome for five minutes. Estimates of CV fitness are determined from the 15 second recovery exercise heart rate.

Correlation coefficients for validity are not given, however, it is assumed the test has face validity since it is a modification of the Harvard Step Test. The Harvard Step Test has been validated by Brouha (1943) with running performance of 2200 male cross country runners (r = .63) and is reported to have test-retest reliability of r = .82. The step test modifications made by Sharkey include lower stepping bench heights for men and women and newer scoring norms to estimate CV fitness. It is probable that the Sharkey Stepping Test is reliable between repeat administrations if the examinee follows the pretesting protocol designed to reduce variability in the heart rate response to the exercise bout.

Threats to the test's validity include examinee motivation to complete the test, leg strength of the examinee to lift the body up and down a bench for five minutes, willingness of the examinee to follow the pretest protocol, and the ability of the tester to measure the test duration and recovery heart rate accurately.

The step test is easy to conduct and requires a variable height plywood box, a watch with a sweep second hand, and a metronome or a tape recording of a metronome. Personnel should know how to read a stopwatch or calculate the passage of time from a digital watch, palpate the radial artery to record the pulse rate, and ensure the examinees are stepping in time with the metronome. Examinees are required to step up and down on the plywood box in time with the metronome for a period of five minutes. The test is objectively scored by measuring the 15 second exercise recovery pulse rate and applying it to gender, age, and body weight specific norms. CV fitness levels range from superior to very poor in ranking and are reported to represent an accurate estimate of the maximal oxygen intake; however, correlation coefficients for the validity of these rankings are not given.

A possible source of error in the Sharkey Step Test is in the inaccurate measurement of the recovery heart rate. The test protocol cautions examinees that the test should not be taken after engaging in activities which are known to elevate the heart rate independent of the test (e.g., following strenuous physical activity or immediately after drinking coffee or smoking). Other sources of error may be an inaccurate measurement of the heart rate, failure to step in time with the metronome, presence of heart arrhythmias that interfere with counting the recovery heart rate, and failure of the tester to read a stopwatch or time the event properly.

SUMMARY

Major Strengths:

1. The test is simple and may be used in most school settings. It is good for testing several people at a time. It does not require knowledge of laboratory testing methods or the use of expensive equipment.

2. It does not require the examinee to learn complex motor skills.

3. The test is easy to score and has age, gender, and body weight specific norms.

Major Weaknesses:

1. Test validity is dependent on the examinee's complying with the pretest protocol of abstaining from activities known to elevate the heart rate and on the tester to measure the recovery pulse rate accurately.

2. It cannot be used for individuals taking medications that modify the heart rate or for those with orthopaedic problems that limit their ability to perform bench stepping.

The Sharkey Step Test is an acceptable test of cardiovascular fitness for teaching and screening purposes. The potential for variability in the heart rate due to pretesting behaviors and measurement error may limit this test for research purposes. While validity and reliability coefficients are not reported, the test has good face validity since it is a modification of the Harvard Step Test. The test includes age, gender, and body weight specific norms for the recovery heart rate which allow an estimate of the examinee's level of aerobic fitness. Aside from the risk of muscle soreness following five minutes of bench stepping, the Sharkey Step Test seems to be a safe, acceptable, indirect assessment tool of CV fitness that may be applied to large groups for screening and instructional purposes.

REVIEW REFERENCE

Brouha, L. (1943). The step test: A simple method of measuring physical fitness for muscular work in young men. *Research Quarterly,* 14:31-36.

SICONOFI STEP TEST

References.
Siconofi, S. F. et al. (1985). A simple valid step test for estimating maximal oxygen uptake in epidemiological studies. *American Journal of Epidemiology,* 121(3):382-390.

Kirkendall, D. R. et al. (1987). *Measurement and evaluation for physical educators.* Champaign, IL: Human Kinetics, pp 181-182.

Additional Sources.
None.

Purpose.
To estimate the maximal oxygen consumption of an examinee through bench stepping.

Objectivity.
Not reported.

Reliability.
Not reported.

Validity.
r's = .89 to .98 were obtained between the step test and a submaximal cycle ergometer test.

Age and Sex.
Females and males, age 19 - 70.

Equipment.
A bench or wooden box 25.4cm (10") high, stopwatch, and heart rate monitor.

Space Requirements and Design.
A clear, level area approximately 2m (6') square with the bench and the examinee in the center.

Directions.
The examinee steps for three minutes per stage for a maximum of three stages. After each three minute stage, the examinee is allowed one minute of sitting rest. The examinee follows stepping cadences of 17, 26, and 34 steps per minute for stages 1, 2, and 3, respectively. Heart rates are recorded at 2:30, 2:45, and 3:00 minutes during each stage of stepping. The examinee goes to stage two if the average heart rate during stage one does not exceed 65 percent of the age predicted maximum heart (PMR) rate [i.e., PMR = .65 (220 - age in years)]. The examinee goes to stage three if the average heart rate does not exceed 65 percent of the age predicted maximum heart rate during stage two. The test is completed after stage three.

Scoring.
Maximal oxygen consumption is predicted with the following equations:

Stage 1: VO^2 (l/min) = 16.287 x Wt (Kg)/1000
Stage 2: VO^2 (l/min) = 24.910 x Wt (Kg)/1000
Stage 3: VO^2 (l/min) = 33.533 x Wt (Kg)/1000

This computed value is then placed into (X1) in one of the two equations listed below to adjust maximal oxygen consumption for sex and age.

Females: y = 0.302 (X1) - 0.019 (X2) + 1.593

Males: y = 0.348 (X1) - 0.035 (X2) + 3.011

Where y = VO^2 (l/min), X1 = VO^2 (l/min) from one of the three stages of the step test, and X2 = age in years.

Norms.
Not reported.

REVIEW

BLANCHE W. EVANS, Ed.D.

Exercise Physiologist
Indiana State University
Terre Haute, IN 47809

As currently reported, the Siconofi Step Test has limited scientific merit. The test's validity ranges from .89 to .98, when compared with a submaximal cycle ergometer test. A better indicator of the validity of the test would be its comparison to another step test or to a treadmill test, since both require upright exercise as opposed to seated exercise. More appropriately, the comparison of values determined from this step test with values obtained from a test measuring VO^2max would be more meaningful. No reliability, objectivity, nor test norms are reported. Administration requires one tester, but the influence of the tester on the results is minimal. The use of a metronome or tape recording of the selected cadences provides consistency in step rate, and the use of a heart monitor decreases the error involved with palpation techniques for determining pulse. These two techniques should allow for reproducible test results.

Some advantages of the test include its simplicity in administration, requirement for minimal expertise, use of a small space, and need for little sophisticated equipment. It can be administered to a large group, used in a school, laboratory or clinical setting, and administered simultaneously to young and old. With three levels of difficulty, the test is appropriate for examinees in a wide age range and in varying states of physical condition. In addition, the increases in step rate per minute are reasonable. The 17 steps/minute pace is slow and boring for the conditioned examinee but is appropriate for others less fit, such as the elderly or obese. The 34 steps/minute pace is fast but is offset by the step height, which is lower compared to other step tests. The lower step height reduces the leg strength required to perform the test and minimizes the balance problems encountered with higher benches.

One disadvantage of the test is that the number of test stages completed is based on multiple heart rate measurements taken within a short time interval at the end of each stage, making a manual determination of pulse impossible. Therefore, the purchase of a good heart rate monitor is required, limiting the successful administration of the test to only those with such monitors. Another major problem with the test is that the target heart rate of 65 percent of age predicted HR max is very low, 130 beats/minute for a 20 year old and 104 beats/minute for a 60 year old. This level of intensity is safe for the age range proposed for the test, but is minimal when attempting to stress the cardiorespiratory system and estimate maximal oxygen uptake. Some examinees may be at their target heart rate of the first stage prior to the test due to emotional or stress related responses. In addition, the heart rate response to the workload is used to determine whether the examinee progresses to the next stage. It is not considered in the calculation of the estimated VO^2max values. Although the formulas used to estimate VO^2max do take into account differences in sex, body weight, and age, they do not provide a means of differentiating beyond three categories - first stage, poor; second stage, average; third stage, above average. Highly conditioned examinees with low body weights cannot obtain high estimated VO^2max values from this test protocol. A 22 year old male with a body weight of 150 pounds, for example, would have an estimated VO^2max of 3.0 liters or 44.5 milliliters per kilogram of body weight regardless of the heart rate response to the final work bout.

SUMMARY
Major Strengths:

1. The test is simple and requires minimal assistance to administer with the results providing a gross estimate or category of level of fitness.

2. The lower step height decreases the fatigue factor and stresses encountered by the quadriceps compared to tests with a higher step height.

Major Weaknesses:

1. The low target heart rate results in poor test results in examinees who are anxious or excited.

2. The use of three stages with a rest between each stage makes the test long and boring, but adds to its safety.

In its current form, the Siconofi Step Test is unacceptable for research. Numerous submaximal tests that require less equipment and less time to complete are available with objectivity, reliability, and validity reported. In addition, they provide norms for various populations. Further research should be conducted to provide the missing data and to examine further the relationship of the test results to other known methods of determining maximal oxygen uptake. The test is acceptable as an educational tool to be used in teaching test administration and for demonstration purposes.

THREE MINUTE HEIGHT-ADJUSTED STEP TEST

Reference.
Frances, K., & Cuipepper, M. (1988). Validation of a three minute height adjusted step test. *The Journal of Sports Medicine and Physical Fitness,* 28(3):229-233.

Additional Sources.
None.

Purpose.
To measure the cardiorespiratory endurance of an examinee through a height adjusted step test based on leg length.

Objectivity.
r = .89 between college women and ECG measurement to determine recovery heart rate.

Reliability.
r = .86 was obtained on college women using a subject count measurement to determine recovery heart rate.

Validity.
r = .70 between VO_2max determined by recovery heart rate following stepping and following a maximal exertion treadmill test.

Age and Sex.
Women, age 19 - 35.

Equipment.
A height adjustable bench, electric metronome, and stopwatch.

Space Requirements and Design.
A clear, level area approximately 2m (6') square with the height adjustable bench and the examinee in the center.

Directions.
The examinee assumes a standing position facing the height adjustable bench. The step height of the bench is based on the height of the examinee's foot when the hip is flexed at 73.3 degrees. On command, "Ready, Go," the examinee steps up and down on the bench to the cadence of an electric metronome which is set at 120 beats per minute or 30 steps per minute. The examinee steps at this pace for a three minute period. Following the stepping, the examinee remains standing while the heart rate is taken.

The heart rate measurement is started 5 seconds after the step test and stopped 15 seconds later. The heart rate is measured by a partner through palpitation of the carotid artery.

Scoring.
The score is the examinee's recovery heart rate measured during the period 5 to 20 seconds after the cessation of stepping.

Norms.
Frances & Cuipepper (1988, p. 231) mean and standard deviation for a small group of college women.

REVIEW

MARGARET J. SAFRIT, Ph.D.
Henry-Bascom Professor
University of Wisconsin-Madison
Madison, WI 53706

The Three Minute Hight Adjusted Step Test is another variation of the familiar step test. It is proposed as a more appropriate measure of the Harvard Step Test in that the step height is based on the height of the foot when the hip is flexed at 73.3 degrees. This step height was derived from the geometric relationship between stature height and femur length. The hip angle of 73.3 degrees was the value determined to yield the highest correlation between heart rate after stepping and VO_2max. The test appears to have substantial logical validity. However, the evidence of concurrent validity is not so impressive. The 15 second recovery heart rate was correlated with VO_2max determined by a maximal exertion Bruce Treadmill Test. The validity coefficient was .70, indicating that the two measures shared approximately 50 percent of the total variance. Although there is some commonality between the two tests, they are also measuring different attributes. Other estimates of validity have also been reported as low. Validity coefficients ranging from -.35 to .77 have been reported for the Harvard Step Test when VO_2max was used as the criterion test. Values ranging from 0.47 to 0.57 were reported for the

Ohio State University Step Test. The Three Minute Height-Adjusted Test is probably measuring sub VO^2max, at least in part.

The validity and objectivity of the test are satisfactory. However, the reliability will always be affected by test objectivity. If performance varies from one time to another, this may be due to a lack of objectivity rather than to unreliability. If a partner assesses heart rate, this can affect the score of the examinee.

The space requirements are minimal to test one examinee. The equipment may pose a problem. While the adjustability of the bench height enhances the logical validity of the test, it requires a more complicated piece of equipment than the standardized bench heights used in other tests. Furthermore, to test more than one examinee at a time would require additional benches with adjustable bench heights.

The test is easy to administer, but not so easy to score. An accurate measure of heart rate response can probably be obtained if the tester has been trained previously. Administration of the test requires determining the appropriate bench height for each examinee. This procedure could make the test excessively time consuming to administer, although a nomogram could be developed to estimate the height easily.

As the examinee is putting forth maximal effort in taking this test, one trial should be sufficient. Using the test as a practice device would probably not be motivating to the examinee.

The test is suitable for college women; however, younger age groups, including males, should be studied. The test is probably safe to administer to this age group, but should not be administered to an older group without a physician's permission.

Due to the moderate size of the validity coefficient, the test is probably not precise enough to estimate VO^2max in a research setting, but may be adequate in an instructional setting. The standard error of estimate is reasonably small. No norms were presented.

SUMMARY

Major Strengths:

1. It is a useful test for general screening of aerobic capacity in an instructional setting.

2. It can be administered with reasonable reliability and objectivity, and has logical validity in that the bench height is adjusted according to the length of the femur and total height of the subject.

3. It is easy to administer - it is a familiar type of test to practitioners in the field.

Major Weaknesses:

1. It does not correlate substantially with VO^2max.

2. The equipment is not readily accessible to the practitioner.

3. Only college women have been used in studying the test statistics.

4. Cross validation procedures were not used in developing the regression equation, despite the test constructors' contention that this was done.

Overall, the test is acceptable for teaching if used with college women. It resolves some of the problems found in earlier step tests and can be administered in numerous settings. It should not be used in research settings in which aerobic capacity must be estimated with precision.

YMCA 3-MINUTE STEP TEST

Reference.
Golding, L. A. et al. (eds.) (1989). *Y's way to physical fitness: The complete guide to fitness testing and instruction.* Champaign, IL: Human Kinetics, pp 106-108, 113-124.

Additional Sources.
None.

Purpose.
To measure cardiorespiratory endurance of an examinee using a bench stepping exercise.

Objectivity.
Not reported.

Reliability.
Not reported.

Validity.
Not reported.

Age and Sex.
Females and males, age 18 - 65 +.

Equipment.
A sturdy bench 30.48cm (12") high, a metronome, a stopwatch, and a stethoscope.

Space Requirements and Design.
A clear, level area approximately 3m (10') square with the bench positioned in the center.

Directions.
The tester sets the metronome at 96 beats per minute to produce the proper cadence of 24 steps per minute. The tester then demonstrates the proper stepping cadence by placing one foot on the bench with the first beat of the metronome, placing the second foot on the bench with the second beat, returning the first foot to the floor with the third beat and returning the second foot to the floor with the fourth beat. This sequence equals one step and is completed 24 times per minute for three minutes. The examinee may lead with either foot and he/she may switch the lead foot during the test.

The examinee assumes a standing position facing the bench and listens to the cadence of the metronome. When ready, the examinee starts stepping and the tester starts the stopwatch. The tester should observe the stepping cadence and correct it when needed. The tester should also announce the time after 1 and 2 minutes of stepping. When 20 seconds remain, the tester should remind the examinee to sit down on the bench immediately after cessation of stepping. Once the examinee is seated after three minutes of stepping, the tester places the stethoscope on the examinee's chest and starts counting the pulse for one minute. The pulse count must be initiated within five seconds of the cessation of stepping. The first pulse is counted as zero.

Scoring.
The score is the pulse count for the one minute after stepping.

Norms.
Corbin & Lindsey (1983, p. 38) boys, girls, men and women; Corbin & Lindsey (1985, p. 44) age and sex not stated; Getchell (1983, p. 56) men and women (variation); Golding, et al. (1989, pp. 113-124) men and women;

Hoeger (1986, pp. 16, 20) men and women (variation); Hoeger (1989, pp. 23, 27) men and women; Pollock & Wilmore (1990, pp. 672-683) men and women; Van Gelder & Marks (1987, p. 173) men and women.

REVIEW

DARLENE YEE, Ed.D.
Associate Professor
Health Education
San Francisco State University
San Francisco, CA 94132

The validity of the YMCA 3-Minute Step Test is difficult to evaluate given the limited information provided. There are a number of unanswered questions. For example, have studies been performed comparing step test results to maximal oxygen consumption? What was the age of the population tested? What should one do about medications the examinee may be taking?

The reliability of the YMCA 3-Minute Step Test will be affected by (1) the method of measuring heart rate, including the skill of the tester, and the specific heart rate value; and (2) variations in the setting, such as the condition of the examinee, time of day, and other relevant variables.

The YMCA 3-Minute Step Test is not as reliable, safe, and useful as the Astrand-Ryhming Test for measuring cardiorespiratory fitness. The Astrand-Ryhming Test is a better evaluation tool for the following reasons: (1) the tester is easily able to monitor blood pressure, heart rate, EKG, and other symptoms during exercise since the examinee is fairly stationary; (2) the length of the test is such that most examinees are able to complete the test and yet it allows for a steady state to be reached; (3) the examinee cannot be easily injured since the activity does not require "mass movements," is non weight bearing, and balance/coordination are not important; and (4) considerable data (normative) and validity/reliability studies have been performed on the test.

Since the bench height is greater than the typical stair step, walk/run tests are also better evaluation tools to measure cardiorespiratory endurance. Walk/run tests offer the advantages of being easy to administer and inexpensive. In Addition they allow many examinees to be tested at one time as opposed to individual testing with cycle or step tests.

SUMMARY

Overall, the YMCA 3-Minute Step Test is a poor evaluative tool for cardiorespiratory endurance for any age group because of the short time frame.

To evaluate cardiorespiratory endurance accurately, the test should be at least 5 to 15 minutes in length. In addition, blood pressure measurements should be taken during any evaluation of cardiac function, especially with an elderly population. It is nearly impossible to measure blood pressure response during a stepping test. Finally, a step test is not appropriate for the elderly because of the increase in potential injury from falling, musclulotendonous injury, and muscle soreness.

MISCELLANEOUS TESTS OF CARDIORESPIRATORY ENDURANCE

30 SECONDS ROPE JUMPING TEST

Reference.
(Hawaii) Aizawa, H. M. (1989). Memo to district superintendents, principals and physical education department heads. Honolulu, HI: Department of Education.

Additional Sources.
None.

Purpose.
". . . measure cardiovascular fitness, leg strength and agility" (Hawaii, 1989, p. 17).

Objectivity.
Not reported.

Reliability.
Not reported.

Validity.
Not reported.

Age and Sex.
Females and males, grades K - 3.

Equipment.
A jump rope and a stopwatch.

Space Requirements and Design.
A clear, level area approximately 3m (10') square with the examinee in the center and a ceiling high enough to permit rope jumping.

Directions.
The examinee assumes a standing position with an end of the rope in each hand. Upon the signal, "Ready, Go," the examinee begins jumping the rope as fast as possible for 30 seconds. In addition to operating the stopwatch, the tester counts the number of times the examinee clears the rope in the 30 seconds. The number of trials is not stated.

Scoring.
The score is the number of times the examinee clears the rope in 30 seconds.

Norms.
Hawaii (1989, pp. 19-20) boys and girls.

REVIEW

REGINALD T-A. OCANSEY, Ph.D.
Assistant Professor
Physical Education
State University of New York,
College at Brockport
Brockport, NY 14420

The 30 Seconds Rope Jumping is used as a test for physical fitness (cardiovascular fitness and leg strength) and motor fitness (agility). There is no information for the test's validity, objectivity, or reliability. It is, therefore, difficult to assess the relationship between the test item and the types of fitness it purports to measure.

Minimal equipment and time are required for administering the test. It does not require the active participation of another individual. The test can be administered in any clear, open area. The directions and procedures for test administration are easy to follow, but do not contain any information regarding practice trials or number of trials per testing session. The test is physically safe and targeted to kindergarten through third grade females and males. The test can be used for training or conditioning purposes for the type of fitness it purports to measure.

Norms are available for the 50th, 80th, and 85th percentiles for both boys and girls in grades kindergarten through three. The scoring system is objective. The tester simply counts the number of times the examinee clears the rope within 30 seconds. An examinee standing in front of a clock with a second hand can use the test for self evaluation.

SUMMARY

Major Strengths:
1. Testers require minimal to negligible training.
2. The test is cost effective and also time efficient.
3. The test requires minimal personnel to administer.

4. The test has clear directions for administration.

Major Weaknesses:

1. The test lacks important information for judging the test's validity, reliability, and objectivity.

2. The relationship between the test item and agility is not clear.

The test is not suitable for research purposes. It can be used for teaching or conditioning purposes for a clearly defined type of fitness. The research of Fleishman (1964), Falls et al. (1965), and Zuidema and Baumgartner (1974) contributed significantly to current understanding of physical fitness. However, in all these studies, 30 seconds of rope jumping did not appear as a relevant item for measuring physical fitness (cardiovascular fitness and leg strength) or motor fitness (agility).

Agility is the ability to change the whole body direction and body segment directions quickly and accurately in a coordinated manner (Kirkendall et al., 1982). Jumping rope as an indicator of the ability to move the body rapidly and alter directions in a coordinated manner presents major validity and congruency concerns. The relationship between jumping rope and agility is not clear. In addition, the extent to which this test measures leg strength is not clear.

Researchers and test users must exercise great caution in using this test as a tool for collecting data or measuring leg strength.

The test may be suitable for the purpose of measuring cardiovascular fitness if it is used in conjunction with validated test items for measuring health related fitness.

12-MINUTE SWIMMING TEST

References.

Cooper, K. H. (1982). *The aerobics program for total well-being.* New York: M. Evans and Co., p 142.

Miller, D. K. (1988). *Measurement by the physical educator: Why and how.* Indianapolis: Benchmark Press, pp 148-149.

Additional Sources.

None.

Purpose.

To measure the cardiorespiratory endurance of an examinee through swimming.

Objectivity.

Not reported.

Reliability.

Not reported.

Validity.

Not reported.

Age and Sex.

Females and males, age 13 - 60.

Equipment.

A swimming suit, stopwatch, and whistle.

Space Requirements and Design.

Swimming pool of known length.

Directions.

The examinee should be allowed to warm up prior to the swimming test. On command, "Ready, Go," the examinee swims in an individual lane as great a distance as possible for a 12 minute period. During the test, the examinee may use any stroke and may rest whenever necessary. The laps are counted and the exact location of the examinee when the whistle is blown to stop is noted. The examinee continues to swim after the test to cool down.

Scoring.

The score is the distance in meters (yards) the examinee swims within the 12 minute period.

Norms.

Barrow et al. (1989, p. 137) boys, girls, men and women; Cooper (1982, p. 142) boys, girls, men and women; Kirkendall et al. (1980, p. 302)

women; Kirkendall et al. (1987, p. 175) boys, girls, men and women; Miller (1988, p. 149) boys, girls, men and women.

REVIEW

MICHAEL MANGUM, Ph.D.

Assistant Professor
Physical Education and Leisure Management
Columbus College
Columbus, GA 31933

The 12-Minute Swim has been presented by Cooper (1977) as a field measure for cardiorespiratory endurance and has developed fitness classifications based on the same performance measure. The rationale for the use of the 12-Minute Swim is apparently similar to that of the 12-Minute Run/Walk, that is the time requirement of the task ensures that the aerobic energy mechanisms of the muscle and the capacity of the cardiovascular system play an important role in task performance. Data that provide evidence for scientific validation of the test are sparse. However, recent unpublished data from Columbus College and from the University of Georgia provide some insight into this question.

This reviewer tested 15 active officers of the U.S. Army for peak aerobic power on the treadmill and arm crank ergometer. Peak values for VO^2 while running ranged from 43.5 to 67.0 ml/kg/min. Three subjects of the sample swim trained whereas the others utilized running as the primary CV conditioning modality. Peak arm crank values showed a strong correlation to the treadmill values and averaged 69 percent of the treadmill values. Correlations between peak VO^2 while running or cranking and 12-Minute Swim distance were .34 and .38, respectively.

Conley et al (1990) at the University of Georgia also examined the question of 12-Minute Swim validity. Their research design was different from the above in two important ways. First, they chose to test a group of recreational swimmers, who could be expected to have better swimming skills. Second, they measured peak VO^2 during tethered swimming, which is more specific to the training mode as well as to the treadmill peak VO^2. Correlations between the tethered swim VO^2 and 12-Minute Swim distance and between the treadmill VO^2 and 12-Minute Swim distance were reported to be .40 and .38, respectively.

These data, compiled independently and in fact without concurrent knowledge, fail to support the validity of the 12-Minute Swim as a predictor of aerobic power. This lack of validity apparently is so when peak VO^2 from tethered swimming, running, or arm cranking is utilized as the criterion measure. An explanation for these findings likely resides in the grossly apparent differences in mechanical efficiency while swimming. One might argue that the Columbus College sample was poorly skilled, since many did not swim train. However, the sample is representative in that a wide range of skills is seen in the general population. Further, the University of Georgia sample did not suffer the skills limitation and did not result in substantially superior correlations. One might also agrue that the samples were too homogeneous and therefore were biased toward low correlations. However, the range of VO^2 noted was 23.5 ml/kg/min in the Columbus College sample, certainly not a narrow range.

SUMMARY

It is concluded that the 12-Minute Swim is not an acceptable field test for predicting aerobic power while swimming. Given this conclusion, the questions of reliability and administrative feasibility are moot.

REVIEW REFERENCES

Conley, D. S., et al. (1990). Validation of the 12 minute swim as a field test of maximal aerobic power. Paper presented at the annual meeting of the Southeast Chapter of the American College of Sports Medicine. Columbia, South Carolina.

Cooper. K. (1977) . *The aerobic way*. New York: Bantam.

Mangum, M. (1989). Unpublished data. Columbus College.

Chapter 5

COORDINATION

ALTERNATE HAND WALL TOSS TEST

References.

Yuhasz, M. S. (1967). The western motor ability test. In Campbell, W. R., & Tucker, N. M. (1967). *An introduction to tests and measurement in physical education.* London: G. Bell and Sons, pp 141, 143.

Harrison, P. W., & Bradbeer, P. A. (1982). Battery tests for the assessment of physiological fitness norms. *Athletics coach,* 16(21):6-12.

Additional Sources.

None.

Purpose.

To measure the coordination of an examinee while throwing and catching a tennis ball.

Objectivity.

Not reported.

Reliability.

r = .89 by test-retest method (Campbell & Tucker, 1967, p. 141).

Validity.

Not reported.

Age and Sex.

Not reported, but suitable for females and males, age 10 - adult.

Equipment.

Twelve tennis balls, a box or other suitable container to hold the balls, marking tape, a stopwatch, and a tape measure.

Space Requirements and Design.

A clear, level area approximately 3m (10') square near a wall that has a clear flat surface. A restraining line is marked off 2m (6.56') from the wall. The container of balls is placed on this restraining line.

Directions.

The examinee takes one ball and assumes a standing position behind the restraining line next to the container of extra balls so he/she can quickly get another ball should he/she lose control of the one in use. On command, "Ready, Go," the examinee throws the ball underhanded against the wall with one hand and catches the ball with the other hand. This procedure is continued for a period of 30 seconds. If the examinee commits any infringement of the rules, that particular catch should not be counted. The rules require that the ball be thrown underhand, that the ball be caught cleanly in the hand (i.e., not trapped against the body), and that the examinee remain behind the restraining line. The examinee is given a one minute practice trial and two legal trials.

Scoring.

The score is the total number of successful catches made during a 30 second test. The better of the test scores is recorded.

Norms.

Campbell & Tucker (1967, pp. 215-218) Canadian boys and British men physical education students.

REVIEW

LINDA R. BARLEY, Ed.D.

Professor
Health and Physical Education
York College-CUNY
Jamaica, NY 11451

Alternate Hand Wall Toss is a test to measure coordination, specifically by throwing a tennis ball against a clear, smooth surface and catching it with the opposite hand. While coordination is abundantly covered in the literature, this test, in its particular form, is not. The usefulness of the Alternate Hand Wall Toss is limited in the following fashion: (1) the test lacks validity, (2) baseline data is not available for adult populations, and (3) while identified as a test of coordination, the test, may in fact, measure motor educability more effectively than it measures hand eye coordination.

Campbell and Tucker (1967, p. 141) report a test-retest reliability of $r = .89$. While the test is suitable for both females and males, there are no reported age norms with the r score.

The practical aspects of the test are such that (1) the test is easily administered, requiring little time and a minimum of 3m (10 square feet) near a wall that has a clear flat surface; (2) equipment needs are limited to a stopwatch, scoring tablet, one dozen tennis balls and a suitable container for the tennis balls.

Scoring is easily managed, the examinee is given one 60 second practice trial and two legal trials. The better of the two scores is recorded; the score is the total number of successful catches made in the 30 second test. Unsuccessful catches include: (1) stepping over the restraining line, (2) trapping the ball against the body, (3) two handed catches, and (4) over handed throws/catches.

SUMMARY

Major Strengths:

1. Easy to administer.

2. Requires little time, limited space and equipment.

3. Requires little training of the tester.

4. Is useful in promoting motor educability and accurate judgement of speed and direction of a moving object.

Major Weaknesses:

1. Lacks validity for research purposes.

2. Lacks norms for age, physical ability, and general health status.

3. May not measure hand eye coordination, but offers an opportunity for motor educability and practice in judging the speed and direction of a moving object.

Acceptable test for motor educability and limited measurement of hand eye coordination.

CABLE JUMP TEST

Reference.
Fleishman, E. A., (1964B). *The structure and measurement of physical fitness*. Englewood Cliffs: Prentice Hall, pp 115, 128, 169-170.

Additional Sources.
None.

Purpose.
To measure an examinee's gross body coordinated performance as a whole body movement.

Objectivity.
Not reported.

Reliability.
r = .70.

Validity.
Construct validity was established.

Age and Sex.
Suitable for females and males, age 14 - adult.

Equipment.
A piece of rope 61cm (24") long.

Space Requirements and Design.
A clear, level area approximately 2m (6') square with the examinee in the center.

Directions.
The examinee stands and holds the rope parallel to the floor just forward of the knees. The rope is gripped with one hand on each end and the arms so positioned that the rope sags in the middle. The examinee then jumps into the air and moves the feet and legs over the rope. In order to be credited with a correct jump, the examinee must maintain her/his grip on the rope, jump through the arms over the rope, land on the feet without losing balance, and not touch the rope with the feet.

A total of five trials are given.

Scoring.
The score is the number of correctly executed jumps out of the five trials.

Norms.
Fleishman (1964B, p. 115) boys and girls.

REVIEW
RAY R. REIDER, M.Ed.

Assistant Professor
Health and Physical Education
Gettysburg College
Gettysburg, PA 17325

Researchers and other users of the Cable Jump Test should feel concerned about the use of this test to measure gross body coordination. Since the examinee must hold, in front of her/him, a short rope in each hand, one may wonder if this test indeed measures gross body coordination, or is it a test of balance and a measurement of equilibrium.

Since the objectivity of the test was not reported, one wonders if different testers could be consistent in scoring the test and if its results can be used as a measurement of body coordination.

The reliability of r = .70 does indicate a moderate correlation, and the Cable Jump Test is a measure of the true differences among the examinees in measuring whole body movement. Since construct validity has been established, it is suggested that this test falls under this parameter and is a test that indicates that those who score higher have a higher level of coordinated performance of a whole body movement.

From a practical view, the Cable Jump Test may fit the needs and purposes of many testers in a group setting. The amount of equipment, cost, space allocation, time, and expertise in administering the test is within the scope of many testers and could be used to indicate a specific area of fitness. National norms for the test have been established, but one may question why the age categories for boys and girls are different. Also, the national norms indicate that the results are negatively skewed because of the great difference in percentile ranking between the four scores of four and five. Even though this test may be suitable for both females and males of adult age, one should be concerned and be extremely cautious in using this test among the adult population because of potential injuries. A big plus for this test may lie in the fact that a classroom teacher could probably train her/his classes to help in administering this test and a large class size would not be detrimental in administration. If there were a sufficient number of ropes, one tester, with very simple instructions, could handle a test site without undue problems.

SUMMARY

Major Strengths:

1. This test is an excellent way to measure gross body coordination within a group setting that requires very little in-depth training.

2. Since national norms have been established and fall within the parameters of fitness testing, the Cable Jump Test can serve as an indicator of one aspect of physical fitness.

Major Weaknesses:

1. No mention of a time factor to complete the five trials is taken into account.

2. Also, exactly what occurs if an examinee does not meet all the requirements of a correct jump? Does an examinee get the chance to start over, or is he/she indeed finished at the point in time when a correct jump is not completed properly.

3. Can children of ages before 14 do this test or is it beyond the realm of being an attainable goal?

This test can be used as an addition to a battery of tests, but it should not be considered a bona fide instrument of measurement in physical fitness.

CORBIN BALL HANDLING TEST

Reference.
Corbin, C. B., (1977). A ball handling test for elementary school children. *Physical Educator,* 34(1):48-50.

Additional Sources.
None.

Purpose.
To measure an examinee's hand eye coordination and ball handling ability.

Objectivity.
Not reported.

Reliability.
Test-retest reliability correlations ranged from r = .60 for fourth graders to r = .94 for sixth graders. For all 121 children, grades 1 to 6, the reliability coefficient was r = .91.

Validity.
Not reported.

Age and Sex.
Females and males, grades 1 - 6.

Equipment.
A tape measure, chalk or a felt-tip marker, stopwatch, and two 20cm (8") diameter rubber playground balls.

Space Requirements and Design.
A clear, level area approximately 3m (10') square with two circles 61cm (2') in diameter drawn on the surface 15cm (6") apart. One ball is placed 30cm (12") from the outside edge of one circle on a straight line extended through the centers of the circles (Figure 5-1).

Directions.
The examinee holds the second ball and stands between the two circles and as close to the circles as possible without touching them. Upon the signal, "Go," the examinee bounces the ball first in one circle and then in the other circle. The examinee must use both hands to catch and bounce the ball. If the first ball is not caught and gets away, the examinee should pick up the second ball and bounce it alternately in the circles. If the examinee loses control of the second ball, he/she must retrieve it and resume bouncing it. A five second practice trial is allowed followed by two 15 second trials. The stopwatch is started when the ball strikes the surface the first time and is stopped on the command, "Stop." If the examinee repeatedly bounces the ball on a line or at less than knee high, a caution is given and the trial retaken.

Scoring.
The score is the total number of times the ball is bounced in the circles during the two trials. One point is subtracted from the score for each time the examinee stepped on either circle while bouncing the ball.

Norms.
Corbin (1977, p. 50) boys and girls.

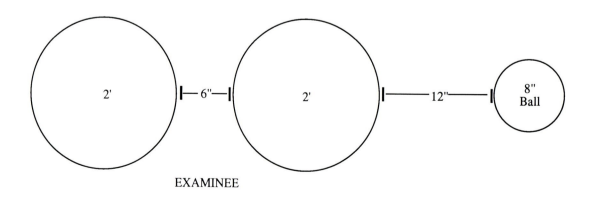

EXAMINEE

Figure 5-1. Corbin Ball Handling Test.

REVIEW

JAMES DECKER, Ph.D.

Assistant Professor
Health, Physical Education,
Recreation, and Safety
East Carolina University
Greenville, NC 27858-4353

The Corbin Ball Handling Test is purported to be an assessment of hand eye coordination of examinees in grades one through six. While the test content is logically derived, no evidence of construct, concurrent or predictive, validity is provided. Without such data the test's validity remains undetermined. Furthermore, the ball handling experience of the examinees may largely determine the results of this test.

Provisions for a test retrial create conditions of questionable tester objectivity. The test instructions state, "If the examinee repeatedly bounces the ball on a line or at less than knee height, a caution is given and the trial retaken." The lack of defined parameters for a retrial can result in a lack of standardization of test procedures.

The overall test-retest reliability correlation is based on a relatively small sample of 121 children. Similarly, the provided means and standard deviations for females and males were based on small samples ranging from 14 to 31 examinees.

The test requires a minimum of physical space and equipment, and only one tester with minimal observational abilities is required. Feasibly, cross age tutors (i.e., secondary students) could be employed to assist in testing large groups. The test requires a relatively small amount of time and a simple data recording mechanism; therefore, it can be used to screen hand eye coordination of small groups of examinees quite efficiently.

The five second practice period would seem to require examinees to begin the actual test before the task is fully understood. A practice period equaling a full trial would be preferable. While this test can be quickly administered, relatively short trial periods create potential reliability problems, especially for younger examinees. Increased trial periods of 30 seconds would be preferable. Also, the results of the test may be more reliable if the mean score of two trials were recorded. Of course, normative data would need to be reanalyzed should this scoring system be employed.

Also problematic is the stipulation that only two balls be used, and that if both balls "get away," the examinee must retrieve one and continue the remainder of the trial. Perhaps a better procedure is to score only ball bounces that result in the ball being caught and to provide numerous balls. If two or more balls get away, the examinee could then grab another ball and continue with the trial.

This test could be used as a basic ball handling activity in which examinees could keep their own score or could take turns counting for a partner. The Corbin Ball Handling Test is suitable for screening of basic hand eye coordination for examinees in grades one through six, however several test parameters (e.g., examinee positioning, retrial procedures, demonstration procedures, and tester verbiage) would need to be enhanced for this test to be utilized for research purposes.

SUMMARY

Major Strengths:

1. Easy to administer.

2. Minimum space and equipment required.

3. Applicable for examinees in grades one through six.

Major Weaknesses:

1. No validity data provided.

2. Tester objectivity questionable.

3. Reliability and normative data based on a small sample.

The Corbin Ball Handling Test is an acceptable test for hand eye coordination screening of examinees, grades one through six, in field settings. Testers can enhance the objectivity and reliability of the test by delineating precise retrial procedures, lengthening practice and trial periods, and using the mean score of two trials. As the test is constructed it is unacceptable for research purposes, however modifications are employable which increase its feasibility for research.

STICK BALANCE TEST

References.
Beunen, G. P. et al. (1988). *Adolescent growth and motor performance.* Champaign: Human Kinetics, p 65.

Renson, R. et al. (1980). Description of motor ability tests and anthropometric measurements. In Ostyn, M. et al. (1980). *Somatic and motor development of Belgian secondary schoolboys: Norms and standards.* Leuven: Leuven University Press, p 31.

Additional Sources.
None.

Purpose.
To measure an examinee's hand eye coordination.

Objectivity.
Not reported.

Reliability.
Not reported.

Validity.
Not reported.

Age and Sex.
Not reported, but suitable for females and males, age 6 - adult.

Equipment.
A stopwatch and an aluminum tube 2cm x 2cm x 30cm (.79" x .79" x 11.81") with both ends closed by rubber stoppers.

Space Requirements and Design.
A clear, level area approximately 3m (10') square with the examinee standing in the center and the tester at the examinee's side.

Directions.
The examinee assumes a comfortable standing position and extends the hand of her/his preference on which to balance the stick. The examinee must close the hand except for the pointer (i.e., index) finger. The examinee positions the aluminum tube vertically on the palm side of the distal phalanx of the chosen pointer finger and holds it in position with the opposite hand. When ready, the examinee removes the opposite hand from the tube and the tester starts the stopwatch. The examinee tries to balance the stick on the pointer finger for as long as possible. The stopwatch is stopped when the tube touches the examinee's body, the tube falls, or the examinee moves her/his feet. One practice trial and three legal trials are given.

Scoring.
The score is the greatest length of time, measured to the nearest tenth of a second, that the tube is balanced on the finger during the best of the three trials.

Norms.
Not reported.

REVIEW

JANET A. SEAMAN, P.E.D.
Professor of Physical Education
California State University
Los Angeles, CA 90032

The Stick Balance Test purportedly measures hand eye coordination which, on face, appears valid. One definitely cannot perform it with the eyes closed! It does not, however, measure the parameter in the customary way, as most hand eye coordination tests require accuracy in making contact with the hand (finger) or an implement and a target or object. There is some element of tactile perception involved, but to what extent is unknown. Validity is not reported, but is presumed to be good with other similar tasks. Neither is reliability reported, it would be expected to be low over three trials since performance will improve to a point with practice. This test is easy to score with a stopwatch measuring tenths of a second. The beginning and ending of the task is clear and the duration of balancing time is easy to discern by any experienced tester.

The space required to perform the test is minimal. The standardized equipment is problematic since it is based on metric units. Obtaining the materials in these dimensions would be difficult. The closure for the two ends is not described in enough detail to know whether they could be replicated. Since there are no norms available, the size and weight of the implement used are inconsequential for most applications.

The test is very easy to administer in terms of time, personnel, space and set up. There should probably be several timed trials until the examinee's performance reaches a plateau. That is, until there is little variance in time between trials. This will reduce the learning effect and increase the reliability of the scores obtained.

Examinees can be given this novel task, assuming there are enough implements for each, and test themselves, drill or in other ways entertain themselves while preparing to test. Even though there are no norms available, the Stick Balance Test would discriminate over a wide range of abilities and would be appropriate for use in research.

SUMMARY

Major Strengths:

1. This test is economical in terms of space, personnel, time and cost of equipment needed.

2. Even without norms, it has value as a pre and post instructional tool for measuring the effects of training on hand eye coordination.

3. It is a novel task and would capture the interest and enthusiasm of all ages.

4. It has the potential to discriminate among a wide range of abilities.

Major Weaknesses:

1. There are not enough practice trials to allow for learning.

2. Standardized equipment is measured in metric units.

3. There are no norms and the external validity, reliability, and objectivity have not been established.

The Stick Balance Test could serve as a useful tool for measuring the effects of instruction or some other intervention in either a teaching or research context. It should be used with standardized equipment that is indigenous to the environment with norms developed locally based on that equipment. As many trials as needed should be provided to allow for a learning plateau, then the best of three trials would have a level of reliability in which the tester could put some confidence. The space needed for testing is not large and should be safe and free of obstacles.

Chapter 6

FLEXIBILITY

ANGULAR/ROTARY MEASURES OF FLEXIBILITY

ANKLE FLEXION* AND EXTENSION** TEST

*Also known as dorsiflexion.

**Also known as plantar flexion.

Reference.
Jensen, C. R., & Hirst, C. C. (1980). *Measurement in physical education and athletics.* New York: MacMillan, pp 119-120.

Additional Sources.
Bosco & Gustafson (1983, pp. 108-109); Johnson & Nelson (1986, pp. 460-461).

Purpose.
To measure the range of motion in an examinee's ankle and foot regions.

Objectivity.
Not reported.

Reliability.
Not reported.

Validity.
Not reported.

Age and Sex.
Not reported, but suitable for females and males, age 6 - adult.

Equipment.
A table, paper pad, pencil, and a protractor.

Space Requirements and Design.
A clear, level area approximately 3m (10') square with the table in the center.

Directions.
The barefoot examinee sits on the table with the legs extended and together. The examinee then extends one ankle as far as possible while keeping the heel of the foot and the back of the knee on the table. The tester then places the pad of paper in a vertical position next to the medial side of the foot. A dot (a) is marked by the tester on the paper at the end of the toenail of the large toe. The examinee then flexes the ankle as far as possible and another dot (b) is marked on the paper at the end of the toenail of the large toe. Finally the examinee relaxes the foot and a third dot (c) is marked on the paper where the ankle bends at the top of the instep.

Scoring.

A line is drawn from the dot (c) representing where the ankle bends at the top of the instep to each of the other two dots (a and b) on the paper. Measurement of the angle for each of the lines from the horizontal is done through the use of a protractor.

Norms.

Johnson & Nelson (1986, pp. 456, 461) boys, girls, men and women for ankle extension only.

NOTE: The range of motion may also be calculated by the angle determined by the vertex being at the point where the ankle bends at the top of the instep (c) and the sides formed by lines drawn to the points representing flexion (b) and extension (a) of the ankle.

REVIEW

JOANNE ROWE, Ph.D.

Assistant Professor
Physical Education
University of Louisville
Louisville, KY 40292

The test does measure flexion and extension of the ankle. There is no indication as to whether this test has been used in research. Reliability is based on the ability of the tester to make the appropriate marks on the score sheet.

Space, facilities and equipment: The Ankle Flexion and Extension Test is easy to administer and requires very little space. A table is needed, as is a protractor.

The major problem seen with this test would be scoring it correctly. The tester holds a sheet of paper next to the medial side of the ankle while marking a dot at the end of the toenail of the large toe. The paper may move as the examinee extends and flexes the ankle. Caution should be taken to ensure correct measurement. If there is normal dorsiflexion, the examinee should be able to dorsiflex between 15 and 20 degrees.

There are no norms established for this test.

SUMMARY
Major Strengths:
1. Good indicator of ankle flexion and extension.

2. Easy to administer.

3. Little equipment needed.

4. Little time required to administer.

Major Weakness:
1. Scoring correctly may present problem.

GONIOMETER TEST

Reference.

Moore, M. L. (1978). Clinical assessment of joint motion. In Basmajian, J. V. (ed.). *Therapeutic exercise.* Baltimore: Williams and Wilkins, pp 151-190.

Additional Sources.

Hastad & Lacy (1989, pp. 215-216); Verducci (1980, p. 254).

Purpose.

To measure the range of motion in each major joint of an examinee's body.

Objectivity.

+/- 1 to 7 degrees depending on skill of tester and joint being measured (Moore, 1978, p. 184).

Reliability.

r = .50 and r = .58 at wrist and r = .85 to r = .99 on 13 motions of the upper extremity (Moore, 1978, p. 182).

Validity.

Face validity is accepted.

Age and Sex.

Females and males, age 6 - adult.

Equipment.

A goniometer and a bench or table large enough for the examinee to recline or sit on. The goniometer has either a 180 degree or 360 degree dial with two arms attached - one arm that rotates about the dial's axis and the other arm fixed so that its baseline is even with the zero mark.

Space Requirements and Design.

A clear, level area approximately 3m (10') square with the bench or table in the center.

Directions.

Since the goniometer can be used to measure the range of motion of every major joint in the body, only the general procedures for using the goniometer are described here. The axis of the goniometer is temporarily positioned over the joint's axis. The arms of the goniometer are placed along and parallel to the longitudinal axis of each segment which forms the joint being measured. The movable arm of the goniometer is placed over the more movable body segment while the fixed arm of the goniometer is placed over the more stationary body segment. The goniometer should be held slightly away from or lightly on the examinee as the movement is executed. At the end of the range of motion, the tester should readjust the goniometer so that its axis is perfectly aligned with the joint's axis and its two arms are properly aligned with the longitudinal axis of each body segment.

Scoring.

The score is the number of degrees the body segment is moved.

Norms.

American Academy (1963); American Academy (1965); Moore (1978, pp. 158-159) nine major joints and a number of movements at each joint.

REVIEW

BARRY A. FRISHBERG, Ph.D.

Associate Professor
Health and Physical Education
South Carolina State College
Orangeburg, SC 29117

The goniometer is the least expensive of a number of reliable methods for measuring a joint's range of motion. Its reliability and validity are dependent upon a number of factors with the two most important being the type of joint measurement being taken and the experience of the tester. When the joint's axis of rotation is clearly identified between two bones with lengthy longitudinal axes and the movement is easily completed in only one plane of motion, then the tester's task is relatively simple and should have a high resultant reliability. When the longitudinal axis of the moveable segment is not easily discerned and/or the movement is not easily stabilized to one plane of motion, then the reliability of the measurement will be significantly lower. For large joints, such as the hip, a goniometer with large arms should be used while smaller goniometers will yield greater reliability when used with smaller joints like the fingers.

As with most instruments, the reliability of the measurement is dependent upon the tester's expertise. Fortunately, the concepts needed to use the goniometer are simple and easy to master. Any undergraduate student should be capable of being trained in a relatively short period of time. It is important that standardized techniques be used since the position and/or the movement of other joints can significantly affect the measurement to be taken. Standardized techniques not only explain the placement of the arms of the goniometer and the movement of the appropriate body segments, but also the position and stabilization of the adjacent body segments.

The environmental conditions, as well as the condition of the examinee, will affect the measurements taken and should be controlled as much as possible to maximize reliability. Actual positions of measurement vary but they should allow freedom of movement while attempting to decrease the probability of compensatory motion. The tester should be sensitive to the fact that requiring the examinee to maintain a given position for a prolonged period of time may cause muscular fatigue, which could result in decreased range of motion. While the measurement should be taken as quickly as possible, it is important that the eyes of the tester are level with the scale to assure accuracy when reading the goniometer.

When compared to other measurement techniques, the goniometer is almost always easier and less restrictive to use. The Leighton Flexometer, for example, has greater reliability, is not affected by the length of segments, but its attachment to the segment makes it more restrictive to movement and extremely sensitive to movements out of the primary plane of action. It is a more expensive instrument, and like the goniometer,

can only be used for static end positions. The electrogoniometer can measure the range of movement dynamically and in all three planes of motion but is more restrictive to examinee movement and much more expensive. Range of motion measurements taken from film or video have other inherent problems but their primary difference with the goniometer would be the cost of the equipment. While the utility of static end position flexibility measurements have been questioned with regard to predicting athletic success or injury susceptibility, their use in therapeutic modes and general population screenings have been well established. Due to the goniometer's popularity, most traditionally defined populations have readily available published normative data.

SUMMARY

Major Strengths:

1. The instrument is relatively inexpensive.

2. The instrument requires minimal space and little supplemental equipment making it adaptable for almost any setting.

3. An undergraduate student in an appropriate field should have the expertise necessary to utilize the instrument.

4. The instrument has acceptable validity for research purposes and an abundance of comparative data available.

Major Weaknesses:

1. The reliability of the instrument is dependent upon the specific joint being measured.

2. The instrument cannot measure the joint's range of motion dynamically.

3. Deviations from standardized techniques can cause significant errors that a novice tester would not recognize.

LEIGHTON FLEXOMETER TEST

References.

Leighton, J. R. (1955). An instrument and technique for the measurement of range of joint motion. *Archives of Physical Medicine and Rehabilitation,* 36:571-578, September.

Montoye, H. J. (ed.) (1978). *An introduction to measurement in physical education.* Boston: Allyn and Bacon, pp 126-141, 358-369.

Additional Sources.

Bosco & Gustafson (1983, p. 111); Hastad & Lacy (1989, pp. 216-217); Verducci (1980, pp. 254-257).

Purpose.

To measure the range of motion in each major joint of an examinee's body.

Objectivity.

Not reported.

Reliability.

r = .90 to r = .98 for test-retest method of 30 different measures by Forbes (1950) cited in Montoye (1978, p. 126).

Validity.

Face validity.

Age and Sex.

Females and males, age 8 - adult.

Equipment.

A Leighton flexometer, low back arm chair, and a bench or table large enough for the examinee to recline or sit on. The flexometer is an instrument which consists of a strap used to secure the instrument to the examinee, a 360 degree dial, and a pointer. Both the dial and the pointer are weighted and thus rotate under the influence of gravity. The dial and the pointer each have their own locking mechanisms and operate independently of each other.

Space Requirements and Design.

A clear, level area approximately 3m (10') square that has a wall with a projecting corner nearby. The arm chair or table is positioned in the center of the floor space.

Directions.

Since the flexometer can be used to measure the range of motion of over 25 different joints, only the general procedures for using the flexometer are described here. The instrument is strapped to the more moveable body segment of the two segments which form the joint being measured. Each joint's range is measured by the examinee moving the involved body segment to one extreme of its range (e.g., full flexion). At this extreme, the dial and pointer should coincide and point upward to the zero mark and the dial is locked in place with the pointer left free to move. The examinee then moves the segment through its full range of motion to the opposite extreme (e.g., full extension). When the body segment is at this opposite extreme, the pointer is locked in place. A direct reading, in degrees, can then be taken from the dial.

Scoring.

The score of a joint is the number of degrees indicated on the dial.

Norms.

Forbes (1950) boys; Leighton (1955, p. 577) boys; Montoye (1978, pp. 358-369) boys, girls, men and women.

REVIEW

PHILLIP BISHOP, Ed.D.

Associate Professor
Health and Human Performance
University of Alabama
Tuscaloosa, AL 35487

The Leighton Flexometer provides one of the simplest and most useful means of measuring flexibility. Although some potential users may find its cost prohibitive, inexperienced testers will find that it is more easily mastered than goniometers or arthrodial protractors because its accuracy does not require that the tester locate the exact joint center.

Leighton's original paper (1955) provides very clear instructions for measuring various joints and offers cautions with regard to sources of error. Directions for use, along with photographs and norms for 6 to 18 year olds, are available for most major joints for both sexes in Montoye (1978) and in Volume 4 of Montoye (1970). Additional norms are available from the following physical therapy references: Hoppenfeld (1976) and Daniels and Worthingham (1986).

SUMMARY

Major Strengths:

1. Simplicity of operation.

2. Does not require identification of joint center.

3. Measurements are independent of segmental length.

Major Weaknesses:

1. The flexometer is quite expensive.

2. Unlike electrogoniometers, the flexometer cannot readily provide a continuous output during movement.

3. Use on small body segments such as fingers is impractical.

4. For body segments that are not straight (e.g., the trunk), the location of the flexometer will influence the results.

5. The body segments measured must be positioned so that gravity acts to move the pointer.

The Leighton Flexometer provides a good means of accurately assessing flexibility of major joints when examinees are stationary. Although more expensive than simple mechanical goniometers, the Leighton Flexometer is probably easier and more accurate to use, particularly for novices. The best source of norms may be a hospital's physical therapy department.

REVIEW REFERENCES

Hoppenfeld, S. (1976). *Physical examination of the spine and extremities*. New York: Appleton-Century-Crofts.

Daniels, & Worthingham (1986). *Muscle testing.* Philadelphia: W. B. Saunders.

Montoye, H. J. (ed.). (1978). *Introduction to measurement in PE.* Boston: Allyn and Bacon.

WRIST FLEXIBILITY TEST

Reference.
Bender, J., & Shea, E. J. (1964). *Physical fitness: Tests and exercises.* New York: Ronald Press, pp 42-44.

Additional Sources.
None.

Purpose.
To measure the range of flexion and extension of an examinee's wrist joint.

Objectivity.
Not reported.

Reliability.
Not reported.

Validity.
Not reported.

Age and Sex.
Not reported, but suitable for females and males, age 6 - adult.

Equipment.
A sheet of paper with a straight line drawn in the center the length of the sheet, a ruler, masking tape, a pencil, a chair, and a table.

Space Requirements and Design.
A clear, level area approximately 2m (6') square with the chair and table positioned in the center.

Directions.
The sheet of paper is taped to the table's top. The examinee sits in the chair and places one hand on the table's top perpendicular to the sheet of paper. The little finger and wrist are aligned on and parallel to the drawn line. The examinee then extends the wrist backward as far as possible and the tester draws a line even with the back edge of the hand. The examinee then flexes the wrist forward as far as possible and the tester draws another line even with the back of the hand. The procedure can be used for either or both wrists.

Scoring.
The line representing flexion of the wrist should almost be perpendicular to the center line originally drawn on the paper. The line representing extension should also be almost perpendicular, but seldom is. Failure to achieve these results would indicate a need for flexibility exercises.

Norms.

Not reported.

NOTE: An alternate form of scoring the test is to use a protractor to measure the angles in degrees between the center line and the lines drawn indicating the range of extension and the range of flexion.

REVIEW

DEBRA A. BALLINGER, Ph.D.
Assistant Professor
Health, Physical Education and Recreation
Old Dominion University
Norfolk, VA 23529-0196

The measurement of flexibility, the capacity of a joint to move through its full range of motion (ROM), has been given renewed attention with an increase in adaptive and therapeutic physical education programs, and with scientific evidence supporting its role in injury prevention in sport settings. Field tests have become simplified with the design of portable and inexpensive goniometers, thus the need for the paper ruler test has decreased significantly. If more scientific measurements are not possible, the Wrist Flexibility Test could be of limited practical use such as to compare progress following therapy, or for an individual to utilize at home between visits to specialists. It is not, however, recommended for group or individual assessment, due to weaknesses in objectivity, reliability, and validity.

Flexibility is known to be influenced by such factors as age, sex, physical activity, and soft tissue composition in and around the joint areas. The test should be compared with goniometer measurements in a controlled laboratory setting to establish age appropriate guidelines for ROM, validity and reliability.

The test directions suggest that flexion and extension lines should approximate 90 degrees (perpendicular lines). Most references checked suggest flexion should approximate 80 degrees from anatomical position (i.e., 0 degrees), and extension should be about 70 degrees. A protractor should be used to measure these angles. Directions should also note that when measuring wrist flexion the fingers will extend, and during extension, the fingers will flex. No attempt should be made to limit this natural movement.

Flexibility is also affected by internal joint temperature. Care should be taken to include instructions for warm up and multiple trials, with the best score being recorded. Test directions need to be standardized procedures. An example might be to include a warm up activity simulating the testing motion for one minute per wrist, allowing three trials, and then recording the greatest ROM. Factors such as time of day, external temperature, and humidity should be recorded, and subsequent test conditions should closely approximate previous assessment conditions to add to the test-retest reliability. Objectivity is also a critical factor, and the tester should practice until high reliability can be achieved. Typical flexometer and goniometer reliability coefficients range from .90 to 98. Care should be taken to ensure stability of the forearm throughout the test, and to avoid rotational movements which could affect the measurements.

Flexibility is highly specific, varying not only between but also within joints. Examinees should be informed that each joint needs to be measured separately, and exercises should involve working ROM throughout all joints. It is also recommended that adduction and abduction measurements be included in wrist flexibility assessment. This test could also be adapted for such estimates, with suggested standards of 35 degrees (adduction) and 20 degrees (abduction) being included in test directions.

SUMMARY

Major Strength:

1. The Wrist Flexibility Test has very limited usefulness, and is only recommended for individuals to monitor progress on a day to day basis if no goniometer is available. With plastic goniometers available at a low cost, this reviewer does not see the need for the use of this test in physical education or field settings.

Major Weaknesses:

1. Lack of normative data for age, sex, body composition, etc.

2. Lack of standardized test administration procedures.

3. No reliability, objectivity, or validity criteria.

4. No consideration for abduction, adduction, or rotational flexibility measurements for wrist flexibility.

Unacceptable test, except as a self test for day to day flexion and extension estimates. Suggest use of inexpensive goniometer - which is less costly than the table and chair in the physical education setting.

DYNAMIC FLEXIBILITY TEST

FLEISHMAN DYNAMIC FLEXIBILITY TEST

Reference.
Fleishman, E. A. (1964B). *The structure and measurement of physical fitness.* Englewood Cliffs: Prentice Hall, pp 112, 128, 134, 162-163.

Additional Sources.
None.

Purpose.
To measure the ability of an examinee to make repeated movements through a range of motion.

Objectivity.
Not reported.

Reliability.
r = .92.

Validity.
Construct validity was established.

Age and Sex.
Suitable for females and males, age 8 - adult.

Equipment.
Tape or a piece of chalk and a stopwatch.

Space Requirements and Design.
A clear, level area approximately 2m (6') square located next to a clear wall. An "X" is marked on the wall at the height of the examinee's shoulders. Another "X" is marked on the floor just far enough from the wall so that the examinee, when standing with her/his back in front of the "X" on the wall, can bend forward and touch the "X" on the floor without the buttocks touching the wall. The "X" on the floor should be marked between the examinee's feet.

Directions.
The examinee stands next to the wall with her/his hands held together (i.e., by interlocking the thumbs) in front of the body. The feet are shoulder width apart. On the command, "Ready, Go," the examinee bends forward and touches the "X" between the feet, straightens up, and twists to the left to touch the "X" on the wall behind. This counts as one cycle. The cycle is repeated, with alternate twists to the right and to the left, as many cycles as possible in 20 seconds. Each "X" must be touched with both hands.

Scoring.
The score is the number of cycles executed in the 20 seconds.

Norms.
Fleishman (1964B, p. 112) boys and girls; Fleishman (1964A, p. 47) boys and girls; McCaughan (1975, p. 14) boys.

REVIEW

DAVID R. HOPKINS, P.E.D.

Associate Professor
Physical Education
Indiana State University
Terre Haute, IN 47809

The Dynamic Flexibility Test is a field test designed to measure the ability to make repeated movements through a range of motion. In essence, the test is a dynamic equivalent of two common static stretch tests (i.e., trunk rotation and standing toe touch). Ballistic stretching of the trunk and hip region is required in the test movement.

Because the test is a measure of resistance to movement (i.e., dynamic flexibility) rather than static flexibility (i.e., range of motion), it can provide an indication of physical performance and inclination for injury. Inherent in the movement for the test is a chance of injury during ballistic stretching. The ballistic movement requires jerky, rapid, and bouncy movements. These actions can hyperextend the joint capsule, stretch ligaments of the knee, and cause excessive pressure of the intervertebral disc in the lower back as well as lead to increased muscle soreness and injury due to small tears in the soft tissue. Performance of the test by unconditioned examinees increases the probability of injury.

The directions are unclear as to whether the examinees may bend at the knees during the floor touch. The diagram in Fleishman (1964) describes a straight knee position during the floor touch. In many cases, examinees will not be able to touch the floor without bending the knees. No allowance is made for this situation in the test administration.

It would also appear that the test movement could create an inherent bias against taller examinees due to the extended range of movement. The degree of validity would be affected by the unclear directions and height bias. No statistical estimates of validity are provided and only construct validity was established. A reliability estimate of .92 is provided which is an acceptable level.

SUMMARY

Major Strength:

1. The test measures resistance to movement in the trunk and hip region which provides information on physical performance and potential for injury.

Major Weaknesses:

1. While the above may be a strength, it can be a weakness in that the potential for injury to unconditioned examinees is increased during the performance of the test.

2. The directions are unclear as to how the floor touch phase can be performed.

3. There is a height bias in performance. The unclear directions and height bias can diminish the validity of the test.

Most authorities do not recommend ballistic exercises for flexibility development of the general population. Thus, while this test may be appropriate for well conditioned athletes, hamstring and low back injuries may result from its administration to the general population concerned with health related physical fitness.

ANKLE LINEAR MEASUREMENT FLEXIBILITY TESTS

ANKLE EXTENSION* TEST

*Also known as plantar flexion.

Reference.
Johnson, B. L., & Nelson, J. K. (1986). *Practical measurements for evaluation in physical education*. Edina, MN: Burgess, pp 97-99.

Additional Sources.
None.

Purpose.
To measure the range of extension in an examinee's ankle.

Objectivity.
r = .99 experienced tester correlated with an inexperienced tester.

Reliability.
r = .88 test-retest method.

Validity.
Face validity was accepted.

Age and Sex.
Females and males, age 6 - college.

Equipment.
A flexomeasure case with a meterstick (yardstick) and the ruler guide inserted.

Space Requirements and Design.
A clear, level area 3m (10') square with the examinee in the center.

Directions.
The barefoot examinee takes a sitting position on the floor with the right leg as straight as possible. The tester holds the meterstick vertical with the zero end on the floor and slides the case downward until the ruler guide rests across the lowest point of the shin bone. The examinee then extends the ankle and the measurement is repeated at the highest point of the foot (either the toes or instep) during maximum extension. The procedures are repeated for the left foot. The difference between the upper foot line during maximum extension and the lower shin bone line is measured to the nearest .5cm (1/8") for each foot and recorded.

Scoring.
The score is the average of the differences in height for both feet.

Norms.
Johnson & Nelson (1986, p. 99) college men and women.

NOTE: An alternate method of scoring the test is to measure the vertical distance from the bottom of the big toe to the floor.

REVIEW

PAUL A. ANDERSON, Ph.D.
Assistant Professor
Physical Therapy
University of Maryland
Baltimore, MD 21201

Professional communication is a two sided word. The communicator needs to use language appropriate to the audience and the topic to insure there is no misunderstanding of intent. Additionally, the audience has the responsibility to be conversant in the language and familiar with the topic. This test description falls short of adequately communicating the topic Ankle Extension.

Knowing the range of motion (ROM) permitted at any joint is of value to the health professional. The physical educator could utilize this information to help maximize performance whereas the physical therapist needs joint ROM for joint evaluation and progress of the rehabilitation. Ranges of motion for all joints and for both genders are needed. The ability to measure or document ROM for the ankle joint has merit. Unfortunately, this test and its methodology are fraught with error.

This test is designed to examine ankle joint extension, or as indicated by an asterisk, plantar flexion. However, ankle joint extension is dorsiflexion (Hollishead, 1985). The reader now encounters a dilemma. Does this test measure ankle joint extension (its title, but correctly known as dorsiflexion) or the asterisked plantar flexion which is properly identified as ankle joint flexion; in which case the title needs to be corrected. Reading the test directions yields little insight into the test constructor's intent. The directions seem to ask the examinee to move her/his ankle joint away from the shin bone. If this is true, the movement is ankle joint flexion or plantar flexion (Hobart, 1984).

The terminology could be tightened in order to eliminate any misunderstanding by correctly identifying body parts and joint positions. Within the anatomical, kinesiology, and biomechanical disciplines a jargon exists that precisely tells the tester what to do within the realm of any given test (Poland et al, 1981). For example, test directions read hold the "right leg as straight as possible." The lower extremity is made up of the "thigh" from the hip to the knee joints; the "leg" from the knee to ankle joints and the "foot" from the ankle distally. The test constructor also employs a term of upper foot, implying there a lower foot. These body part phrases are used incorrectly. Also, terms that precisely describe the desired position of the joints could be used. The test constructor could say to the examinee to extend the knee when he/she is sitting on the floor or dorsiflex the ankle prior to measuring the ROM.

The measuring of the ankle joint ROM has some problems. First, a flexomeasure case in this test could be replaced by a simple goniometer that physical and occupational therapists employ with excellent accuracy. When employing a goniometer, the tester can refer to the normative data for all of the joints of the body (Clarkson, & Gilwich, 1988). Second, this test does not describe accurately the starting position of the examinee's ankle joint raising the question whether the examinee is in full dorsiflexion moving into full plantar flexion. It is not clear if the examinee starts with the ankle joint in the neutral position and then moves it into full plantar flexion. Third, the test description does not tell the reader if the ROM is active or passive. Active ROM is undertaken by the examinee and reflects a functional ROM; whereas passive ROM is when the tester moves the joint through its ROM indicating the joint's ROM. Perhaps measuring both would be valuable. Fourth, the

scoring of the test can be more precise. This test example is in centimeters or a fraction of an inch; however, joint motion is rotational, thus units of measure should be in degrees or radians.

The test constructor states that the face validity of the test was accepted. The above comments raise serious doubts, thus placing the face validity in question. A correlation coefficient of $r = 0.9$ or greater is the rule of thumb for reliability thus this test of a $r = 0.88$ is close to reliable but room for improvement exists. The test constructor reports an $r = .99$ for objectivity. An intraclass correlation, as reported by Shrout and Fleiss (1982), comparing more than two performances would give a better indication of objectivity.

SUMMARY

Major Strength:

1. This test can be administered by a single tester, in a small area and relatively quickly.

Major Weaknesses:

1. Questionable validity.

2. Test reliability by one or more testers not demonstrated.

3. Which specific ankle joint movement is being examined; plantar flexion or dorsiflexion?

4. Incorrect use of terminology leading to unclear directions to examinees and testers.

5. Imprecise measurement tool and units.

This Ankle Extension Test is unacceptable.

REVIEW REFERENCES

Clarkson, H. M., & Gilwich, G. B. (1988). *Musculoskeletal assessment: Joint range of motion and manual muscle strength*. Baltimore: Williams and Wilkins.

Hobart, D. J. (1984). *A dissector of human anatomy*. Medical Examination Publishing, Co.

Hollishead, W. H. (1985). *Textbook of anatomy*. New York: Harper and Row.

Poland, J. L., Hobart, D. J., & Payton, O. D. (1981). *The musculoskeletal system*. Medical Examination Publishing Co.

Shrout, P. E., & Fleiss, J. L. (1979). Intraclass correlations: Uses in assessing rater reliability. *Psychological Bulletin*, 86:420-428.

ANKLE FLEXION* (STANDING) TEST

*Also known as dorsiflexion.

Reference.
Johnson, B. L., & Nelson, J. K. (1986). *Practical measurements for evaluation in physical education.* Edina, MN: Burgess, pp 97, 99.

Additional Sources.
None.

Purpose.
To measure the range of flexion in an examinee's ankle joint.

Objectivity.
r = .99 experienced tester correlated with an inexperienced tester.

Reliability.
r = .88 test-retest method.

Validity.
Face validity was accepted.

Age and Sex.
Females and males, age 6 - college.

Equipment.
A meterstick (yardstick) or tape measure.

Space Requirements and Design.
A clear, level area approximately 3m (10') square next to a clear wall.

Directions.
The examinee stands facing the wall and back from it about .5m (20"). While keeping the heels flat on the floor, the examinee places the hands on the wall and then leans forward, touching the chin and chest to the wall. If the examinee is not successful at touching her/his chin and chest to the wall while keeping the heels flat on the floor, the examinee repeats the same procedure at a distance closer to the wall. If the examinee was successful at the initial distance, he/she moves back from the wall. A total of three trials are given to determine the maximum distance of success. The examinee's body and knees must be kept straight while touching the chin and chest to the wall. The tester measures the distance between the toe line and the wall after the best lean forward is made with the heels flat on the floor. The tester then measures the height from the floor to the examinee's chin while he/she is standing erect.

Scoring.
The score is the measured distance from the floor to the examinee's chin minus the measured distance from the wall to the examinee's toes during the lean.

Norms.
Johnson & Nelson (1986, p. 99) men and women.

REVIEW
CHERYL NORTON, Ed.D.
Associate Professor
Human Performance
Metropolitan State College
Denver, CO 80204

The Ankle Flexion Test is a field test designed to measure the amount of flexion in the ankle. As such, it does not require extensive equipment or technical training to administer. Consequently, the test can be performed in any environment, by minimally trained personnel and can be used on a wide variety of age groups.

Because the Ankle Flexion Test is a measure of static flexibility, it provides information on range of motion rather than resistance to movement (i.e., dynamic flexibility). Thus, the test may not be as indicative of physical performance or as highly related to the likelihood of injury as a measure of movement resistance would be.

While the scores on the test indeed reflect the amount of ankle flexion, they are given on a linear scale (i.e., inches or centimeters) rather than in angular units (i.e., degrees). Angular measures indicate directly the range of motion in a joint and the health of an articulation. A linear measure cannot be as translated easily into a meaningful range of motion measure. Thus, this test would not be as effective in determining recovery of ankle flexion after an injury as if range of motion were measured directly in degrees of movement. In addition, there is not sufficient normative data given in a linear scale to indicate minimal acceptable scores for all age groups and both sexes. Thus, the use of these test scores, in most cases, would be limited to pretest and posttest comparative data analysis (i.e., to show improvement).

Performance of the test itself may be somewhat discomforting for some examinees. Although the test appears to require little effort on the part of the examinee, placing the chin and chest flat against a wall and placing the feet some distance from the wall creates a pressure point along the spine. The farther the feet are placed from the wall (i.e., the examinee with more ankle flexion), the further down on the wall the chin/chest must be placed and the greater the hyperextension of the spine. At some point, this examinee may be forced to arch the neck in order to keep the chin/chest in contact with the wall as the feet are placed farther from this surface. Since not all joints of the body have equal flexibility, it is possible that: (1) true flexion of the ankle cannot be measured because of inadequate flexibility of the spine, or (2) in determining flexibility of the ankle, the spine could be injured. The second possibility would have more potential occurrence if the examinee were excessively fat in the trunk. Thrusting the chest forward would displace this weight from over the examinee's weight center and in essence "suspend" it from the spine.

Finally, although there is a starting position given, the true distance indicating maximal ankle flexion would be determined by trial and error.

With only three attempts given, it is possible that a true measure would not be determined in this number of trials, especially if the tester were proceeding cautiously.

SUMMARY

In summary, the Ankle Flexion Test provides an acceptable measure of ankle flexibility, especially if pretest and posttest scores are required. Absolute measures on this test, however, may have little relationship to performance or injury. Although it is not a test an examinee could score herself/himself, the equipment is inexpensive, space requirements are minimal, and administration of the test does not require any technical skills. Consequently, it is a reasonable test for a school or recreational environment. Caution should be given to using this test with people who have back problems, are excessively fat or have inflexible spines. The test does not require a lengthy testing period, however, consideration may be given to using more trials, especially for an examinee who differs significantly from the average (i.e., exhibits extreme ankle flexibility or limited flexibility) in order to obtain a realistic measure. Research using this test should be limited to developing better normative data for the wide age groups it is proposed for (i.e., six years old to adult) and relating these measures to a health standard.

HIP LINEAR MEASUREMENT FLEXIBILITY TESTS

FRONT-TO-REAR SPLITS TEST

References.
Johnson, B. L. (1978). Flexibility assessment. In Blair, S.N. (ed). *SDAAHPER proceedings,* pp 63-69.

Johnson, B. L., & Nelson, J. K. (1986). *Practical measurements for evaluation in physical education.* Edina, MN: Burgess, pp 90-92, 455.

Additional Sources.
None.

Purpose.
To measure the range of flexion and extension in an examinee's hip joints from front to rear.

Objectivity.
r = .99 experienced tester correlated with an inexperienced tester.

Reliability.
r = .91 test-retest method.

Validity.
Face validity was accepted.

Age and Sex.
Females and males, age 6 - college.

Equipment.
A flexomeasure case with a meterstick (yardstick) and ruler guide inserted. The flexomeasure case and ruler guide should be positioned close to the zero end of the meterstick (yardstick).

Space Requirements and Design.
A clear, level area approximately 3m (10') square with the examinee in the center.

Directions.
From the standing position, the examinee slowly and steadily moves the legs as far apart front to rear as possible (i.e., flexion at one hip joint and extension at the other hip joint). The use of the hands for balance during the test is permitted. As the examinee's crotch is lowered toward the floor, the tester holds the instrument vertical directly behind the examinee with the zero end on the floor. When the examinee reaches the lowest point and with the knees still locked, the flexomeasure case is moved upward until the ruler guide rests under the crotch. The score is then recorded. Three trials are given.

Scoring.
The score is the smallest vertical distance during the three trials measured to the nearest .5cm (1/4").

Norms.
Johnson & Nelson (1986, pp 92, 455) boys, girls, men and women.

REVIEW

SUE W. WHITE, M.Ed.

Assistant Professor
Physical Education
Black Hills State University
Spearfish, SD 57999
and
JANELLE BRAATZ. M.S.

Assistant Professor
Physical Education
Black Hills State University
Spearfish, SD 57999
and
LARRY M. LANDIS, Ph.D.

Professor of Social Science
Black Hills State University
Spearfish, SD 57999

The purpose of this test is to measure the range of flexion and extension of the hips from front to rear. By definition, the test has face validity. Test objectivity was measured using a split-half reliability test comparing the results obtained by an experienced practitioner and student participants on test-retest. A reliability coefficient of .973 was obtained. As the manner in which the splits are performed (i.e, left leg forward and right leg back or right leg forward and left leg back) can significantly affect the measure of flexibility, it is important that the test-retest procedure be administered with splits being performed in a consistent manner.

The measurement instrument (Flexomeasure) is inexpensive and readily available. The instrument is a simple device that can be used easily. The test is easily administered with a minimal amount of explanation required for even an inexperienced tester. One tester can successfully administer the test but to ensure a proper measurement, it is helpful if an assistant is present to help stabilize the Flexomeasure. Space is not a problem and as the reliability measure reported above indicates, the test can be administered successfully by inexperienced testers. The scoring is easy to do and it is objective. The test is normed.

SUMMARY

Major Strengths:

1. The test is easily set up, and readily administered, measured, and scored.

2. It demonstrates both flexion and extension in a convincing fashion.

3. The test differentiates effectively the abilities of examinees being tested. As such, the test seems a useful teaching or demonstration device and would appear to be useful as a research tool in those instances where the measurement of these abilities are required (e.g., gymnasts, hurdlers, and ice skaters).

Major Weakness:

1. The test is highly reliable but the utility of the results of this test is quite limited.

This test is an acceptable test. It appears adequate for demonstration, teaching, and research purposes. While the results of this test may be dramatic in the ability to demonstrate an examinee's hip flexibility, its utility to the general practitioner is probably limited.

HIP ADDUCTOR FLEXIBILITY TEST

Reference.
Tomita, P. H. (1989), Take the flex test. *Shape,*
8(11):88-89.

Additional Sources.
None.

Purpose.
To measure the range of abduction in an
examinee's hip joints.

Objectivity.
Not reported.

Reliability.
Not reported.

Validity.
Not reported.

Age and Sex.
Not reported, but suitable for females and males,
age 6 - adult.

Equipment.
A ruler.

Space Requirements and Design.
A clear, level area approximately 2m (6') square
with the examinee in the center.

Directions.
The examinee assumes a sitting position with the
legs relaxed. The knees are positioned out away
from and to the sides of the body. The heels of
the feet as positioned next to the buttocks with
the soles of the feet together. The hands grasp
the ankles. The examinee should use the elbows
to gently press against the knees until resistance
is encountered. The vertical distance between
the mid point of the kneecap and the floor is then
measured for each leg.

Scoring.
The score is the shortest vertical distance
recorded for each leg. The distance between
these points is recorded as a negative score.

Norms.
Not reported.

REVIEW

FRANK SMITH, Ph.D.
Dean, School of Education
St. Edward's University
Austin, TX 78704

No evidence has been presented to demonstrate
that this test will measure the component of hip
adductor flexibility as commonly defined in the
literature. In fact, this reviewer was unable to
find a "common" definition of what constitutes
flexibility of the hip adductor muscles.

True hip abduction occurs when the body is in
the anatomical position and the hip is in extension. When the hip is flexed and rotated laterally,
as it is in this test, the ligaments that might
restrain the action of abduction (i.e., the
iliofemoral and ischiofemoral ligaments) are
relaxed. Thus, the only limiting factor to passive
abduction in this position appears to be the musculature of the medial femoral region: the hip
adductors. However, it should be noted that the
adductor longus and adductor magnus muscles
also serve as medial rotators at the hip and are
therefore placed under stretch when the hip is
laterally rotated.

No evidence has been presented to demonstrate
that the test will provide consistent results. Test
scores could improve with replication due to the
repeated stretching of the hip adductor muscles.

No evidence has been presented to demonstrate
that the test can be administered by various
testers and consistent results be obtained. However, since the directions are simple and direct,
there is no reason to believe that objectivity does
not exist.

Both age and sex are significant factors in determining the flexibility of the hip adductors.
Women and youths tend to be more flexible in
this aspect. The equipment is inexpensive and
easy to obtain. The nature and dimensions of the
area are well defined and present no difficulty.

The directions require that the examinee make
a subjective evaluation on how far to "gently"
press the legs into abduction. Some examinees
will cease pressing at the onset of discomfort,
while others may press on through the pain. Also,
if both legs are not tested simultaneously, the
examinee may tend to narrow the gap between
the knee tested and the floor by simply tilting the
pelvis toward that side.

A stretching protocol involving the hip adductors should be introduced before testing to reduce the chance of injury to this sensitive area.

The scoring method is easy to follow; however, a limit on the number of trials should be given. This should increase reliability.

The test results are not very meaningful to the tester or the examinee since no norms are reported.

SUMMARY

Major Strengths:

1. The test appears to truly measure hip adductor muscle flexibility by eliminating the inhibiting effect of the accessory ligaments of the hip.

2. Flexibility in the medial femoral region is desirable, since overstretching injuries of this musculature are painful, slow to heal, and awkward to treat and support.

Major Weaknesses:

1. No rationale is presented which would substantiate the validity, reliability, or objectivity of the test.

2. Test directions require that the examinee make subjective evaluations on flexibility limits.

3. Examinees could "cheat" by tilting the pelvis toward the leg tested.

4. Apparently, no norms have been developed which give the test results meaning.

In its present form, the aforementioned test is acceptable for teaching and casual evaluation purposes.

HIP ADDUCTOR STRETCH TEST

Reference.
Hagerman, F. C. et al. (1989). Effects of a long term fitness program on professional baseball players. *The Physician and Sportsmedicine*, 17(4):101-104, 107-108, 115-119.

Additional Sources.
None.

Purpose.
To measure the range of abduction in an examinee's hip joints.

Objectivity.
Not reported.

Reliability.
Not reported.

Validity.
Not reported.

Age and Sex.
Not reported, but suitable for females and males, age 6 - adult.

Equipment.
A felt tip marker and a short, soft tape measure.

Space Requirements and Design.
A clear, level area approximately 3m (10') square with the examinee in the center.

Directions.
The examinee should perform a warm up of general flexibility exercises. Using the felt tip marker, the tester clearly marks the examinee's medial femoral epicondyles. The examinee, while sitting with the upper body erect and the hands flat on the floor at the sides of the body, spreads the legs as far apart as possible while keeping the knees extended. The tester then uses the tape measure to determine the horizontal distance between the two marked epicondyles. Three trials are administered.

Scoring.
The score is the distance between the two epicondyles, measured to the nearest inch, for the best of three trials.

Norms.
Hagerman et al. (1989, p. 108) major league baseball team over a period of seven years.

REVIEW

KATHLEEN TRITSCHLER, Ed.D.

Assistant Professor
Sport Studies
Guilford College
Greensboro, NC 27410

The Hip Adductor Stretch is one of five flexibility tests administered to professional baseball players as part of an overall physical fitness assessment (Hagerman et al., 1989). It was noted by the researchers that "injuries to the hamstring and adductor muscles are common among baseball players" (Hagerman et al., p. 117), thus providing the rationale for this specific test in the overall flexibility battery.

The Hip Adductor Stretch test can be categorized as a field test of relative flexibility, reported by a linear measurement (Johnson & Nelson, 1986). It is a field test because it requires no specialized equipment (just a soft tape measure), and little specialized training on the part of the tester (just knowledge of how to locate the bony landmarks of the medial femoral epicondyles). It is a relative measure of flexibility, because the measurement reflects to some degree the length of the examinee's femur. And, the measurement is linear (i.e., scored in inches) rather than rotary (i.e., scored in degrees of rotation).

From the perspective of this reviewer, the field nature of this test is clearly a plus. It is extremely quick, easy, and inexpensive to administer. Furthermore, if the examinee performs the test with careful attention to keeping the knees extended and testing only after the recommended "warm up of general flexibility exercises" (Hagerman et al., p. 104), the Hip Adductor Stretch Test is likely to be highly reliable. The best of three trials scoring also contributes to high test reliability. Validity would appear to be high when the test is used for the purpose of assessing change within the same examinee over time (e.g., as a result of a specific training program).

There is, however, a distinct problem from the perspective of test validity when the test scores are used for inter-examinee comparisons. The problem derives directly from the relative nature of this flexibility test. There is an inherent test bias against examinees with short femurs. Imagine two examinees with equal adductor flexibility, but having a difference of several inches in the length of their femurs; clearly by this testing procedure the short femured examinee would receive a lower score. Since the score is not modified in any way to account for femur length, the validity of the flexibility measure is called into question.

It is recommended that Hagerman and colleagues consider applying McCloy's quotient (McCloy & Young, 1954) to this and the other four items in their battery of flexibility tests. McCloy's quotient was developed specifically to take into account the lengths of influencing body parts in flexibility measures.

SUMMARY

Major Strength:

1. The test's excellent practicality in terms of time, equipment, and tester training.

Major Weakness:

1. The test's failure to account for the influence of femur length on the flexibility score.

REVIEW REFERENCES

Hagerman, F. C. et al. (1989). Effects of a long term fitness program on professional baseball players. *The Physician and Sportsmedicine,* 17(4):101-104, 107-108, 115-119.

Johnson, B. L., & Nelson, J. K. (1986). *Practical measurements for evaluation in physical education.* Edina, MN: Burgess Publishing.

McCloy, C. H., & Young, N. D. (1954). *Tests and measurements in health and physical education.* New York: Appleton-Century-Crofts.

HIP FLEXOR TEST

Reference.
Tomita, P. H. (1989). Take the flex test. *Shape,* 8(11):88-89.

Additional Sources.
None.

Purpose.
To measure the range of flexion in an examinee's hip joints.

Objectivity.
Not reported.

Reliability.
Not reported.

Validity.
Not reported.

Age and Sex.
Not reported, but suitable for females and males, age 6 - adult.

Equipment.
A ruler and a table.

Space Requirements and Design.
A clear, level area approximately 3m (10') square with the table positioned in the center.

Directions.
The examinee assumes a supine position on the table with her/his legs, bent at the knees, hanging over the edge of the table. The examinee begins the test by pulling both knees up toward the chest until the lower back is flat against the table. While continuing to hold onto the left leg, the examinee releases the right leg and allows it to return to the table. When the leg reaches its lowest point, the perpendicular distance between the back of the knee and the table top is measured. The lower back must remain in contact with the table throughout the test. This same procedure is repeated for the left leg.

Scoring.
The score is the vertical distance between the back of the knee and the table top. The score is recorded as a negative number. If the leg is even with the table top, a score of zero is recorded.

Norms.
Not reported.

REVIEW

RONALD K. HETZLER, Ph.D.
Assistant Professor
Health, Physical Education and Recreation
University of Hawaii at Manoa
Honolulu, HI 96822

This test is an adaptation of the Thomas Test of hip flexor flexibility. Both are passive tests of the length of the hip flexors. Normal flexibility would result in a score of zero on the Hip Flexor Test. The major difference between the two tests is that this test quantifies a lack of flexibility in the hip joint. The Hip Flexor Test is a simple test to conduct and appears to be both valid and reliable. Furthermore, the objectivity of the test is adequate and with suitable training similar results should be obtainable between even novice testers. Since no special equipment is needed and space requirements are minimal, this test could serve as a good field test of the flexibility of the hip flexors.

The test is safe and easy to administer and would require only minimal training of the tester. Only a few minutes would be required to test each examinee. However, maximal flexibility usually increases with the number of trials. This was not addressed in the Hip Flexor Test. The examinee should be allowed to repeat the test until no further increase in flexibility is noted. Additionally, the test does not allow for the quantification of exceptional flexibility. Exceptional flexibility could be assessed by having the examinee move closer to the edge of the table and measuring the distance from the bottom of the knee (below the horizontal plane) to the table top. Normative data would help in the interpretation of the results.

SUMMARY

Major Strength:

1. The test allows for quantification of a lack of flexibility, which provides a basis for determining improvement over time.

Major Weaknesses:

1. The test lacks normative data.

2. Increasing the number of trials until no improvement occurs is recommended.

In summary, the Hip Flexor Test is an acceptable test to assess the flexibility of the hip flexors.

SIDE SPLITS TEST

References.

Johnson, B. L., & Nelson, J. K. (1986). *Practical measurements for evaluation in physical education.* Edina, MN: Burgess, pp 91, 93, 456.

Johnson, B. L. (1977). *Practical flexibility measurement with the flexomeasure.* Portland, TX: Brown and Littleman Company.

Additional Sources.

None.

Purpose.

To measure the range of abduction in an examinee's hip joints by spreading the legs apart.

Objectivity.

r = .99 experienced tester correlated with an in-experienced tester.

Reliability.

r = .92 test-retest method.

Validity.

Face validity was accepted.

Age and Sex.

Females and males, age 6 - college.

Equipment.

A flexomeasure case with meterstick (yardstick) and ruler guide inserted. The flexomeasure case and ruler guide should be positioned close to the zero end of the yardstick.

Space Requirements and Design.

A clear, level area approximately 3m (10') square with the examinee in the center.

Directions.

From a standing position, the examinee slowly and steadily spreads the legs (i.e., abduction at the hip joints as far apart side to side) as possible. The use of the hands for balance during the test is permitted. As the examinee's crotch is lowered as close to the floor as possible, the tester holds the instrument vertically behind the examinee with the zero end on the floor. When the examinee's crotch reaches the lowest point, with the knees still locked and the hips not shifted past vertical, the tester slides the flexomeasure case up until the ruler guide rests under the crotch. The score is then recorded. Three trials are given.

Scoring.

The score is the smallest vertical height achieved during the best of three trials measured to the nearest .5cm (1/4").

Norms.

Johnson & Nelson (1986, p. 93, 456) boys, girls, men and women.

REVIEW

LORRAINE REDDERSON, Ed.D.

Professor of Physical Education
Lander College
Greenwood, SC 29646

The Side Splits Test was administered to 10 volunteers from a movement class. Results of the test were correlated with results of the Sit and Reach Test (South Carolina Physical Fitness Test). The correlation coefficient was r = .85. Assuming that the two tests had enough similar characteristics, it can be said that the Side Splits Test is valid.

The 10 students took the test twice. The correlation coefficient for the test-retest was r = .91. It can therefore be pronounced reliable. This reviewer administered the test both times.

The space requirements for this test are excellent because very little space is required. Whatever type room is used, it should provide some privacy to the testing. The equipment required may cause some problems due to the lack of alternatives. One tester is enough and the time consumed in administration makes the test practical. Three trials are sufficient.

The test is suitable for college students and does discriminate among users due to body structure, and female and male differences in flexibility. The test is not dangerous. Examinees cannot score themselves. Test results could be used for research purposes.

SUMMARY

Major Strengths:

1. A test for measuring hip abduction flexibility.

2. The use of a flexomeasure.

Major Weaknesses:

1. Difficulty in obtaining accurate measures.

2. Difficulty in maintaining same body position.

3. Wearing apparel can interfere with scores and testing.

The Side Splits Test is acceptable in its present form. It would be helpful if examinees would wear leotards or some other tight clothing when taking the test. It would also be good to control some related factors such as leg length or width of the spreading of the feet. It is difficult for the examinees to keep their knees locked when abducting at the hips.

HIP AND SPINAL COLUMN LINEAR MEASUREMENT FLEXIBILITY TESTS

FORWARD BEND OF TRUNK TEST

Reference.
Jensen, C. R., & Hirst, C. C. (1980). *Measurement in physical education and athletics.* New York: Macmillan, pp 117-118.

Additional Sources.
Bosco & Gustafson (1983, pp. 106-107); Safrit (1986, pp. 338-339); Safrit (1990, p. 508).

Purpose.
To measure the range of motion in an examinee's trunk and hips.

Objectivity.
Not reported.

Reliability.
Not reported.

Validity.
Not reported.

Age and Sex.
Not reported, but suitable for females and males, age 6 - adult.

Equipment.
A table and a small tape measure.

Space Requirements and Design.
A clear, level area approximately 3m (10') square near a wall. The table should be positioned with one of its edges against the wall.

Directions.
The examinee assumes a sitting position on the table with the legs extended perpendicular to the wall. The feet are placed flat against the wall, hip width apart. The examinee then bends forward and downward as far as possible moving the hands toward the heels of the feet. This position is held and the vertical distance from the table to the top of the examinee's sternum (i.e., suprasternal notch) is measured.

Scoring.
The score is the vertical distance from the table top to the examinee's suprasternal notch, measured to the nearest .5cm (1/4").

Norms.
O'Connor & Cureton (1945, p. 314) girls for forehead to floor.

NOTE: Another method of scoring the test is to measure the distance between the fingertips and the back, bottom edge of the heels.

REVIEW

WILLIAM F. CLIPSON, Ed.D.

Emeritus Professor
Physical Education
University of Alabama
Tuscaloosa, AL 35486

The purpose and description of the test as stated can be interpreted to mean that the range of motion is not to be limited by the hamstrings. If the knees are to remain straight throughout the test, then it should be stated in the directions. With the knees straight, the range of motion in the hips and trunk is limited by the hamstrings which should be stated in the purpose. For example, the purpose is to measure the range of motion in the trunk and hips with extended hamstrings.

Although no reliability or objectivity coefficients are reported, the test should be both reliable and objective at a high level. However, the directions should specify whether the test should be given with, or without a warm up to maintain consistency.

Face validity can be accepted for this test, but it will be influenced by the sitting height of the examinee. When dealing with individual improvement rather than comparing individuals, sitting height has little impact on the results.

This test is economical in time required for administration and the equipment needed. It is suitable for any age and sex and can be scored by most examinees except those in the lower three or four elementary grades.

Scoring from the sternum to the table top is a little more difficult than from the fingertips to the back of the heels. Smaller children can learn the latter method more quickly.

There are no norms reported for the test when measures are made from the sternum. However, the American Alliance for Health, Physical Education, Recreation and Dance (AAH-PERD) and the President's Council for Physical Fitness and Sports (PCPFS) have developed norms for the Sit and Reach Test and the Modified Sit-Reach Test where measuring is done from the fingers.

SUMMARY

Major Strengths:

1. The test is easy to administer and takes little time or equipment.
2. It is applicable to all ages and both sexes.

Major Weaknesses:

1. There are no norms when measures are taken from the sternum.

2. Short sitting height results in a more positive score.

This is an excellent test for research when there are no comparisons to be made between individuals. The results can be used for determining individual improvement and for comparing similar groups. Of course, a decision must be made about allowing a warm up prior to testing.

For teaching situations, either of the tests developed by the AAHPERD or the PCPFS should be better because of available norms. Both of these tests are valuable for encouraging students to give attention to flexibility as a part of one's health or sports fitness.

KRAUS-WEBER FLOOR TOUCH TEST

References.

Kraus, H., & Hirschland, R. P. (1954). Minimum muscular fitness tests in school children. *Research Quarterly,* 25(2):178-188.

Willgoose, C. E. (1961). *Evaluation in health education and physical education.* New York: McGraw Hill, pp 153-154.

Additional Sources.

Hastad & Lacy (1989, pp. 212-213); Safrit (1986, pp. 336-337); Safrit (1990, p. 506).

Purpose.

To measure the range of motion in an examinee's back and hip joints.

Objectivity.

Not reported.

Reliability.

Not reported.

Validity.

Not reported.

Age and Sex.

Females and males, children through young adults.

Equipment.

A ruler.

Space Requirements and Design.

A clear, level area approximately 3m (10') square with the examinee in the center.

Directions.

The six Kraus-Weber tests are given on an individual basis. No warm up is permitted. Test 6, the test of the length of back and hamstring muscles, is performed in the following manner. The examinee stands erect in bare feet or in her/his socks, feet together and the hands at the sides of the body. While keeping the knees straight, the examinee leans down slowly and tries to touch the floor with her/his fingertips. The examinee holds the position for a count of three. Bouncing is not permitted.

Scoring.

The touch (T) is given only when the floor touch is held for three seconds. Less than T is marked by the vertical distance between the floor and the fingertips and is recorded as a negative score.

Norms.

Not reported.

REVIEW

B. DON FRANKS, Ph.D.
Professor of Kinesiology
Louisiana State University
Baton Rouge, LA 70803

This test is an indicator of the flexibility of the low back and hamstring muscles. Flexibility of low back and hamstring muscles is one important aspect of a healthy low back - one of the major physical fitness components. This test has content validity and can be administered in a reliable and objective manner. The Sit and Reach Test (AAHPERD, 1988) is the preferred test in this area since it is done in a sitting position, thus reducing pressure on the back. The inclusion of warm up (AAHPERD, 1988) is appropriate both for safety and a more accurate score of flexibility.

This test can be used in any testing situation. It does not require much space, tester skill, or time. The test can be improved by having the examinee sit, rather than stand, and by including a warm up. These modifications have been made in the Sit and Reach Test (AAHPERD, 1988).

SUMMARY

Major Strengths:

1. The test is an indicator of an important aspect of physical fitness.

2. The test can be administered easily in any fitness setting.

Major Weakness:

1. The test is administered to the examinee in the standing position without warm up.

The Kraus-Weber Floor Touch Test is acceptable for those situations where a quick estimate of low back/hamstring muscle flexibility is desired. The Sit and Reach Test with warm up is a better test of low back and hamstring muscle flexibility.

REVIEW REFERENCE

AAHPERD (1988). *Physical Best.* Reston, VA: American Allance for Health, Physical Education, Recreation and Dance.

MODIFIED SIT AND REACH TEST

References.
Johnson, B. L., & Nelson, J. K. (1986). *Practical measurements for evaluation in physical education*. Edina, MN: Burgess, pp 88-89, 455.

Johnson, B. L. (1977). *Practical flexibility measurement with the flexomeasure*. Portland, TX: Brown and Littleman Co.

Additional Sources.
Barrow et al. (1989, pp. 139, 141); Baumgartner & Jackson (1991, p. 250); Hastad & Lacy (1989, pp. 285-286); Kirkendall et al. (1980, pp. 321, 323); Kirkendall et al. (1987, p. 401).

Purpose.
To measure the range of motion in an examinee's hips and back along with extension of the hamstring muscles of the legs.

Objectivity.
r = .99 between the scores of experienced and inexperienced testers.

Reliability.
r = .94 test-retest method.

Validity.
Face validity.

Age and Sex.
Females and males, age 6 - college.

Equipment.
A flexomeasure case, meterstick or yardstick, and tape.

Space Requirements and Design.
A clear, level area approximately 2m (6') square. The meterstick (yardstick) is placed on the floor so that the 38cm (15") mark is even with a line on the floor and the flexomeasure case is face down. Each end of the meterstick (yardstick) is taped to the floor.

Directions.
The examinee sits on the floor and straddles the meterstick (yardstick) with the heels no further than 12.70cm (5") apart. The heels are placed even with the line indicating the 38cm (15") mark. The buttocks are positioned beyond the zero end of the stick. An assistant should stand and brace her/his toes against the examinee's heels while two other assistants hold the knees down to keep them locked. When ready, the examinee slowly stretches forward and uses the fingertips of both hands to push the flexomeasure case as far down the stick as possible. The reading at the near edge of the flexomeasure case is then recorded. The test can also be administered without the use of a flexomeasure case by having the examinee run her/his fingers as far down the meterstick (yardstick) as possible.

Scoring.
The score is the greatest distance reached during the best of three trials measured to the nearest cm (1/4").

Norms.
Alabama (1988, pp. 13-15, 20-21) boys and girls; Barrow et al. (1989, pp. 139-140) men and women; Baumgartner & Jackson (1991, p. 251) men and women; Brown et al. (no date, p. 14) boys and girls; Hastad & Lacy (1989, p. 284) boys and girls;

Hoeger (1989, p. 84) men and women; Johnson & Nelson (1986, p. 89, 455) boys, girls, men and women; Kirkendall et al. (1980, pp. 328-330) boys and girls; Kirkendall et al. (1987, pp. 402-403) boys and girls, normal and special populations;

Miller (1988, p. 234) boys and girls; Pollock & Wilmore (1990, pp. 672-683, 685) men and women; President's Council (1985, pp. 3, 7) boys and girls; President's Council (1989, p. 8) boys and girls; Virginia (1988, pp. 17, 21) boys and girls.

REVIEW

JOYCE GRAENING, D.A.

Assistant Professor
Physical Education
University of Arkansas
Fayetteville, AR 72701

Face validity of this test is accepted because it is assumed that an examinee must have good flexibility in the lower back, hips, and posterior thighs in order to score well. The test appears to be consistent on a repeated trial basis and the directions are clear even to a novice tester. However, this test is dependent upon three assistants: one to brace the examinee's heels and two to lock the examinee's knees down. These assistants could affect the performance of the examinee. The validity and reliability of the test could be improved by giving examinees sufficient instruction and warm up. Warm up should include slow, sustained, static stretching of the lower back and posterior thighs.

This test may be administered using a partner system and with other flexibility tests. Many examinees can be tested within a typical class period. A small area with adequate floor space is all that is needed for testing. Equipment needs are minor. A flexomeasure case could be easily built.

Although this is a reasonably practical test, it is not without problems. Flexibility is measured in centimeters or inches rather than degrees. Performance on the test is somewhat dependent on the ratio of trunk length to lower body length.

The test also allows examinees to reach with one hand ahead of the other if the hands are not held together. Furthermore, it requires little equipment, is inexpensive and easy to administer, and requires little time to administer.

SUMMARY

Major Strengths:

1. Fast and easy to administer.

2. Does not require expensive equipment.

3. Can be administered to both sexes and a wide age range.

4. Has strong reliability and objectivity.

Major Weaknesses:

1. Test is dependent on three assistants.

2. Test is unsuitable for examinees who cannot reach their toes.

Overall, this test is acceptable remembering that it does have dependent variables. Allowances are not made for those examinees who cannot reach their toes or the flexomeasure case and therefore cannot score at all. It appears that a similar test using a sit and reach box might be more appropriate in these cases. The box fits against the wall and allows for a negative score.

SIT AND REACH TEST

References.

AAHPERD (1980). *AAHPERD health related physical fitness test manual.* Reston, VA: American Alliance for Health, Physical Education, Recreation and Dance, pp 19-21, 34-35.

AAHPERD (1984). *AAHPER technical manual: Health related physical fitness.* Reston, VA: American Alliance for Health, Physical Education, Recreation and Dance, pp 23-24.

Wells, K. F., & Dillon, E. K. (1952). The sit and reach - A test of back and leg flexibility. *Research Quarterly,* 23(1):115-118.

Additional Sources.

Barrow et al. (1989, pp. 107, 110-111, 143); Baumgartner & Jackson (1982, pp. 264-266); Baumgartner & Jackson (1987, pp. 300-302, 305); Baumgartner & Jackson (1991, pp. 281-283, 287); Bosco & Gustafson (1983, pp. 109-110);

Clarke & Clarke (1987, p. 173); Hastad & Lacy (1989, pp. 209-212, 231, 234-235, 237); Johnson & Nelson (1986, pp. 86-88, 457); Kirkendall et al. (1980, pp. 250, 299-300); Kirkendall et al. (1987, pp. 126, 169-170); Miller (1988, p. 157); Safrit (1986, pp. 241-244); Safrit (1990, pp. 372-376, 506); Verducci (1980, pp. 257, 282).

Purpose.

To measure the range of motion (flexion) in an examinee's hips and trunk.

Objectivity.

Not reported.

Reliability.

r = .84 to r = .98 with one exception being r = .70 (AAHPERD, 1984, p. 24).

Validity.

Logical validity and r = .90 correlated with the standing-bobbing test (Wells & Dillon, 1952, p. 118).

Age and Sex.

Females and males, age 5 - adult.

Equipment.

A sit and reach box, 30.5cm x 30.5cm x 30.5cm (12" x 12" x 12") with a 53cm (21") long scale attached on top. The scale is marked off in centimeters with the 23cm mark even with one side of the box.

Space Requirements and Design.

A clear, level area approximately 2m (6') square near a wall with the sit and reach box positioned against the wall.

Directions.

The examinee sits on the floor with the knees straight and the feet shoulder width apart. The feet are pressed firmly against the sit and reach box. The examinee extends the arms with the palms downward and one hand on top of the other in a forward horizontal motion along the top of the scale. While using this movement, the examinee bobs forward four times and holds the maximum reach position on the fourth forward movement. At this point the score is recorded. During the test, the knees must remain straight, the hands must remain even and the position of maximum reach must be held for one second.

Scoring.

The score is the most distant point touched, measured to the nearest centimeter (1/2").

Norms.

Alabama (1988, pp. 13-15, 22-23) boys and girls; Alexander et al. (1985, p. 9) Canadian women; American Alliance (1980, pp. 34-35) boys and girls; American Alliance & Pate (1985, pp. 11-13, 17, 20-21) college men and women; American Alliance (1988, pp. 28-29) boys and girls; American Alliance (1990, pp. 10-11) boys and girls;

Arizona Association (1983, pp. 3-28) boys and girls; Barrow et al. (1989, pp. 105, 130, 143) boys, girls, men and women; Baumgartner & Jackson (1982, pp. 265-266) boys and girls; Baumgartner & Jackson (1987, p. 301) boys and girls; Baumgartner & Jackson (1991, pp. 267, 282, 287-289) boys and girls; Beunen et al (1988, pp. 35, 84, 96) boys; Canadian Association (1985, p. 9) women;

Canadian Minister (1979, p. 20) men and women; Chrysler - AAU (1990, p. 6) boys and girls; Clarke & Clarke (1987, p. 162) boys and girls; Corbin & Lindsey (1983, p. 85) age and sex not stated; Corbin & Lindsey (1985, p. 67) men and women;

Fitness Canada (1986, p. 38) boys, girls, men and women; Fitness Institute (1981, no page number) boys, girls, men and women; Franks (1989, pp. 42-47) boys and girls; Getchell (1983, p. 50) men and women; Greenberg & Pargman (1989, p. 81) men and women;

Harrison & Bradbeer (1982, pp. 24-25) boy and girl athletes; Hastad & Lacy (1989, p. 211) boys and girls; Hoeger (1986, p. 48) men and women; Jackson & Ross (1986, p. 33) men and women; Johnson & Nelson (1986, pp. 88, 203-205, 458) boys, girls, men and women;

Kirkendall et al. (1987, pp. 126, 174) boys, girls, men and women; Lindsey et al. (1989, p. 9) men and women; Maryland (1986, p. 16) boys and girls; Miller (1988, p. 159) boys and girls; Ostyn et al. (1980, pp. 99, 127-140) boys; Prentice & Bucher (1988, p. 159) men and women; President's Council (1988, pp. 3, 7) boys and girls;

President's Council (1989, p. 8) boys and girls; Pyke (1985, p. 10) boys and girls; Rhode Island (1989, pp. 23-26) boys and girls; Ross et al. (1985, p. 65) boys and girls; Ross et al (1987, p. 68) boys and girls; Safrit (1986, p. 243, Appendix A-37) boys and girls; Safrit (1990, pp. 342, 345, 347, 352, 374-376, Appendix A-38) boys and girls; Simons et al. (1990, pp. 103, 129, 142-145) girls; South Carolina (1983, pp. 15, 30-38) boys, girls, men and women; Stephens et al. (1986, p. 15) men and women; Stokes et al. (1986, p. 169) men and women; Stone (1987, pp. 75-76) age and sex not stated; Van Gelder & Marks (1987, p. 190) men and women; Virginia (1988, pp. 41-42) boys and girls; Zuti & Corbin (1977, p. 499) men and women.

REVIEW

ROBERT KOSLOW, P.E.D.

Chair and Professor
Physical Education and Sport
James Madison University
Harrisonburg, VA 22807

The Sit and Reach Test has commonly been used to assess flexibility of the lower back and hamstrings. Although this test has been readily accepted as a measurement tool, there does exist some concerns regarding several aspects of the test. The question has been raised concerning the validity of the Sit and Reach Test as it relates to torso/limb ratios. However, problems seem to arise in only those cases where outlying ratios exist (Jackson & Baker, 1986). A more alarming factor to be considered stems from the fact that, for years, the test was considered to have logical validity. Jackson and Baker (1986), in an attempt to examine relationships between test scores and measures of lower back and hamstring flexibility, found a moderate relationship between sit and reach scores and measures of hamstring flexibility, and a very low relationship between test scores and lower back flexibility. Therefore, any judgements concerning lower back flexibility and Sit and Reach Test scores must be made with caution.

It has been hypothesized that the amount of pretest stretching can become a factor in the assessment of reliability and objectivity. However, there exists limited research which has examined potential confounding due to fluctuations in warm up procedures. More data is needed in order to assess the objectivity of the Sit and Reach Test. Some concern can be expressed about the number of pretest trials (three) allowed. No evidence was found to support this number of pretest trials. Thus, one can only speculate as to the effects of the three pretest trials on performance. Reliability measures pertaining to examinees four years of age through adulthood are in the acceptable range.

The Sit and Reach Test is a reasonably easy test to administer. The test apparatus (a measuring box constructed to specific dimensions as expressed in the AAHPERD Test Manual) can be purchased or constructed by the tester. A single tester can handle all testing procedures with little difficulty. The amount of time needed to administer the test can become burdensome due to the fact that a specific piece of equipment is needed. Thus, the testing is done one examinee at a time. The quality of each examinee's performance may be easily monitored by the tester, thus assuring accurate and reliable data.

SUMMARY

Major Strengths:

1. National norms are current and readily available through the AAHPERD.

2. The test is relatively easy to administer.

3. There is limited need for equipment. Thus, this test is often an included segment of overall fitness assessment.

Major Weaknesses:

1. It has not been proven that this test should be considered an acceptable measure of lower back and hamstring flexibility. If the test is used, caution must be employed when interpreting just what muscle groups are being assessed.

2. There is a possibility of problems associated with the objectivity of the test.

3. There is a potential for confoundment due to uncontrolled pretest warm up activities.

If the ability to reach past one's feet while keeping the legs extended is considered an important aspect of fitness, then the Sit and Reach Test is an appropriate measurement tool. In sum, the Sit and Reach Test has been commonly deemed an acceptable means of assessing flexibility.

REVIEW REFERENCES

AAHPERD (1980). *AAHPERD health related fitness manual.* Reston, VA: American Alliance for Health, Physical Education, Recreation and Dance.

Jackson, R., & Baker, A. (1986). The relationship of the sit and reach test to criterion of hamstring and back flexibility in young females. *Research Quarterly for Exercise and Sport,* 57(3):183-186.

KNEE LINEAR MEASUREMENT FLEXIBILITY TEST

KNEE FLEXION TEST

Reference.
Tomita, P. H. (1989). Take the flex test. *Shape,* 8(11):88-89.

Additional Sources.
None.

Purpose.
To measure the range of flexion in an examinee's knee joint.

Objectivity.
Not reported.

Reliability.
Not reported.

Validity.
Not reported.

Age and Sex.
Not reported, but suitable for females and males, age 6 - adult.

Equipment.
Ruler.

Space Requirements and Design.
A clear, level surface approximately 2m (6') square with the examinee in the center.

Directions.
The examinee assumes a prone position with the left knee bent. With the help of the tester, the examinee's left ankle is moved toward her/his buttocks until a slight resistance is felt. The vertical distance between the edge of the heel and the buttocks is then measured by the tester. The examinee cannot lift the buttocks or arch the lower back during the test. The procedures are repeated for the right leg.

Scoring.
The score is the vertical distance between the examinee's heel of the foot and the buttocks. The score is recorded as a negative number. If the examinee's heel touches the buttocks, it is recorded as a zero.

Norms.
Not reported.

REVIEW

JACQUELINE A. DAILEY, Ed.D.
Program Coordinator
Health, Physical Education and
Recreation
University of Wisconsin-Whitewater
Whitewater, WI 53190

This is but one of five flexibility tests included in Tomita's (1989) Flex Test program suggested to "help maintain freedom of movement," (p. 88). What is not made clear is why one would need to have flexibility of the knee (quadriceps) - the test constructor notes that the function of the quadriceps is to extend the knee and this test measures flexion. The Knee Flexion Test is a measure of static flexibility, not dynamic flexibility as commonly defined in the literature. It would seem that a dynamic measure would be much more appropriate here for both the aerobic exerciser and/or strength trainer. Further, it is an indirect measure of static flexibility in that the score is obtained through linear movement. Acceptable test-retest reliability coefficients can never be achieved with such imprecise measurement along with the fact that performance on this test can be significantly improved with practice. The establishment of objectivity will also suffer in that no exact degree of measurement in inches (i.e., to the nearest 1/4 in.) is required. Having an assistant stretching and measuring will also impact on objectivity.

The space and equipment requirements of the test do not seem to pose problems. Test design and directions, however, pose several problems for the tester. First, as with any flexibility test, a thorough warm up must be provided. The test constructor suggests these tests should be performed after the workout, succeeding the cool down stretch. The major limitation to both static and dynamic flexibility has been found to be the tightness of soft tissue structures (Heyward, 1984), 57% of which are composed of nonelastic connective tissue. Thus, waiting this long to ensure adequate warm up and stretching out procedures seems to be carrying things a bit too far.

Second, with safety of the knee in mind, the assistant/tester who is to take the measurements is encouraged to use gentle movements and not to force the stretch beyond the natural, comfortable range of motion. Certainly, this would not be the same for everyone. This action has been seriously questioned by Lindsey and Corbin (1989) because of the stress put on the knee joint. An added element of stress could enter here with an assistant doing the stretching and the measuring. None of the other tests in the battery requires such an action.

An equally serious consideration is that the examinee's gluteal size would influence performance on this test - another problem with linear measurement. Those examinees less endowed would exhibit more negative inches. Fourth, there is no mention of more than one trial being assessed. Most all published tests for static flexibility require the administration of three trials and the recording of the best score.

Suggested procedures for the administration of this test within the battery seem inappropriate. A suggestion to rectify this would be to administer the battery after the warm up and stretch out, but prior to the workout. A test alternative would be to observe participants exercising in all five areas of concern (i.e., the shoulders, hip flexors and adductors, quadriceps, lower back, and hamstrings) with appropriate prescription to follow.

Since the Knee Flexion Test, as described by the test constructor, is a field test of static flexibility, it obviously is not intended to meet the scientific rigor demanded of the researcher. Of utmost concern for the general practitioner is determining whether this test is a necessary component of the battery. If it is, establishing the desired criterion levels of performance for the intended examinees would come next. No norms or criterion levels have been established for the test.

SUMMARY

Major Strengths:

1. This test of static flexibility requires no special equipment.

2. Significant improvement may be noted in a short period of time.

Major Weaknesses:

1. Physical activities require activity specific types of flexibility, the validity of which must be statistically established.

2. This test is not reliable (stability) because of the learning effect, test length (one trial), and lack of consideration for the buttocks size in assessment.

3. Objectivity for this test cannot be established due to its reliance on linear measurement and the influence of the tester.

4. Other factors that may be involved in static flexibility (e.g., strength and balance) have yet to be identified.

5. This test is not sophisticated enough for the laboratory researcher to use - tests using the Leighton flexometer (a direct measurement taken in degrees) offer much more promise.

An unacceptable test for the practical assessment of abilities in specific activities requiring the measurement of the capacity of a joint to move fluidly through its full range of motion as described by the test constructor. Because scores on this test are not absolutes, they cannot be used to predict, classify, or diagnose. The establishment of this test's validity is the first priority for its user.

REVIEW REFERENCES

Heyward, V. H. (1984). *Designs for fitness: A guide to physical fitness appraisal and exercise prescription*. Minneapolis, MN: Burgess Publishing Company.

Lindsey, R., & Corbin, C. (1989). Questionable exercises - Some safe alternatives. *Journal of Physical Education, Recreation and Dance*, 60(8):26-32.

SHOULDER LINEAR MEASUREMENT FLEXIBILITY TESTS

SHOULDER FLEXIBILITY TEST

Reference.
Scott, M. G., & French, E. (1959). *Measurement and evaluation in physical education.* Dubuque: Wm. C. Brown, pp 318-319.

Additional Sources.
None.

Purpose.
To measure the range of motion in an examinee's shoulder joint using three different test items.

Objectivity.
Not reported.

Reliability.
r = .81 for each arm in the "Reach Down the Back," r = .88 for the right arm and r = .83 for the left arm in the "Reach Across the Chest and Down" and r = .94 for the right arm and r = .96 for the left arm in the "Opposite Arm Across the Chest" by Nicoloff (1955), cited in Scott and French (1959, pp. 318-319).

Validity.
Not reported.

Age and Sex.
Not reported, but suitable for females and males, age 6 - adult.

Equipment.
A felt tip marker and a ruler.

Space Requirements and Design.
A clear, level area approximately 2m (6') square that includes a projecting wall, corner, or a vertical pole.

Directions.
Before the testing is initiated, the prominence of the seventh cervical vertebra is marked on the examinee's back with a felt tip marker.

Reach Down the Back :

The examinee stands with the left hand on the hip and her/his nose, chest, and abdomen against the projecting corner. The examinee then raises the right arm over the right shoulder and extends it down along the spine as far as possible in a steady movement while keeping the shoulders horizontal. This position is held until the vertical distance from the seventh cervical vertebra to the end of the fingertips is measured. The same procedure is repeated with the left arm.

The score is the vertical distance from the seventh cervical vertebra to the end of the fingertip farthest down the back measured to the nearest .5cm (1/4").

Reach Across the Chest and Down:

The examinee stands erect and extends the right arm over the left shoulder and down the back as far as possible. The vertical distance is measured between the mark on the seventh cervical vertebra and the end of the fingertip furthest down the back. The same procedure is repeated with the left arm.

The score is the vertical distance between the seventh cervical vertebra and the end of the fingertip furthest down the back measured to the nearest .5cm (1/4").

Opposite Arm Across Back :

The examinee stands facing the projecting corner or vertical pole with her/his nose, sternum, and abdomen touching. Raising the right arm and bending the elbow, the examinee reaches across the back as far as possible. Simultaneously the left arm is brought behind the back and with the elbow bent up the back, an effort is made to touch the fingers of one hand with the fingers of the other hand. A measurement of the vertical distance between the middle fingers is then taken. Overlapping of the fingers results in a plus score while failing to touch the fingers together results in a negative score. A zero score is recorded if the ends of the fingers just touch. The test is repeated with the positions of the arms reversed.

The score is the vertical distance measured to the nearest .5cm (1/4").

Scoring.

See each of the three tests presented above.

Norms.

Corbin & Lindsey (1985, p. 67) men and women; Greenberg & Pargman (1989, p. 81) men and women.

REVIEW

CONNIE FOX, Ed.D.

Assistant Professor
Physical Education
Northern Illinois University
DeKalb, IL 60115

The test appears to have face validity in terms of measuring shoulder flexibility. The test actually consists of three measurements at three different angles for both sides of the body. It is important to note that there is not a single test of flexibility, but the measurement is specific to the joint. Also, joints on opposite sides of the body may differ in range of motion. While shoulder flexibility is not a high priority for fitness, it may be important to measure for sport potential.

The test has marginal reliability for all but the third angle tested, "reach opposite arm across the chest."

No estimates of objectivity are reported. Due to the directions of the test, the inaccuracy of locating the correct vertebra, and of the inability of examinees to hold the reach, objectivity is suspect.

Space and equipment requirements are not difficult, except for the requirement of a projecting corner. This concept is not understood. Some care must be taken to assure that examinees do not lean while being tested.

The test does require marking on the back of the examinee and of measuring a distance below the mark. This seems to call for a dress requirement of perhaps a bathing suit. One tester must measure the entire group, so the process may be slow.

The test is not suitable for a drill, but may be appropriate for partner stretches during warm up or cool down. It appears to be suitable for all

school age children. Caution should be taken when measuring inflexible adults or following injury.

Scoring is as objective as the directions allow. It may be difficult to accurately mark the vertebra and to measure a reach to a shoulder instead of along the spine. It is not clear whether the score is the distance between the vertebra and the fingertip or if the score is the difference between the vertebra and the fingertip height moved in a horizontal line to the lowest vertebra (absolute distance or distance in a vertical direction along the spine). It would seem that the length of the fingers would have an impact on the score.

The test is not recommended for research purposes, nor for self evaluation since it cannot be self administered. The "opposite arm across back" may be an exception.

SUMMARY

Major Strengths:

1. The test examines the specific shoulder joint when flexibility of that joint is of importance.
2. Also, the use of three angles has the potential to measure the angle of most importance.

Major Weaknesses:

1. It is not clear that there is a need to measure this shoulder flexibility. Perhaps another test can predict this flexibility.
2. The lack of objectivity is of concern. Inaccuracy of locating the measuring point and of locating the reach point introduces error.
3. Influence of finger length introduces more error, further reducing objectivity.

Overall, the test is unacceptable for use in research and in teaching. An exception would be the third test (opposite arm across back) used for stretching before or after exercise. The other two tests may be used for partner stretches. Another possible use for the test is for athletes in sports where shoulder flexibility is highly desired. The use of the test for conditioning the shoulder is acceptable. The test may have some value in a sports rehabilitation program following an injury.

SHOULDER FLEXIBILITY FACTOR TEST

Reference.
Greipp, J. F. (1982). The assessment of shoulder flexibility. *Pennsylvania Journal of Health, Physical Education and Recreation,* Fall, pp 19-20.

Additional Sources.
None.

Purpose.
To measure range of motion in an examinee's shoulder joints.

Objectivity.
Not reported.

Reliability.
Not reported.

Validity.
r = .97 between the shoulder flex factor test and angle degree measurements of the shoulder.

Age and Sex.
Females and males, age not reported.

Equipment.
An incline bench and a tape measure or a folding carpenter's rule. The incline bench should be approximately 28cm (11") wide with a minimum height of 71cm (28") at the high end and a minimum height of 58cm (23") at the low end. The bench should be long enough for an examinee to lie on in a supine position.

Space Requirements and Design.
A clear, level area approximately 3m (10') square with the incline bench and the examinee in the center.

Directions.
The examinee assumes a supine position with her/his head on the higher end of the incline bench. The examinee's arms should be held straight out to the sides parallel to the floor, with palms down (i.e., facing the floor). The examinee then permits the arms to fall toward the floor without undue pain. The arms must be maintained perpendicular to the trunk (i.e., abducted 90 degrees) when the measurement is taken. When the examinee is unable to move the arms closer to the floor (i.e., closer together), a measurement is taken. With the use of a tape measure or a folding carpenter's rule, the distance between the wrists is measured to the nearest cen-

timeter (1/4") at the styloid processes (i.e., the prominent bumps) on the little finger side of the wrists. To adjust for the differences in arm length among examinees, the height of the examinee is measured.

Scoring.
The score is the distance measured between the wrists divided by the standing height of the examinee. This score is the shoulder flex factor. To convert the shoulder flex factor to degrees, the following formula is used:

Angle in Degrees = (264 x shoulder flex factor) - 74.23.

Norms.
Not reported.

REVIEW

JIMMY H. ISHEE, Ph.D.

Associate Professor
Physical Education
University of Central Arkansas
Conway, AR 72032

Flexibility does not exist as a general characteristic; thus, great differences can occur within a single individual at various joints. This need for specific tests of flexibility and appropriate interpretation is well documented in the literature. This test, similar to other flexibility tests, does not possess a high degree of validity as a measure of general flexibility.

The test uses a relative approach to the measurement of flexibility by incorporating the height of the examinee in the scoring procedure. This is a commonly used technique in evaluating flexibility when absolute standards are not necessary. Evidence of validity is presented in the form of a relationship between the test and angle degree measurements of shoulder flexibility. There was a substantial correlation between the two measures of shoulder flexibility. There are no indices of reliability nor objectivity provided for the test. It is important to note that a test cannot be a valid measure unless it is reliable. Due to this, the validity estimate of the test is questionable.

The test requires minimum space and equipment and can be administered by a single tester. The time to administer the test is relatively short but only one examinee can be tested at a time. The test directions do not indicate the number of trials that should be performed. Warm up would probably have a significant effect upon an examinee's scores. In flexibility tests, a number of trials are typically used to facilitate warm up and guard against injury. The test would be suitable for both sexes but difficult for some age groups. Self scoring would not be possible and the lack of normative data limits interpretation of the test scores.

SUMMARY

Major Strength:

1. Requires minimum space and equipment.

Major Weaknesses:

1. Questionable validity.

2. Absence of reported reliability or objectivity indices.

3. Lack of clarity regarding trials, warm up, and procedures.

4. Absence of reported normative data.

The Shoulder Flexibility Factor Test is an unacceptable test for research or teaching purposes. No test should be employed until all areas of reliability, objectivity, and validity have been addressed. Interpretation of the results would be limited by the lack of normative data. Further investigations are necessary into these areas before this test should be used in practical settings.

SHOULDER FLEXIBILITY - HORIZONTAL ABDUCTION TEST

Reference.
Jensen, C. R., & Hirst, C. C. (1980). *Measurement in physical education and athletics*. New York: MacMillan, pp 118-119.

Additional Sources.
None.

Purpose.
To measure the range of horizontal abduction in an examinee's shoulder joints.

Objectivity.
Not reported.

Reliability.
Not reported.

Validity.
Not reported.

Age and Sex.
Not reported, but suitable for females and males, age 6 - adult.

Equipment.
Tape measure.

Space Requirements and Design.
A clear, level area approximately 3m (10') square located next to a wall.

Directions.
The examinee stands with her/his back against the wall. The arms are raised to a horizontal position with the palms forward. The examinee then moves away from the wall as far as possible while simultaneously horizontally abducting the arms. Throughout the test the arms must remain horizontal and the little fingers must maintain contact with the wall.

Scoring.
The score is the greatest horizontal distance from the wall to the spine at arm level measured to the nearest .5cm (1/4").

Norms.
Not reported.

NOTE: An optional form of this test is as follows. The examinee assumes a sitting position on the floor with her/his back erect and the legs fully extended. The examinee's arms are raised to the side at shoulder height with the palms of the hands facing forward. The examinee then moves the arms back as far as possible. Throughout the test, the trunk must remain erect, the palms must face forward and the arms must remain at shoulder level. The score is the horizontal distance measured between the fingers of the two hands.

REVIEW

BRENDA LICHTMAN, Ph.D.
Associate Professor
Health and Kinesiology
Sam Houston State University
Huntsville, TX 77340

Since no objectivity, validity, or reliability was reported, the scientific aspects of the Shoulder Flexibility-Horizontal Abduction Test are unacceptable. Without norms being available, it is impossible for the users to compare their results with others who are of similar age and gender.

From a practical standpoint the procedures require very little equipment. Unfortunately, the directions are not clear. One of the most troublesome aspects is that left and right sides should be measured independently, as bilateral horizontal flexion might not be present due to unequal use of the shoulder joints. Additionally, it is impossible to horizontally abduct the arms with the little fingers touching the wall while the palms are facing forward.

Most flexibility tests provide some outside resistance or force (e.g., gravity) which the examinee can use to help herself/himself move through the joint's range. Neither is present in these procedures. It is extremely important that the tester not allow the examinee to flex the cervical region of the spine. Should this occur, scores would reflect greater passive flexibility. While the test is said to be appropriate for children as young as six years old, it would seem difficult for an examinee of that age to follow directions explicitly making certain that the arms did not drop from the horizontal. In fact, this judgment adds to the degree of subjectivity the tester must exhibit.

The directions do not specify whether the examinee is permitted to warm up through some type of stretching routine. This would be advisable to prevent cramps from occurring in the rhomboid and trapezius muscles. While no information is provided regarding the number of trials which are to be given, most flexibility tests select the best attempt from two or three trials. Such a procedure should be used when administering this test as the position which the examinee will be trying to achieve is both awkward and unusual.

SUMMARY

Major Strengths:

1. Since no elaborate equipment is required, the test would be feasible in any setting.

2. Logical validity would seem to be present.

3. Even though objectivity was not reported, the scoring requires only a small degree of subjectivity.

Major Weaknesses:

1. No test properties were provided.

2. The directions are unclear. It is impossible to horizontally abduct the arms with the little fingers touching the wall while the palms are facing forward.

3. In both forms of the test, no static resistance, pressure from some outside source or momentum generated through speed of action is used. This is not typical of most flexibility tests. Individuals who possess well developed rhomboid and trapezius muscles would be impeded even though the anterior portion of their shoulder joints are not placed on a significant stretch.

4. Technically, the scoring should reflect the horizontal distance from the little finger to the spine, not from the wall to the spine.

5. Testers should measure this horizontal distance on both the left and right sides independently, as bilateral horizontal flexion might not be present. The term "the greatest horizontal distance" implies this, but it should be stated more directly.

Unacceptable test: Since no test properties were reported, users cannot judge its validity and reliability. The directions are not clear, as, it is impossible to have the little fingers touch the wall while the palms face forward during horizontal abduction. Such a position requires that the shoulders be rotated medially (forward). Examinees must move their arms through horizontal abduction without the assistance of an external static or dynamic resistance. This is not typical of most flexibility tests and seems to discriminate against those who have well developed rhomboid and trapezius muscles. Without external force application, such examinees would have difficulty moving through their full range of horizontal abduction, even though the anterior portion of the shoulder joint would be under relatively little stretch.

SHOULDER ROTATION TEST

References.
Hoeger, W. W. K. (1986). *Lifetime physical fitness and wellness.* Englewood, CO: Morton Publishing Co., pp 51-52.

Johnson, B. L., & Nelson, J. K. (1986). *Practical measurements for evaluation in physical education.* Edina, MN: Burgess, pp 96-97, 456.

Additional Sources.
None.

Purpose.
To measure the range of motion in an examinee's shoulder joints.

Objectivity.
r = .99.

Reliability.
r = .97 for test-retest, (Johnson & Nelson, 1986, p. 96).

Validity.
Face validity.

Age and Sex.
Females and males, all age groups.

Equipment.
A large caliper (or three yardsticks which can be used to construct caliper) and 1.5m (60") measuring tape glued on an aluminum, plastic, or wooden stick. Johnson and Nelson (1986) recommend a rope be used instead of the stick.

Space Requirements and Design.
A clear, level area approximately 3m (10') square with a height clearance of 3m (10') and the examinee in the center.

Directions.
The examinee assumes a standing position with the stick being held behind the back with both hands. The examinee uses a reverse grip (i.e., forearms pronated) to hold the stick with the right hand on the zero mark of the tape and the left hand on the other end of the stick. The examinee must keep the arms straight and attempt to bring the stick over the head, making sure that the grip remains in place and the elbows remain locked. Johnson and Nelson (1986, p. 96) recommend that the examinee begin the test with

the hands gripping the rope in front of the body and then move the rope overhead to a position in back of the body. The examinee is then instructed to repeat the test after moving the left hand in a short distance on the stick. This procedure of decreasing the distance between the hands is continued until the examinee is no longer able to rotate the stick overhead without bending the elbows or modifying the grip. The shortest distance between the two hands is measured to the nearest cm or 1/2".

To obtain the biacromial width, the examinee stands erect with the arms at the sides. The tester places the caliper against the lateral edge of the acromion processes of the shoulders. The horizontal distance between the acromion processes is measured to the nearest cm (.25").

Scoring.
The score is the measurement of the shortest distance on the rotation test minus the biacromial width.

Norms.
Hoeger (1986, p.52) men and women; Hoeger (1989, p. 88) men and women; Johnson & Nelson (1986, pp. 97, 456) boys, girls, men and women.

REVIEW

DALE E. DEVOE, Ph.D.

Associate Professor
Exercise and Sport Sciences
Colorado State University
Fort Collins, CO 80523

Flexibility is a measure of the range of motion available at a joint or group of joints. The concept of flexibility includes both static and dynamic factors. The quantitative assessment of overall flexibility is complicated because flexibility is joint specific. There seems to be relatively little evidence that test scores on one item of flexibility reflect flexibility on another. Concern should exist for the problematic aspects governing flexibility measurements. The Shoulder Rotation Test purports to measure shoulder rotation. Specifically, the test is intended to measure primarily the extent to which the shoulders will rotate with as narrow a grip as possible.

The movements of the shoulder joint are similar as those of the hip joint but with larger magnitudes. In contrast to the hip joint, the shoulder joint sacrifices stability for a remarkable degree of mobility. The movements of the shoulder girdle accompany those of the shoulder joint to increase the range of motion. The assessment of the composite movements of the shoulder complex (i.e., shoulder girdle plus shoulder joint) are complicated due to its musculature. Factors limiting shoulder range of motion vary according to the specific movement (e.g., rotation and abduction). The test is acceptable as a general assessment of medial rotation.

It would be impossible in large group testing to utilize the precise and individual methods of physiological assessment of flexibility. The Shoulder Rotation Test would be time consuming due to the number of trials and difficulty of getting examinees to achieve the correct position, especially elementary school aged children. The test would be of little practical value if administered to preschool aged children.

The stated test-retest reliability provides suitable precision for research purposes and the test's objectivity allows for administration by experienced and inexperienced testers. An adequate number of trials is provided for in the protocol; the facility and space requirements are minimal; the test contains no inherent dangers. Percentile norms are published, based on the scores of 100 college men and 100 college women. There is a need for more comprehensive norms and scoring scales.

It appears important to determine how the end results of flexibility measurement should be utilized. There is little scientific evidence to indicate how much flexibility is optimal. The relationship between flexibility and proficiency is not exact. However, the test could serve as a motivational device.

Flexibility is viewed as an important health related fitness component. Properly administered, this test has applicability to sport participants (e.g., swimmers) who require shoulder flexibility for powerful strokes. The Shoulder Rotation Test is good; it requires minor specialized equipment which is explained; the action is described; the scoring method is objective, clearly specified, and can be followed simply.

SHOULDER AND WRIST ELEVATION TEST

Reference.
Johnson, B., & Nelson, J. K. (1986). *Practical measurements for evaluation in physical education.* Edina, MN: Burgess, pp 91-94, 456-458.

Additional Sources.
Bosco & Gustafson (1983, p. 107); Miller (1988, pp. 160-162).

Purpose.
To measure the range of flexion in an examinee's shoulder joints and the range of extension in the wrist joints.

Objectivity.
r = .99 experienced tester correlated with an inexperienced tester.

Reliability.
r = .93 test-retest method.

Validity.
Face validity was accepted.

Age and Sex.
Females and males, age 6 - college.

Equipment.
Flexomeasure case with a meterstick (yardstick) and ruler guide inserted and an extra meterstick (yardstick). The flexomeasure case and ruler guide should be positioned close to the zero end of the meterstick (yardstick).

Space Requirements and Design.
A clear, level area approximately 3m (10') square with the examinee in the center.

Directions.
The examinee assumes a prone position with her/his arms fully extended overhead. The examinee then grips the extra meterstick (yardstick) with the hands about shoulder width apart. The examinee raises the stick upward as high as possible through flexion at the shoulders and extension at the wrists while keeping the chin on the floor and the elbows straight. As the stick is raised, the flexomeasure should be positioned vertically in front of the examinee with the zero end of the meterstick on the floor. When the examinee's arms reach the highest point, the tester raises the case of the flexomeasure upward

until the ruler glide rests under the stick at the midpoint between the hands. The reading to the nearest .5cm (1/4") is taken. Three trials are given.

The tester should then measure the examinee's arm length from the acromion process (i.e., top of the arm at the acromioclavicular joint) to the tip of the middle finger while he/she is standing erect. Using the flexomeasure, the tester places the zero end of the meterstick (yardstick) next to the middle fingertip (as the arm hangs down) and raises the flexomeasure case until the A-B line rests on the acromion process. The reading is taken to the nearest .5cm (1/4").

Scoring.
The score is the examinee's arm length minus the greatest height the arms are raised during the best of three trials. The closer the height the arms are raised to the examinee's arm length, the better the score. A score of zero is perfect.

Norms.
Johnson & Nelson (1986, pp. 94, 456, 458) boys, girls, men and women; Miller (1988, p. 161) men and women; Prentice & Bucher (1988, p. 159) men and women; Stokes et al. (1986, p. 169) men and women.

NOTE: Although some individuals are so flexible that they can move the stick beyond the vertical position, the measurement must be taken at the highest vertical point.

REVIEW

PHYLLIS T. CROISANT, Ph.D.

Associate Professor
Physical Education
Eastern Illinois University
Charleston, IL 61920

This test gives an objective and reliable assessment of an examinee's ability to hyperflex at the shoulder, indicating limitations to range of motion in the sagittal plane. Due to the task of grasping a meterstick, wrist extension is also included with the forward flexion or elevation movement. Scoring is relative to limb length, with an elevation equal to arm length considered to be perfect. This appears to be an arbitrary standard as no norms are available to indicate the amount of shoulder elevation needed by a gymnast or swimmer, for example. Shoulder flexibility required of athletes certainly varies by activity.

The Shoulder and Wrist Elevation Test requires little equipment or space, and is easily administered with minimal training. The test can be given using only two metersticks, if a flexomeasure case is not available (Johnson & Nelson, 1986, pp. 457-458).

Since flexibility is joint specific, this test would be an appropriate assessment tool for individuals involved in activities that require shoulder hyperflexion, such as gymnastics, swimming, and wrestling. The test is somewhat time consuming as examinees are tested individually. However, since shoulder flexibility is not a health-related item and it is unlikely that large groups will be tested, the time element is relatively unimportant.

Warm up exercises or stretching can substantially improve flexibility scores, so examinees should be permitted several practice trials in addition to a general warm up before being tested.

SUMMARY

Major Strengths:

1. It requires little equipment or space.

2. Scores are highly objective with minimal tester training.

3. Scores are reliable provided a warm up is permitted.

Major Weaknesses:

1. Norms are not available for middle school, junior high, and high school age students.

2. Norms are not available for athletes, such as gymnasts, who really are the population of interest.

Coaches and teachers will find the Shoulder and Wrist Elevation Test an acceptable measure for evaluating shoulder flexibility of students and athletes, and for determining changes due to training or injury.

SPINAL COLUMN LINEAR MEASUREMENT FLEXIBILITY TESTS

BRIDGE-UP TEST

References.
Johnson, B. L., & Nelson, J. K. (1986). *Practical measurements for evaluation in physical education.* Edina, MN: Burgess, pp 88-90, 455, 458-459.

Johnson, B. L. (1977). *Practical flexibility measurement with the flexomeasure.* Portland, TX: Brown and Littleman Co.

Additional Sources.
Jensen & Hirst (1980, p. 121).

Purpose.
To measure the range of motion in an examinee's spine during a backward movement.

Objectivity.
r = .99 between the scores of an experienced tester and an inexperienced tester.

Reliability.
r = .97 for test-retest method.

Validity.
Face validity is admissible when the examinee has enough strength to extend the body from the floor.

Age and Sex.
Females and males, age 6 - college.

Equipment.
A mat and a flexomeasure case with a meterstick (yardstick) and ruler guide inserted. The flexomeasure case and ruler guide should be positioned closest to the zero end of the stick.

Space Requirements and Design.
A clear, level area approximately 3m (10') square with the mat and the examinee in the center.

Directions.
The examinee assumes a supine position on the mat. When ready, the examinee tilts the head back and begins arching the back while walking the hands and feet toward each other. During the arching movement, the thumbs should be next to the ears. The head may remain on the mat if needed. The tester then places the flexomeasure at the side of the examinee and slides the flexomeasure case upward until the ruler guide contacts the highest point of the arched back. The score is recorded. After three such trials, the examinee assumes a standing position and the tester measures the height of the examinee's navel from the floor.

Scoring.
The score is the best of three trials measured to the nearest centimeter (1/4") subtracted from the height of the examinee's navel. The smaller the difference between the measured height of the navel and the arch, the better the score.

Norms.
Johnson & Nelson (1986, pp. 90, 455, 459) boys, girls, men and women.

REVIEW

CYNTHIA B. BOOK, Ph.D.
Field Research Manager
American Guidance Service
Circle Pines, MN 55014-1796

The purpose of the Bridge-Up Test (Johnson, 1977) is to measure the range of motion of the spine in a backward movement. At face value, the test would seem to measure hyperextension of the spine; however, arm strength (i.e., the ability to raise the body from the floor) and lack of shoulder flexibility could greatly affect the results of the test. Likewise, the position of the head during the backbend might alter the detection of back flexibility; backbend performance is enhanced when the head and neck are also hyperextended. It is unclear whether the alternate method of arching the back while keeping the head on the mat produces results equivalent to the original test. Future research might address the possibility of attaining equal or greater back hyperextension when the head is on the mat and the factors of arm strength and shoulder flexibility are eliminated. It would also be interesting to see radiographic pictures of an "excellent" backbend in order to determine exactly what areas of the spine where involved in the performance and to what degree.

The coefficients provided for reliability and objectivity of the Bridge-Up Test are satisfactory but it is not known if they apply to all age groups and both genders. While the test directions do not include the involvement of another individual in the performance of the test, it would be wise to have someone spot the examinee throughout the backbend. Younger or weaker examinees could become disoriented or simply lack the strength to maintain the testing position and fall.

The actual performance and scoring of the test does not require excessive space, complicated measurement, or tricky recording. While most institutions will have mats or padded areas on which to perform the test, ownership of the flexomeasure is unlikely. The recommended alternative to the flexomeasure is to measure the distance between the hands and feet during the backbend but no information is provided as to the validity of this alternative as it would greatly simplify the measurement procedure.

The Bridge-Up Test is both easy and quick to administer but not feasible for mass testing as examinees are evaluated one at a time. Only one tester is required to administer the test and no special expertise is necessary. If a physical educator were team teaching or had assistants available, the test could be made a station on a circuit.

The directions for administration of the test need clarification on a number of points. First, the feet of the examinee should remain flat on the floor so that no advantage is gained in raising the height of the spine. Second, the tester should be reminded to keep the flexomeasure perpendicular to the floor when measuring the highest point of the arched spine. Third, no guidance is provided as to the rounding of the measure to the nearest quarter-inch; does one round up or down? Last, the tester should be instructed to measure as quickly as possible for safety reasons.

Three trials are recommended but no information is provided as to how that number was chosen. It would be of value to know if or what trend exists across a larger number of trials.

Perhaps two or three trials are necessary for warm up and the actual measurements should be on trials four, five, and six, for example.

The complete administration and scoring of the Bridge-Up Test is not suitable for a classroom drill. However, having students safely practice backbends as a drill for improvement of form and strength is perfectly acceptable.

That the test is recommended for both genders, ages six through college, seems reasonable. Norms which are 12 years old are provided for college age examinees and an adequate amount of discrimination exists among users. The existence of norms for the younger age groups is not known.

While examinees cannot physically score themselves, the test is useful for self evaluation of progress. For example, a gymnast might test herself/himself at the beginning, middle, and end of a season and chart improvement in flexibility.

The test is not of suitable precision for research purposes. The validity of the test is too questionable and the measurement procedure lacks precision.

SUMMARY

Major Strengths:

1. The test appears to be reliable and objective.

2. The test is easy to administer and score.

3. The test may be a good tool for motivating and measuring improvement of flexibility for individual students or members of a sport team.

Major Weaknesses:

1. The validity of the test is questionable.

2. There is probably limited availability of a flexomeasure at most institutions.

3. The test is not suited for mass testing in the classroom.

4. Older norms exist for college age examinees only. More precautions are necessary to make the test safe.

The Bridge-Up Test is an unacceptable test and is inadequate for research and/or teaching. The questionable validity of the test is the most prominent concern. The test is not conducive to mass testing and the norms are old and incomplete for the recommended age groups.

FLEISHMAN EXTENT FLEXIBILITY TEST

Reference.
Fleishman, E. A. (1964B). *The structure and measurement of physical fitness.* Englewood Cliffs: Prentice Hall, pp 78, 111, 128, 134, 161-162.

Additional Sources.
Bosco & Gustafson (1983, pp. 110-111).

Purpose.
To measure the range of rotation in an examinee's spine.

Objectivity.
Not reported.

Reliability.
r = .90.

Validity.
Construct validity was established.

Age and Sex.
Suitable for females and males, age 8 - adult.

Equipment.
Marking tape and a meterstick (yardstick).

Space Requirements and Design.
A clear, level area approximately 2m (6') square located next to a wall. Using the marking tape, a vertical line is made on the wall and continued on the floor perpendicular to the wall. The meterstick (yardstick) is then taped on the wall parallel to the floor with the 30cm (12") mark even with the left edge of the tape line on the wall. The 0 to 30cm (0-12") are positioned to the left of the tape when measuring the right arm and to the right of the tape when measuring with left arm. The meterstick (yardstick) is placed at the height of each examinee's shoulder.

Directions.
The examinee stands, her/his non preferred side next to the wall at a distance of an arm's length with the hand in a fist. The feet are positioned together and parallel to the wall. When ready, the examinee raises her/his preferred arm (i.e., the arm the greatest distance from the wall) to the side until it is parallel to the floor. The palm of the hand should face the floor and the fingers

should be together and fully extended. The examinee then twists back (i.e., clockwise with the right hand and counterclockwise with the left hand) around as far as possible and attempts to touch the meterstick with the outside hand at shoulder level. One practice trial and one legal trial are given.

Scoring.
The score is the greatest distance reached and held for two seconds on the meterstick (yardstick).

Norms.
Fleishman (1964B, p. 111) boys and girls; Fleishman (1964A, p. 45) boys and girls; Hoeger (1986, p. 50) men and women; Hoeger (1989, p. 86) men and women.

REVIEW

KATHLEEN MILLER, Ph.D.
Professor
Health and Physical Education
Associate Dean, School of Education
University of Montana
Missoula, MT 59812

The Fleishman Extent Flexibility Test (FEFT) was originally called the Twist and Touch Test and was one of three tests factored out as Extent Flexibility (Factor V) in a large factor analysis study. This test was retained as the single test used to measure "extent" flexibility, but as such, suggests measuring rotation of the spine and not the broader purpose of "trunk and back flexibility in a forward, lateral, or backward direction."

The FEFT is valid in that it is a measure of flexibility, but is not valid in that it measures much more than the stated purpose. Fleishman (1964B, p. 78) says the test is a measure of rotation of the spine.

The FEFT appears to be a reliable measure and does not require the active participation of another individual. No evidence was presented nor found which established objectivity.

Equipment and space requirements do not cause a problem. The test is relatively easy to administer, can be done with one tester and does not require an excessive amount of time. The use of a practice trial is good, but it may be better to use the best of three trials rather than just one. The test, as proposed, is not suitable for use as a conditioning drill. Age/gender norms are provided, but they were established in 1964, and are therefore, not current.

The FEFT appears suitable for the age and ability levels for which it is intended and the norms presented indicate the test discriminates by age and by gender. The test is not inherently dangerous, but anyone who has a medial, lateral, or anterior cruciate ligament problem in the knee might experience discomfort and would therefore be limited in the amount of turn possible.

The scoring is objective and examinees could use the test for self evaluation. However, the test is not suitable for research purposes. Too many factors are not controlled and the validity of the results must be seriously questioned.

SUMMARY

Major Strength:

1. Ease of administration.

Major Weaknesses:

1. Questionable validity.

2. Out of date norms.

The FEFT is an unacceptable test. It is inadequate for research and/or teaching because of its questionable validity. The test purports to measure rotation of the spine. However, the FEFT, as proposed, measures much more, such as horizontal shoulder abduction and pelvic rotation. The test does not take into consideration that because of anatomical structures, there is a large amount of rotation (approximately 92 degrees) available at A/O - C7/T1 vertebrae, only moderate rotation (approximately 49 degrees) at T1/2 - T12/L1 vertebrae, and very little rotation (approximately 12 degrees) at L1/2 - L5/S1 vertebrae. The test does not take into consideration that differences in body types can also limit the amount of spinal rotation possible.

Spinal rotation is more likely to be assessed accurately when other factors such as shoulder flexibility and hip rotation are controlled. Of the tests found in the literature for rotation of the spine, the rotation test suggested by Leighton comes the closest to eliminating shoulder abduction and hip rotation and is still relatively easy to administer.

If the test is to be used as one of many to assess flexibility and is to be self administered, a diagram, such as the one provided in Fleishman's book, should accompany the directions.

REVIEW REFERENCES

Luttgens, K., & Wells, K. F. (1982). *Kinesiology*. Philadelphia: Saunders College Publishing.

Nordin, M., & Frankel, V. H. (1989). *Basic biomechanics of the skeletal system*. Philadelphia: Lea & Febiger.

Paris, S. V. (1979). *The spine: Etiology and treatment of dysfunction*. Manuscript of course notes used in conjunction with a special class.

Rasch, P. J. (1989). *Kinesiology and applied anatomy*. Philadelphia: Lea & Febiger.

Saunders, H. D. (1982). *Evaluation and treatment of musculoskeletal disorders*. Minneapolis: H. D. Saunders.

White, A. A., & Panjabi, M. M. (1978). *Clinical biomechanics of the spine,* Philadelphia: J. B. Lippincott.

TRUNK AND NECK EXTENSION TEST

Reference.
Johnson, B. L., & Nelson, J. K. (1986). *Practical measurements for evaluation in physical education.* Edina, MN: Burgess, pp 94-95, 459-460.

Additional Sources.
Bosco & Gustafson (1987, p. 107); Hastad & Lacy (1989, pp. 213-214); Jensen & Hirst (1980, p. 120); Miller (1988, pp. 158, 160-161); Safrit (1986, pp. 337-338); Safrit (1990, pp. 507-508).

Purpose.
To measure the range of extension in an examinee's trunk and neck.

Objectivity.
r = .99 experienced tester correlated with an inexperienced tester.

Reliability.
r = .90 test-retest method.

Validity.
Face validity was accepted.

Age and Sex.
Females and males, age 6 - college.

Equipment.
A chair and a flexomeasure case with a meterstick (yardstick) and the ruler guide inserted.

Space Requirements and Design.
A clear, level area approximately 3m (10') square with the chair and the examinee in the center.

Directions.
The tester starts by measuring the examinee's trunk and neck length. To do this, the examinee must assume an erect sitting position in the chair with the chin level (i.e., parallel to the floor). The tester then holds the meterstick vertical, placing the zero end between the examinee's legs on the chair seat. Next, the tester raises the flexomeasure case until the bottom of the ruler guide touches the tip of the examinee's nose. The distance is measured to the nearest .5cm (1/4").

The examinee then assumes a prone position on the floor with her/his hands resting at the small of her/his back and raises the trunk upward as high as possible from the floor. A partner should hold the examinee's hips to the floor by placing her/his hands on the back of the examinee's thighs at the base of the buttocks. The tester, located in front, holds the meterstick vertical with the zero end on the floor and slides the flexomeasure case upward until the upper edge of the ruler guide touches the tip of the examinee's nose. The reading is taken to the nearest .5cm (1/4").

Scoring.
The score is the examinee's trunk and neck length minus the greatest height the trunk and neck are raised during the three trials. The closer the height of the trunk and neck approaches the length of the trunk and neck, the better the score. A zero score is recorded when the height of the trunk and neck equals the length of the truck and neck. A score of zero is considered perfect.

Norms.
Alexander et al. (1985, p. 9) Canadian women; Corbin & Lindsey (1983, p. 85) age and sex not stated; Getchell (1983, p. 50) men and women; Greenberg & Pargman (1989, p. 81) men and women;

Miller (1988, p. 160) men and women; Johnson & Nelson (1986, p. 95, 460) men and women; O'Connor & Cureton (1945, p. 314) girls; Prentice & Bucher (1988, p. 159) men and women; Stokes et al. (1986, p. 169) men and women.

REVIEW

R. A. FAULKNER, Ph.D.

Associate Professor
Physical Education
University of Saskatchewan
Saskatoon, CANADA S7N 0W0

This test purports to measure the extension of the trunk and neck; this is only partly true. It is actually a test of active range of movement that involves contraction of the trunk muscles (in particular the lumbar and cervical extensors). Muscular strength of these extensors is a limiting factor in the test.

The test involves an indirect (linear) measure of the movement. There is no indication of how long the examinee needs to hold the extended position in order to accurately complete the measure. This may be a critical factor in examinees with poor muscular strength; that is they simply may not be able to hold the position long enough for the tester to get an accurate measurement.

The correlation between "experienced" and "inexperienced" testers (measure of objectivity) is reported to be higher (.99) than the test-retest correlation (.90). The description of how these tests were conducted is insufficient to evaluate, but the reported results are puzzling.

An attempt has been made to control for anthropometric differences among examinees by interpreting the score relative to measured "trunk and neck" length. In order to assure accuracy of the "trunk and neck" measure, the head should be held in the standard "Frankfurt plane" (Ross et al., 1978) by aligning the tragion of the ear with the orbitale. An examinee with good neck extension could move her/his head far enough posteriorly to move the nose posterior to the perpendicular line. A better landmark would probably be the cervical notch rather than the nose.

There should be some concern about safety in this test for some examinees (particularly adults). Precautions need to be added indicating that those with acute or chronic back pain should not perform the test; and that if any pain is experienced during the test by examinees they should stop immediately.

There is no rationale for the scoring system used. As in most range of movement tests, in general, the greater the range of motion the better; but there is no documentation in the literature to suggest what is the minimal movement required for basic performance and health benefits. It is suggested that lifting one's trunk and neck off the floor to a distance equal to one's trunk and neck length is "perfect." There is absolutely no rationale for this suggestion. This extensive range of motion might, in fact, be considered abnormal - as it would require the examinee to move to a position of almost 90 degrees at the lumbar/sacral joint.

SUMMARY

Major Strengths:

1. The test is relatively simple to do.

2. It will give an indication of active range of motion of the trunk and neck.

3. An attempt is made to control for anthropometric (length) differences among examinees.

Major Weaknesses:

1. The test is not a "valid" test of trunk and neck flexibility, as muscular strength of the back and neck extensors could be limiting factors.

2. Test reliability may be lower in examinees who have relatively "weak" back extensors, and who cannot hold the extended position long enough to get an accurate measure.

3. Back and neck extension can be measured more accurately using direct techniques (Hubley, 1982).

4. There are safety concerns for some examinees.

5. The scoring description is inappropriate.

The test would be an acceptable "field" test providing the description of the test is changed to reflect what it is measuring, safety precautions are added, and the "scoring" system is modified. It is not an adequate test for research purposes because it does not directly measure range of motion.

REVIEW REFERENCES

Hubley, C. (1982). Testing flexibility. *Physiological testing of the elite athlete.* In MacDougall, J. D., Wenger, H. A., & Green, H. J. (eds.). Ithaca, NY: Movement Publications.

Ross, W. D. et al. (1978). *Kinanthropometric landmarks and terminology.* In Shepard, R. J., & Lavallee, H. (eds.). Springfield, IL: Charles C. Thomas, pp. 44-50.

Chapter 7

KINESTHESIS

KINESTHESIS TESTS OF FORCE PRECISION

BALL THROW TEST

Reference.
Jensen, C. R. (1970). Unpublished studies of tests of kinesthetic perception, Brigham Young University.
Jensen, C. R., & Hirst, C. C. (1980). *Measurement in physical education and sports*. New York: Macmillan, pp 172-173.

Additional Sources.
None.

Purpose.
To measure the ability of an examinee to imitate a simple coordination task of throwing a ball a specified distance with the eyes blindfolded.

Objectivity.
Not reported.

Reliability.
Not reported.

Validity.
Not reported.

Age and Sex.
Not reported, but suitable for females and males, age 14 - adult.

Equipment.
A softball, measuring tape, blindfold, and marking tape.

Space Requirements and Design.
A clear, level area approximately 12m x 21m (40' x 70'). An X is marked in the center of the 12m width at one end of the 21m length. A target line is placed 15.24m (50') from the X.

Directions.
The examinee stands on the X in a throwing position. With the ball in the dominant hand and a blindfold over the eyes, the examinee tries to develop a sense of the distance to the target line.

The examinee then throws the ball, attempting to cause it to land on the line 15.24m (50') away. The distance, measured to the nearest .25m (foot), the ball lands from the line is recorded. Three trials are given.

Scoring.
The score is the sum of the distances the ball deviated from the line for the three trials.

Norms.
Not reported.

NOTE: The throwing style (i.e., overhand or underhand) to be used is not specified. Nothing is said about giving practice trials. It seems that several practice trials with the eyes open and several with the eyes closed would enhance the reliability of the test.

REVIEW

DAVID E. BELKA, Ph.D.

Associate Professor
Physical Education
Miami University
Oxford, OH 45056

Published accounts of the Ball Throw Test fail to describe the scientific aspects of validity, reliability, or objectivity. The name of the test does not describe what the test measures.

The Ball Throw Test requires little preparation of the test site, can be explained clearly and briefly, and can be administered easily in a short amount of time by one tester with little experience or training. The testing protocol, as well as the scoring system, is feasible in terms of time and tester experience. It is impossible to determine if the test discriminates among its intended users since no information about the type of user was explained. No norms are included. No explanation about why the test distance was selected is included, nor are general warm up or warm up trials discussed. The type of throw (overhand or underhand) is not specified. No comparison of the scores for the blindfold throw to scores for a throw with eyes open is given. This lack, coupled with no validity information, negates any contention that this test might have significant value.

SUMMARY

Major Strengths:

1. This test is practical in terms of time and ease of administration.

2. The directions are simple to understand.

3. The scoring system is simple to administer and the test may be interesting for middle school and high school students.

4. The only possible value of this test is for formative evaluation or for inclusion as a novel task in teaching.

5. Perhaps the test could be used as part of a battery of kinesthetic perception, if adequate information were available.

Major Weaknesses:

1. A complete lack of scientific aspects, coupled with inadequate or no information about applicability and interpretation of results, makes this an unacceptable test.

2. Without validity and reliability support, the test is useless.

3. Lack of norms and scientific aspects make misnamed Ball Throw Test of no value for research and of very little value for instruction use. This test is unacceptable.

BASKETBALL FOUL SHOT TEST

References.
Jensen, C. R. (1970). Unpublished studies of tests of kinesthetic perception, Brigham Young University.

Jensen, C. R., & Hirst, C. C. (1980). *Measurement in physical education and sports.* New York: Macmillan, pp 171-172.

Additional Sources.
None.

Purpose.
To measure the ability of an examinee to imitate a simple coordination task by shooting basketball foul shots accurately with the eyes blindfolded.

Objectivity.
Not reported.

Reliability.
Not reported.

Validity.
Not reported.

Age and Sex.
Not reported, but suitable for females and males, age 14 - adult.

Equipment.
A basketball, blindfold and basketball goal.

Space Requirements and Design.
The free throw lane area by one basketball goal.

Directions.
The examinee stands at the foul line and takes three practice shots. Without the examinee moving from the foul line, the tester places a blindfold over the examinee's eyes. The examinee is then given five shots. Points are awarded in the following manner: 3 points if the ball goes through the rim, 2 points if the ball hits the rim but fails to go through, 1 point if the ball hits the backboard but misses the rim, and 0 points if the ball misses the rim and backboard completely.

Scoring.
The score is the total number of points earned for the five trials.

Norms.
Not reported.

NOTE: It is assumed that any type of shooting style (e.g., overhead or underhand) is acceptable and that the shot must otherwise be legal (e.g., the examinee cannot step over the foul line).

REVIEW

FREDERICK C. SURGENT, Ed.D.

Professor of Physical Education
Frostburg State University
Frostburg, MD 21532
and

KIM CARTER & MATT ADAMS

Undergraduate Students
Department of Physical Education
Frostburg State University
Frostburg, MD 21532

For all practical purposes this test causes little, if any, problems with time, facilities, or equipment. A basketball court with a net, standard basketball rim, backboard, and the appropriate markings are easy to come by. Additionally, this test requires minimal personnel to administer.

Considering the developmental limitations of young performers when dealing with psychomotor skills (attention and organization of cue, perception, sensory feedback, etc.) the test should only be administered to those over the age of 14. This test is suitable for drills that promote learning in those who understand the purpose of the test and those who have developed physiologically to utilize the internal information provided to those intrinsic organs responsible for sensory feedback. Kinesthetic adaptation must take place to perform this skill successfully blindfolded. The more the examinee can adapt kinesthetically to the movements that accomplish the goal, the greater the chances of accurate, consistent results. This test does not present the tester or the examinee with any hazardous situations.

Since the test measures response outcome as opposed to response production, the scoring is objective enough to provide the examinee with adequate feedback for self evaluation.

This test does not provide objectivity, reliability, and validity measures nor does it present the examinee with a novel task. This can lead to misleading results if the examinees have had prior experience in the free throw of a basketball. Since this test is designed to measure kinesthetic adaptation by the examinee, an examinee with prior experience should not be scored with the examinees who are not experienced in the free throw of a basketball. Perhaps a pretest to organize the different skill levels would prove more effective in comparing the results to one another and the scoring method. Specific research on the different styles of foul shooting as they relate to kinesthesis could be undertaken, however, care in selection of the examinees, as detailed above, would need to be considered.

Although there are no objectivity, reliability, or validity scores for this test, the idea behind this test demonstrates that the concept of kinesthesis is definitely measured. Furthermore, the test does seem to meet some aspects of the previously mentioned test criteria. However, in administering this test to examinees slightly familiar with the task, it was noted in the trials that the examinees would retain negative practices following an attempt. For example, when examinees were given three sighted trials and then blindfolded and allowed five attempts to make the basket they would shoot too far to the left, right or not far enough on the second blindfolded shot. With no knowledge of the results, the examinees continued to overshoot to the left, right or short. Perhaps if the examinees were allowed a sighted shot prior to each blindfolded shot they would rely more on positive kinesthetic feedback.

In different arenas with different testers the test remained at a solid constant. Most examinees who shot fairly well enjoyed similar success on the blindfolded shots.

SUMMARY

Major Strengths:

1. This test is very easy to administer and easy for the examinee to understand.

2. The simplicity of the skill tested helps to eliminate error on the part of the tester and the examinee.

3. This test is appropriate as a teaching method and a form of self evaluation.

4. Because the shot may be performed either in an overhand or underhand style, this test has the potential to be a flexible test for the measurement of kinesthesis.

5. Being a closed skill, this skill is an excellent one to develop automatic performance in free throw shooting for practice and game situations.

Major Weaknesses:

1. The test could be improved by allowing the examinee a sighted trial before each blindfolded trial. This would enable the examinee to use positive feedback to make immediate adjustments.

2. Since this skill is not a novel skill, prior practice would affect the performance of the examinee.

Due to the major weaknesses listed previously, this test falls short of excellence. However, with the recommended modifications it could become a good test of kinesthesis and an aid in development of skill in shooting fouls under many different situations.

DISTANCE PERCEPTION JUMP TEST

References.
Johnson, B. L., & Nelson, J. K. (1986). *Practical measurements for evaluation in physical education*. Edina, MN: Burgess, pp 440-441.

Scott, M. G., & French, E. (1959). *Measurement and evaluation in physical education*. Dubuque: Wm. C. Brown, p 396.

Additional Source.
Jensen & Hirst (1980, pp. 168-169).

Purpose.
To measure the ability of an examinee to imitate a simple coordination task by jumping a specified distance.

Objectivity.
r = .99 by Wyatt (1969) cited in Johnson and Nelson (1986, p. 440).

Reliability.
r = .44 for test-retest of seventh and eighth grade boys with total of two trials as score; r = .61 when 10 trials were used (Johnson & Nelson, 1986, p. 440).

Validity.
Face validity (Johnson & Nelson, 1986, p. 440).

Age and Sex.
Females and males, preschool and above.

Equipment.
A blindfold, marking tape, and a ruler.

Space Requirements and Design.
A clear, level area approximately 3m (10') square with two parallel lines 2.54cm (1") in width and 61cm (24") in length, placed 60.96cm (24") apart between their nearest edges. The lines are known as the starting line and the target line.

Directions.
The examinee stands with the toes just behind the starting line. The examinee judges the distance between the two lines and closes the eyes. The examinee then tries to sense the effort required to jump and land with the heels on the far edge of the target line. The examinee then jumps and holds the landing position until the tester has measured the distance from the heel (i.e., the

heel the greatest distance from the far edge of the target line) to the target line. The distance is measured to the nearest half-inch (cm). A total of two trials are given.

Johnson and Nelson (1986, pp. 440-441) recommend a total of 10 trials be given, that a blindfold be used, that the examinee be permitted to view the landing location after each trial, that the distance be measured perpendicularly to the nearest 1/4" deviation from the line to the farthest heel, and that the score be the total distance for the 10 jumps.

Scoring.
The score is the sum of the distances for the two trials.

Norms.
Johnson and Nelson (1986, p. 441) boys.

REVIEW

M. GOLDMAN, Ph.D.
Professor of Physical Education
University of Massachusetts-Boston
Harbor Campus
Boston, MA 02125

This test purports to measure perception. On the surface it would appear that it does do that, or at least does it to some extent. However, more than casual analysis seems to indicate that the Distance Perception Jump combines several skills that may be only peripherally related to perception so that the claim of face validity may be questionable. Most sources agree that face validity may be used to define a test that obviously is measuring what it says it measures, as in the case of some tests of speed. However, face validity is sometimes used when the test defies validation by a more concrete and acceptable method. The Distance Perception Jump does not appear to lend itself unquestionably to a claim of face validity.

The directions for the Distance Perception Jump allow great, and arbitrary, variation in the testing distance used, particularly with younger examinees. The directions are not really clear as to the method to be used in the shielding of vision. The great latitude permitted in these two areas would certainly cast a questionable light on the test's reliability and objectivity. The very high objectivity rating of the Distance Perception Jump belies the test's somewhat flexible directions. The directions further suggest that the reliability of the test will increase from fair to substantial with an increase in the number of trials. While this cannot be questioned as a statistical "given," the size of the increase seems unwarranted for this test.

While norms are provided for the Distance Perception Jump, they were formulated using a limited number of secondary school age boys. No norms are available for any other male age group or for females.

The Distance Perception Jump requires very little in the way of space and equipment save, perhaps, for some kind of blindfold. However, the footwear of the examinee to be tested is not specified, and this lack can further affect the reliability and objectivity of the test adversely. A sneaker shod examinee may have better control over the jump and far more confidence in landing safely than an examinee who is tested in stocking clad feet or similar slippery footwear. There is no mention of a spotter being placed behind the examinee to guard against the examinee falling backward, nor is the use of a safety mat suggested as a possible standardization.

Depending upon the number of trials to be given to each examinee - and there seems to be some discrepancy over whether this should be 2 or 10 - this test can consume an inordinate amount of time. If the examinee is to receive feedback by a personal visual inspection, then removing and replacing the blindfold between jumps will increase the time to test each examinee considerably. The testing time per examinee will also be affected by the type of blindfold used.

The Distance Perception Jump does not lend itself to use as any kind of drill or conditioning item. It cannot be scored by an examinee working alone. Only a second individual can make the measurement required with any accuracy.

This test is exceptionally easy to administer and would require very little training for any assistants assigned to measure the jumps. Beyond making sure that the starting and target lines are the proper distance apart, and parallel to each other, the tester needs only to be able to measure the jump efficiently and accurately. The time constraints of 10 trials with knowledge of results after each precludes the use of only a single testing station with multiple examinees.

SUMMARY

Major Strengths:

1. The strengths of this test lie in its simplicity to set up and administer.
2. It is supremely easy to score.

Major Weaknesses:

1. The validity of this test must be questioned since it also seems to bring elements of balance and, possibly for the younger examinees, leg power, into the equation. One must wonder what the results might be if those latter two elements were eliminated by simply having a blindfolded examinee stand on the target line and point the toes of one foot to a given distance along a rule.

2. Footwear, or the lack of it could be standardized without being a safety factor, and the fear of falling or slipping would be eliminated.

3. The directions for the Distance Perception Jump do not deal with the treatment of trials in which the examinee slips and/or falls and thus gets no score, or an unusable one. Certainly the vagueness of the directions, as well as the omissions that are apparent, do not give one confidence in the reliability and objectivity of the test. Without these it is not valid.

4. Most adults being tested would probably find it difficult, if not impossible, to shut their eyes voluntarily during the entire jump sequence. For small children especially, the occlusion of vision could be traumatic were a blindfold used. For older children, only a kinesthetic blindfold would give some guarantee that perception and not vision was in fact being tested. This is a major stumbling block for this test. While most tests of kinesthetic perception require that a blindfold be used, many of these tests do not require whole body motion as is the case with the Distance Perception Jump.

Perhaps some individual might see in the Distance Perception Jump some potential for measurement that is sorely needed and not answered by another, more valid measure of perception.

And perhaps that individual might find a way to modify the Distance Perception Jump so that the norms are up to date for each of the groups for whom the test is prescribed. Until that can be accomplished, the Distance Perception Jump is unacceptable for research or teaching.

GRIP TO DESIGNATED AMOUNT TEST

Reference.

Scott, M. G., & French, E. (1959). *Measurement and evaluation in physical education*. Dubuque: Wm. C. Brown, p 393.

Additional Sources.

None.

Purpose.

To measure the ability of an examinee to exert a specified force while gripping a dynamometer.

Objectivity.

Not reported.

Reliability.

Not reported.

Validity.

Not reported.

Age and Sex.

Not reported, but suitable for females and males, age 8 - adult.

Equipment.

A grip dynamometer.

Space Requirements and Design.

A clear, level area approximately 2m (6') square with the examinee in the center.

Directions.

While standing with the eyes open, the examinee grips the dynamometer in one hand until its pointer indicates nine kilograms (20 pounds). The examinee then resets the pointer to zero, closes her/his eyes and tries to grip nine kilograms (20 pounds) again. The deviations, in kilograms (pounds), are recorded. One practice and three legal trials are given with each hand.

Scoring.

The score is the sum of the deviations for the six trials.

Norms.

Not reported.

NOTE: The target number of kilograms (pounds) to be gripped should be adjusted according to the age and strength of the group being tested. The target number of kilograms (pounds) should always be a submaximal grip or effort.

REVIEW

LARRY D. ISAACS, Ph.D.

Professor of Health,
Physical Education and Recreation
College of Education and
Human Services
Wright State University
Dayton, OH 45435

This test is designed to serve as a measure of kinesthesis. While researchers are not always in total agreement as to the precise definition of this term, they are in agreement that kinesthesis is not one single entity. For example, Scott (1955) suggested that the kinesthetic sense is made up of the following specific abilities: (1) muscular contractions of a known amount, (2) ability to balance, (3) ability to measure and identify body positions, (4) precise use of the hands, and (5) orientation of the body in space (Oxendine, 1984). Likewise, Johnson and Nelson (1986) have defined kinesthetic perception as "the ability to perceive the position, effort, and movement of parts of the body or of the entire body during muscular action..." (p. 440). Because the kinesthetic sense is not a single entity, it stands to reason that no one test can effectively assess this measure. In fact, kinesthetic perception is body part specific. Therefore, if adequate assessment is to occur, a battery of tests would be more appropriate.

The scientific aspects of the test are not acceptable since neither objectivity, reliability nor validity have been reported. In general, most other tests of kinesthetic perception have reported acceptable levels of objectivity and reliability but validity is generally passed off as face validity. One can speculate that the objectivity and reliability for this test could be made acceptable if several guidelines are followed. First, a quality grip dynamometer should be used. The dynamometer should have an adjustable grip and an easy to read scale. A calibrated digital scale would be most desirable and would undoubtedly result in an acceptable objectivity coefficient. Second, since the test is for both sexes, ages eight to adult, most likely it will be necessary to use a children's size grip dynamometer for some of the younger examinees. Reliability can be further improved by enforcing a standard protocol regarding adjustment of the grip dynamometer prior to testing (i.e., hand position on the grip dynamometer).

Practical aspects regarding test administration are appealing. More specifically, the test can be administered to large groups in very little time, and the only piece of equipment needed is a grip dynamometer. The tester should however, not lose sight of the fact that no matter how easy the test is to administer, if it is not a test which has been proven valid, the results will mean little.

Test directions are somewhat ambiguous. For example, in the directions the tester is instructed to use a target weight of 20 pounds. However, a note accompanying the directions says that the target weight should be adjusted according to the age and strength of the examinee. Unfortunately, no suggestions are offered regarding the most appropriate weight except to say that it should be submaximal.

SUMMARY

Major Strengths:

1. Only equipment needed is an appropriately sized grip dynamometer.

2. The test is easy to administer.

3. Large groups can be assessed in very little time.

Major Weaknesses:

1. The test has not been adequately validated.

2. The test directions are ambiguous.

3. Norms are not available.

Overall, this test is not acceptable for research purposes. The test, can however, be used as a teaching aid in a motor learning laboratory designed to help students better understand this one aspect (i.e., reproduction of force or effort) of kinesthetic perception.

REVIEW REFERENCES

Johnson, B. L., & Nelson, J. K. (1986). *Practical measurements for evaluation in physical education*. Edina, MN: Burgess Publishing.

Oxendine, J. B. (1984). *Psychology of motor learning*. Englewood Cliffs, NJ: Prentice-Hall, Inc.

Scott, M. G. (1955). Measurement of kinesthesis. *Research Quarterly*, 26:324-341.

PUSH-PULL TO DESIGNATED AMOUNT TEST

Reference.
Scott, M. G., & French, E. (1959). *Measurement and evaluation in physical education.* Dubuque: Wm. C. Brown, p 393.

Additional Sources.
None.

Purpose.
To measure the ability of an examinee to exert a specified force while pushing and/or pulling on a dynamometer.

Objectivity.
Not reported.

Reliability.
Not reported.

Validity.
Not reported.

Age and Sex.
Not reported, but suitable for females and males, age 10 - college.

Equipment.
A grip dynamometer with a push-pull attachment.

Space Requirements and Design.
A clear, level area approximately 2m (6') square with the examinee in the center.

Directions.
The test may be given for the push, the pull or both. In using the push and pull tests as measures of kinesthesis, a submaximal target number of kilograms (pounds) is experimentally determined for the pull test and for the push test based on the age and strength of the group being tested. When performing the pull and push tests, the examinee stands erect with the arms positioned parallel to the ground and the elbows bent. The dynamometer is held in front of the chest with one hand on each handle. The dynamometer may not be braced against the chest. Upon command, the examinee either pulls outward or pushes inward in an attempt to achieve the target number of kilograms (pounds). The examinee is not permitted to view the scale on the dynamometer when taking the tests. The devia-

tions from the target amount, measured in kilograms (pounds), is recorded for each trial. The exact number of trials is not stated.

Scoring.
The score is the sum of the deviations, expressed in kilograms (pounds), for all trials of the pull test and/or for all of the trials for the push test.

Norms.
Not reported.

REVIEW

BILL KOZAR, Ph.D.
Associate Professor
Physical Education
Boise State University
Boise, ID 83725

The Push-Pull to Designated Amount is presented as a measure of kinesthetic acuity and memory. Since kinesthesis appears to consist of a number of specific abilities, this test may more appropriately be considered as two tests, each of which represents a specific and limited measure of kinesthesis. The test, as presented, implies, or perhaps assumes, a high correlation between the push and pull components. However, tests of kinesthesis typically exhibit low intercorrelations. Therefore, until the push and pull are shown to measure the same or highly similar kinesthetic ability, they need to be viewed as measuring different abilities.

No validity figures are given. This is not surprising since few valid tests of kinesthesis exist (Sage, 1977; Oxendine, 1984). While no reliability or objectivity measures are given, both should be adequate if good testing procedures are followed.

Measuring the push-pull reproduction capabilities of examinees presents few problems once a dynamometer capable of measuring both components is secured. The nature of the test(s) and equipment are such that several examinees could be tested simultaneously if a number of dynamometers were available. Obviously, the dynamometers should be calibrated periodically to ensure accurate measurements.

There are, however, a number of problems associated with the directions section of the test. Exactly how the submaximal criterion force in kilograms or pounds is arrived at is not explained adequately. While this submaximal criterion force is determined on the basis of the age and strength of the group being tested, does this mean that a maximum force for each examinee is determined, a group mean then calculated, and a percentage of this group mean used as the submaximal force (e.g., 60 percent) or, is a percentage of each examinee's maximal force used? The latter seems obligatory, for years of psychophysical research has generally found that there is a power, rather than a linear, function regarding perception of effort and changes in physical intensity. It is also conceivable that in a group with a wide range of strength scores, a percentage of maximum based on the group mean would make it impossible for some examinees to distinguish the submaximal force from their maximal force because the difference is less than one just noticeable difference (j.n.d.). That is, a submaximal force which is 70 percent of a group mean may be so close to an examinees' maximum that he/she could not differentiate kinesthetically between the two.

The directions also offer no guidelines regarding the manner in which the criterion force is to be achieved. Nor can one tell once the maximal force is arrived at (e.g., 80 lbs.) and the submaximal criteria is determined (e.g., 60 percent of 80 lbs.), if the examinee is told to exert a force of 48 lbs. without having a specific recent reference in memory of this force, or if the examinee receives one visually monitored practice trial to establish a correct reference which he/she now uses in attempting to reproduce the criteria force? It is not made clear whether the examinee is to use a gradual force build up or is to perform the task in a ballistic type manner where the examinee very quickly achieves the criteria. This question is critical, for motor behavior research indicates that quite different control mechanisms are used in each case.

The type of hand grip used on the dynamometer is not addressed. It would seem that all examinees should grip the dynamometer with the palm facing towards or away from them. Viewing the dynamometer scale is not permitted, however subtle visual cues other than the scale may provide valuable information while nonrelevant visual stimuli may cause interference. To control for this, all examinees should take the test blindfolded. It is assumed that since examinees are not allowed to view the dynamometer scale, no knowledge of results (KR) is provided by the tester. This should be spelled out in the instructions. The exact number of trials should be set to avoid fatigue effects. This number would be influenced by the age of the examinee and the amount the submaximal force is relative to the maximal force. The time between trials needs to be specified as well, to control for both memory and kinesthetic after effects.

SUMMARY

Major Strengths:

1. Apparatus relatively inexpensive.

2. Space requirements are minimal.

3. Technical aspects are such that individuals can be trained to administer test quickly and easily.

4. If equipment is calibrated properly and testing procedures are expanded and followed, reliability and objectivity should be adequate.

Major Weaknesses:

1. Validity measures are not provided. Very few valid measures of kinesthesis have in fact been reported.

2. Directions are inadequate. Problems exist in:

a. Exactly how submaximal force is determined.

b. Whether examinee is, or is not, provided with a correct reference of the submaximal force which is to be reproduced/produced.

c. Manner in which submaximal force is to be achieved (i.e., gradual or ballistic).

d. Type of hand grip examinee should use.

e. Examinees should be blindfolded to eliminate effects of any visual cues.

f. Should tester be instructed not to provide knowledge of results (KR)?

g. Number of trials needs to be specified.

h. Time between trials needs to be specified.

3. There appears to be an assumption that the push and pull components are measuring the same kinesthetic ability.

4. No norms are provided.

Push-pull components need to be tested to determine the level of correlation which exists rather than assuming that either one of these components may be used as a measure of the same kinesthetic ability. Directions for administering the test need much more detail to prevent different interpretations and to take into account recent scientific information regarding the measurement of kinesthesis. Norms for different populations need to be established, especially since there is evidence that kinesthetic acuity and memory are age related. Work also needs to be done to establish some validity figures. Until these changes, and additions are made, this test is of minimal value in research and instructional settings.

SHUFFLEBOARD DISTANCE PERCEPTION TEST

References.
Johnson, B. L. (1966). The shuffleboard control of force test. Unpublished study, Northeast Louisiana University.

Nelson, J. K. (1971). Modification of shuffleboard and bean bag kinesthesis tests. Unpublished study, Louisiana State University.

Johnson, B. L., & Nelson, J. K. (1986). *Practical measurements for evaluation in physical education.* Edina: Burgess, p 442.

Additional Sources.
None.

Purpose.
To measure the ability of an examinee to perceive the effort required to push a shuffleboard disk a specified distance.

Objectivity.
Not reported.

Reliability.
r = .71 for seventh and eighth grade boys and r = .66 for fourth grade girls using the test retest method.

Validity.
Face validity.

Age and Sex.
Suitable for females and males, age 9 - adult.

Equipment.
Shuffleboard sticks, disks, chalk or tape, blindfold, and tape measure.

Space Requirements and Design.
A clear, level area approximately 3m x 9m (10' x 30') with three starting lines placed 1.52m (5'), 3.04m (10') and 4.57m (15') from the edge of the target. The target is composed of 19 zones marked off by parallel lines 15.24cm (6") apart. The 10 zones closest to the starting lines are numbered 1 to 10 and the next nine zones are numbered 9 to 1 (Figure 7-1).

Directions.
Initially the examinee is given four or five practice trials away from the target to become acquainted with the pushing motion and the disk surface conditions. Then the examinee goes to the starting line, 1.52m (5') from the target, and

judges to the distance to zone 10. A blindfold is then placed over the eyes, and he/she is given 10 trials. The examinee is permitted to see where the disk stops after each trial. The number of the zone where the disk stops is recorded for each trial. The same procedures are repeated using the starting lines 3.04m (10') and 4.57m (15') from the target.

Scoring.
The score is the total number of points obtained for the 30 trials.

Norms.
Johnson & Nelson (1986, p. 442) men and women.

REVIEW

SHERRY L. FOLSOM-MEEK, Ph.D.

Assistant Professor
Physical Education
University of Missouri
Columbia, MO 65211

This test purports to measure the ability to judge the effort required to push a shuffleboard disk a specified distance, which is one aspect of kinesthetic functioning. Because vision is occluded, there is little doubt that the test has face validity as a measure of effort perception.

Based on test-retest, reliability coefficients are .71 for seventh and eighth grade boys and .66 for fourth grade girls. Four or five practice trials away from the target are allowed for the purpose of learning the shuffleboard pushing movement. Test directions are clear in regard to the following areas: (a) examinee sees the target prior to being blindfolded; (b) examinee is blindfolded for each trial; (c) examinee receives knowledge of results (KR) feedback by viewing where disk stops after each trial; (d) examinee takes 10 trials from each distance - 5 ft., 10 ft., and 15 ft.; (e) zone size and numbering; and (f) scoring. The directions are not clear as to how often disks are removed from the target area.

The tester's presence should not affect the performance of the examinee unless he/she were to reinforce the examinee's performance verbally.

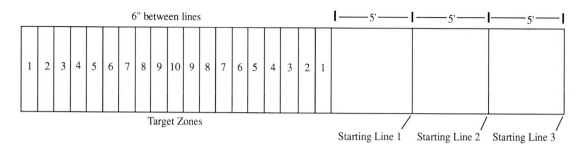

Figure 7-1. Shuffleboard Distance Perception Test.

However, this situation would be highly unlikely because the examinee receives KR feedback by viewing where the disk stops following each trial.

Facility, space, and equipment requirements should pose no problems with this test. An area at least 25 feet long is needed, which could easily be set up in a gymnasium or hallway. There should be additional space beyond the target so disks cannot rebound off a wall back onto the target. A minimum of shuffleboard equipment - one cue (stick) and several (up to 10) disks would be needed.

Because of clarity of test directions, the tester should be able to administer the test with ease. In addition to marking off the target area with tape or chalk, time required for test administration is the time it takes for the practice trials and 30 test trials, with visual inspection of results following each trial. It appears that test time would be approximately 15 to 20 minutes per examinee. Ten trials from each distance are more than an adequate number to measure effort perception. Based on the test-retest reliability coefficients of the normative sample, there may be a learning effect with this number of trials. Because of this learning effect, the test is suitable to use as a drill to promote learning. The test itself should be challenging as a self testing activity.

Normally shuffleboard is not included in elementary and middle/junior high school physical education curricula; it is found in recreational settings, such as summer camps, which many children begin attending at 9 or 10 years of age.

The movement pattern in shuffleboard is underhand with no backswing. The cue is placed directly behind the disk and is then pushed, which is unlike other underhand pattern skills in physical education. The test might be appropriate for the range of upper elementary students through older students in a school setting, but the movement pattern may have to be taught to most students. If the test is intended to discriminate among its intended users, criteria for good and poor kinesthesia and performance by age should be included. It is difficult to interpret results without these criteria. If such criteria were known, the test could be used in therapeutic settings as well as in school settings.

There appear to be no dangerous aspects related to this test. Scoring is objective, and the test could be easily scored by tester, examinee, or another student.

The test is of suitable precision to use for research purposes. It measures a different aspect of kinesthesia than do other commonly used tests of kinesthetic functioning (e.g., finger to nose, angels in the snow, and imitation of postures). This test could be used in conjunction with other measures of kinesthesia to determine a more complete picture of kinesthetic functioning. Norms for the test are not given by age or gender, and there are no criteria for good and poor effort perception.

SUMMARY

Major Strengths:

1. The directions are clear.

2. The test has face validity as a measure of effort to perception, which is one aspect of kinesthesia.

3. The test is practical for use in research and in limited educational settings.

Major Weaknesses:

1. The practice trials are away from the target. One trial from each of the three distances might better acclimate the examinee to the test than practice trials away from the target.

2. The underhand movement pattern with no backswing is unusual to upper elementary and middle/junior high school physical education skills, and, therefore, will have to be taught to most examinees.

3. Scoring criteria for good and poor kinesthetic functioning and performance by age are not reported.

The test is acceptable and adequate for research and teaching with the following qualifications: for both research and educational usage, scoring criteria for good and poor kinesthetic functioning and performance by age are needed. However, use of the test in research settings may produce these criteria. When these criteria are available, the test would be appropriate to use as one measure in determining whether special physical education services are needed. Because the test measures only effort perception, it should be used in conjunction with other measures of kinesthesia in order to determine a more complete assessment of an examinee's kinesthetic functioning. Unless the test is used to measure kinesthetic learning, the learning effect from the 30 trials needs to be controlled in research settings.

KINESTHESIS TESTS OF MOVEMENT PRECISION

ARM RAISING SIDEWARD 90 DEGREES TEST

Reference.
Scott, M. G., & French, E. (1959). *Measurement and evaluation in physical education.* Dubuque: Wm. C. Brown, p 391.

Additional Sources.
None.

Purpose.
To measure the ability of an examinee to move the arms to a specified position.

Objectivity.
Not reported.

Reliability.
Not reported.

Validity.
Not reported.

Age and Sex.
Not reported, but suitable for females and males, age 8 - adult.

Equipment.
A goniometer and a stick figure drawn on posterboard with one arm in a front, horizontal position.

Space Requirements and Design.
A clear, level area approximately 3m (10') square with the examinee in the center.

Directions.
The examinee stands erect and looks at the stick figure, paying specific attention to the position of the arm. The examinee then closes her/his eyes and raises the right arm forward (i.e., flexion at the shoulder) with the palm of the hand facing down, to match the horizontal position of the stick figure. The tester then uses the goniometer to measure the exact angle of the arm and records the degrees of deviation from horizontal. The examinee is given one more trial with the right arm and then two trials with the left.

Scoring.
The score is the sum of the deviations in degrees for all four trials.

Norms.
Not reported.

REVIEW

LINDA BARLEY, Ed.D.

Professor
Health and Physical Education
Gerontological Studies and Services
York College of The City University
of New York
Jamaica, NY 11451

Arm Raising Sideward 90 Degrees is a kinesthetic measurement infrequently covered in the literature. The usefulness of the physical measurement is limited in the following manner: (1) the test lacks validity, (2) baseline data is not available for targeted populations, and (3) while identified as a kinesthetic measurement, the test may, in fact, measure range of motion and/or balance.

The practical aspects of the test are such that the test is easily administered, requiring little time or space. Equipment needs are limited to a stick figure drawing and a goniometer. Scoring is easily managed; but, the recommended two trials are probably insufficient. Given the lack of norms for age, physical ability and general health status, the test should not be used for research efforts. However, the test is useful as a drill to promote learning, conditioning and charting changes in an examinee's performance.

SUMMARY

Major Strengths:

1. Easy to administer.

2. Requires little time, space or equipment.

3. Requires minimal training of the tester.

4. Is useful in promoting learning and conditioning.

Major Weaknesses:

1. Lacks validity for research purposes.

2. Lacks norms for age, physical ability and general health status.

3. May not measure kinesthetic acuity, but range of motion instead.

This is an acceptable test for promoting conditioning and individual learning.

KINESTHETIC OBSTACLE TEST

References.

Johnson, B. L. (1966). A kinesthetic obstacle test. Unpublished study, Northeast Louisiana State University.

Johnson, B. L., & Nelson, J. K. (1986). *Practical measurements for evaluation in physical education.* Edina, MN: Burgess, pp 442-443.

Additional Sources. None.

Purpose.

To measure the ability of an examinee to move in a predictable manner without using the eyes.

Objectivity.

Not reported.

Reliability.

r = .30 for college women and r = .53 for men, test retest method.

Validity.

Face validity.

Age and Sex.

Females and males, age 10 - college.

Equipment.

A blindfold, 12 chairs, marking tape, and a tape measure.

Space Requirements and Design.

A clear, level area approximately 3m x 15m (10' x 50') with a starting line 1.52m (5') from one end of the 15m length and three perpendicular columns of chairs. The middle column of four chairs are placed 1.52m (5'), 6.10m (20'), 9.76m (32'), and 12.20m (40') from the starting line (measured to the center of each chair). The right and left columns of chairs are placed on lines perpendicular to the starting line 40.64cm (16") from the center of the middle column. The four chairs in the right column are placed 2.44m (8'), 4.88cm (16'), 8.54cm (28') and 10.98m (36') from the starting line. The four chairs in the left column are placed 2.44m (8'), 3.66m (12'), 7.32m (24'), and 10.98m (36') from the starting line. The distances for both columns are measured from the edge of the chair nearest the starting line. Two straight lines of tape should be placed to the outside of the right and left columns of chairs

perpendicular to the starting line and 38.10cm (15") from the outside edge of the chairs. These two lines serve as boundary lines (Figure 7-2).

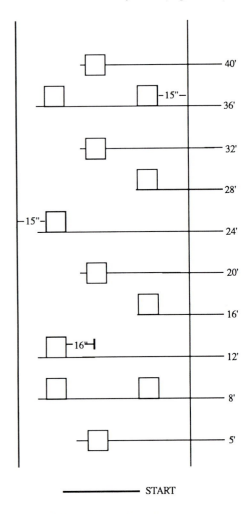

Figure 7-2. Kinesthetic Obstacle Test.

Directions.

The examinee takes a standing position behind the middle of the starting line facing the chairs. A blindfold is placed over the eyes. The examinee then tries to walk between the boundary lines and through the chairs without touching any of them. A 10 point penalty is assessed for touching a chair. When a chair is touched, the tester directs the examinee to the center column, one step ahead of the chair which was touched.

A five point penalty is assessed when the examinee moves outside the boundary lines or outside the pattern of the chairs. The tester directs the examinee back to the center nearest to where he/she went out. One practice trial with the eyes open and one legal trial with the blindfold are given.

Scoring.
The score is 100 minus any penalty points.

Norms.
Johnson & Nelson (1986, p. 443) men and women.

REVIEW

LARRY M. LANDIS, Ph.D.
Professor of Social Science
Vice President for Academic Affairs
Black Hills State University
Spearfish, SD 57999
and
SUE W. WHITE, M.Ed.

Assistant Professor
Physical Education
Black Hills State University
Spearfish, SD 57999

The purpose of this test is to evaluate the ability of the examinee to perceive and maintain her/his relative position during movement through space. Perception and success are defined in terms of visual space, thus the examinee is required to negotiate a familiar mazeway while blindfolded.

By definition, the test has face validity. A reliability coefficient, established through a test-retest methodology, was computed at .51 for all examinees, .49 for women, and .81 for men. Test objectivity was measured using a split half reliability test comparing the results of examinees who were instructed by each of the two testers on both the test and the retest. Coefficients of .29 and .37 respectively were calculated.

The administration of the test requires a large room, the size of which is not uncommon in institutional settings. A diagram of the layout would be helpful. Equipment is in no way esoteric and the set up is easily administered with a minimal amount of explanation required. One tester can successfully administer the test but for safety, scoring, and ease of transition between examinees, two testers are recommended. Considering the instruction, the initial walk through, the blindfolding, and the blindfolded walk through, examinees required from 7 to 10 minutes to complete the exercise. The initial walk through, followed by the blindfolded test is adequate, though many of the examinees wanted to do the test another time.

The test is useful in demonstrating the existence of the kinesthetic sense relative to the positioning of the body in general space. It is a safe test but two cautions seem wise. The examinee should be spotted while blindfolded and the use of cotton balls over the eyes ensures that the examinee cannot see and protects eyes from exposure to infectious diseases when a common blindfold is used. The test is suitable for use by a wide range of examinees in terms of age and sex, and it does demonstrate a range of ability.

The scoring is objective but cumbersome. It is best performed by a scorer who is independent of the trial (i.e., not the examinee and not the tester who is spotting the examinee). While norms have been established for the test, relatively low reliability and objectivity scores suggest that further norming may be needed. With that caveat, the test seems generally suitable for research purposes.

SUMMARY
Major Strengths:

1. The test is easily set up, and readily administered and scored.

2. It demonstrates, in a convincing fashion, the existence of the kinesthetic sense and the differing abilities of examinees to use that sense to maneuver successfully through a mazeway. As such, the test is a useful teaching or demonstration device and would appear to be a useful research device.

Major Weaknesses:

1. Reliability and objectivity coefficients suggest the need for careful norming.

2. The test is somewhat time consuming and, hence, requires scheduled time trials.

3. The test is cumbersome, though not particularly difficult to score.

4. Safety considerations require multiple testers.

This test is an acceptable test. It appears adequate for demonstration, teaching, and research purposes.

While the results of this test may be dramatic in their ability to demonstrate an examinee's kinesthetic capacities, the coefficients of reliability and objectivity reported above suggest a need for further work in the interpretation of these results.

LEG RAISING TEST

Reference.
Scott, M. G., & French, E. (1959). *Measurement and evaluation in physical education*. Dubuque: Wm. C. Brown, p 392.

Additional Sources.
None.

Purpose.
To measure the ability of an examinee to move the legs to a specified position.

Objectivity.
Not reported.

Reliability.
Not reported.

Validity.
Not reported.

Age and Sex.
Not reported, but suitable for females and males, age 8 - adult.

Equipment.
A gravity type goniometer and a stick figure drawn on posterboard illustrating an individual lying on the side of her/his body with the leg raised (i.e., abduction at hip joint) 20 degrees.

Space Requirements and Design.
A clear, level area approximately 3m (10') square with the examinee in the center.

Directions.
The examinee lies on her/his side and looks at the stick figure, paying specific attention to the position of the raised leg. The tester attaches the goniometer to the examinee's ankle. The examinee then closes her/his eyes and raises the leg to match the position of the stick figure. The deviations in degrees are recorded for each trial. Two trials are given with each leg.

Scoring.
The score is the sum of the deviations in degrees for the four trials.

Norms.
Not reported.

NOTE: Another version of this test involves the lower leg. For the lower leg version, the examinee stands with a hand on a table. The examinee then raises the lower leg until it is parallel to the floor, (i.e., a right angle is formed at the knee). Two trials are given with each leg and the score is the sum of the deviations, measured in degrees, from the desired right angle position.

REVIEW

LOUIS BOWERS, Ph.D.
Professor of Physical Education
University of South Florida
Tampa, FL 33620

Scott and French (1959) defined kinesthesis as "that sense which enables the individual to perceive the position and movement of the total body and of its parts." Steinhaus further separated vision from the performance of kinesthesis in his 1966 article entitled "Our Muscles See More Than Our Eyes."

This test claims to assess kinesthesis by measuring the examinee's ability to move the legs to a specified position as indicated on a drawing of a stick figure person. Although the ability to feel, and repeatedly move a body part to the same position constitutes one part of the definition of kinesthesis, it is questionable that correctly perceiving and then duplicating the 20 degree angle represented by a stick figure should be a part of a test of kinesthesis as defined above.

An alternative recommended test procedure would be to have the examinee lift the leg to a desired height and repeat the movement to the same position.

The objectivity and reliability of the test are not stated. When one examines the directions for administration of the test one notes several weaknesses with regard to achievement of either of these criteria. The number of trials, two for each leg, is insufficient to represent consistent performance of kinesthesis. Also, by combining the trials from two legs, a comparison of the performance of each leg is lost. While the gravity type goniometer has the potential to discriminate between performances with a recording to the nearest degree, it is very difficult to obtain an accurate reading of the goniometer due to the unsteadiness of the leg in an abducted position.

The age and sex for which the test would be appropriate is not stated, but it would seem to be appropriate for both females and males from age eight through adulthood. There are unfortunately no norms provided for performance on the test for either group at any age.

The administration of the test is safe. It can be administered either indoors or outdoors, and requires minimal space. Only one tester is required to administer the test; however, sufficient numbers of gravity type goniometers and trained testers would be necessary for large group testing. The specific type goniometer which should be used for the test is not stated.

Examinees cannot accurately test themselves or each other, as the skill needed to use the goniometer accurately requires instruction and experience.

SUMMARY

Major Strengths:

1. The test can be administered both indoors and outdoors and requires very little space.

2. It is a safe test which requires little training for the examinee.

3. This test is appropriate for either females or males from age eight to adulthood.

Major Weaknesses:

1. The validity of the test as a measurement of kinesthesis is questionable due to the use of a stick figure drawing to demonstrate a 20 degree angle.

2. The objectivity and reliability of the test are not given.

3. An insufficient number of trials for each leg are recommended.

4. The need for a number of gravity goniometers and trained testers makes this a time consuming operation when large groups are tested.

The validity of the Leg Raise Test, designed as a test of kinesthesis by measuring the ability to move the legs to a specified position, is compromised by the use of a stick figure to demonstrate the 20 degree target position. Two trials for each leg are insufficient, and the objectivity and reliability are not known; therefore this test is not recommended for either evaluation in teaching or for research purposes.

REVIEW REFERENCES

Scott, M. G., & French, E. (1959). *Measurement and evaluation in physical education.* Dubuque, IA: Wm. C. Brown.

Steinhaus, A. (1966). Your muscles see more than your eyes. *Journal of Health and Physical Education Recreation,* 37(7):38.

PRONATION AND SUPINATION TEST

Reference.
Scott, M. G., & French, E. (1959). *Measurement and evaluation in physical education.* Dubuque: Wm. C. Brown, pp 391-392.

Additional Sources.
None.

Purpose.
To measure the ability of the examinee to move the forearm to a specified position.

Objectivity.
Not reported.

Reliability.
Not reported.

Validity.
Not reported.

Age and Sex.
Not reported, but suitable for females and males, age 8 - adult.

Equipment.
A table, chair and a knob 7.62cm (3") in diameter which is attached to the center of the baseline of a protractor. A pointer is attached to the knob so that it turns as the knob is turned. The protractor and knob apparatus are attached to the edge of the table. A piece of cardboard approximately 40cm (16") square.

Space Requirements and Design.
A clear, level area approximately 3m (10') square with the examinee seated in front of the knob and the protractor.

Directions.
The examinee reaches forward so that the elbow clears the side of the body while grasping the knob. With the pointer set at 90 degrees, the tester turns the knob while using the eyes until the pointer is targeted at the 140 degree mark. The examinee concentrates on the movement required to produce the desired 140 degree mark and releases. The pointer is returned to the 90 degree mark. The examinee is then given four trials at turning the knob to the 140 degree mark while the tester blocks the examinee's view of the protractor by holding the cardboard between the examinee's eyes and the protractor. A practice trial with the use of the eyes is then given in turning the pointer in the other direction to the 40 degree mark followed by four trials with the examinee's view of the protractor blocked. The deviations in degrees from the desired angle are recorded for each trial.

Scoring.
The score is the sum of the deviations in degrees for the eight trials.

Norms.
Not reported.

REVIEW

ELAINE BUDDE, Ph.D.
Professor of Physical Education
Roanoke College
Salem, VA 24153

The test constructors fail to provide information on the scientific aspects of this test. While logical (face) validity may have been considered, it was not claimed. There is a serious problem relative to the stated purpose of the test. Is the purpose really to measure the ability to move the forearm to a specified position, or is it to assess the ability to replicate the forearm's arc of motion using kinesthetic cues, or perhaps to measure "visual memory," since the examinee has just performed the task with the eyes open? These are factors which may strongly influence scores, yet they have, apparently, not been considered. They would also seem intrinsic to a clear statement of purpose of the test. In addition, the reliability and objectivity components of the test were not assessed. Lack of vital statistical information makes it impossible to accept the test without further assessment of its value.

The test requires minimal space, and the equipment needed would be relatively easy to assemble. One tester, without special training or expertise, could administer the test in a short time. The scoring, using degrees of deviation as read directly from the protractor, permits an objective system of scoring. It is impossible to make a judgement as to the adequacy of the number of trials when the question of purpose of the test is so unclear. Why would four trials be better than one if no feedback is given and no learning occurs? If the purpose of the test is to use kinesthetic cues to replicate motion, it is unlikely that kinesthetic recall would persist over four trials. The examinee would tend to remember the motion just completed, not the original sighted one. Using the score of the sum of the deviations in degrees for eight trials precludes any possibility that the score might be influenced by direction of movement. It also may be advisable to have examinees use their dominant arm.

SUMMARY

Major Strengths:

1. The test is easy to administer and requires minimal space and equipment.

2. The scoring system is objective.

Major Weaknesses:

1. The question of validity is not addressed.

2. An assessment of test reliability is not available.

3. The stated directions, scoring, limited use of visual cues, and lack of feedback do not provide information that assists in a clear understanding of purpose.

4. Norms are not available.

The test is unacceptable for research and teaching purposes due to the lack of basic statistical information on validity and reliability.

WALKING A STRAIGHT LINE WITH TURNS TEST

Reference.
Scott, M. G., & French, E. (1959). *Measurement and evaluation in physical education.* Dubuque: Wm. C. Brown, pp 395-396.

Additional Sources.
None.

Purpose.
To measure the ability of an examinee to execute turns and to move the body with precision while blindfolded.

Objectivity.
Not reported.

Reliability.
Not reported.

Validity.
Not reported.

Age and Sex.
Not reported, but suitable for females and males, age 8 - adult.

Equipment.
A blindfold, marking tape and a tape measure.

Space Requirements and Design.
A clear, level area approximately 12m (40') square with a 2.54cm (1") wide line about 5.49m (18') long down the middle.

Directions.
The examinee stands at one end of the line and places the blindfold over her/his eyes. The examinee then takes two steps forward, brings the trailing foot forward parallel to, but not touching, the lead foot. The examinee then executes a complete 360 degree turn in place, being sure to keep the feet apart. The examinee takes two steps and executes another 360 degree turn. After executing a total of eight steps and four turns, the examinee remains motionless until the tester measures the perpendicular distance from the line to the nearest toe. It is suggested that several practice trials be given as well as a minimum of three legal trials.

Scoring.
The score is number of centimeters (inches) from the line to the nearest toe.

Norms.
Not reported.

REVIEW

T. GILMOUR REEVE, Ph.D.
Professor
Health and Human Performance
Auburn University
Auburn, AL 36849-5323

This test, Walking a Straight Line with Turns, is intended to provide a measure of one's ability to execute body turns and to move the body with precision while blindfolded. Because the examinee is blindfolded during the test, emphasis is on kinesthetic awareness and spatial orientation as contributors to efficient performance. Also, the test is based on self paced performance with the examinee selecting her/his own rate of movement. The scientific aspects of the test are not available. Objectivity, reliability, and validity coefficients are not reported. Moreover, although the test may be administered to females and males across a wide range of ages (eight and older), normative data have not been provided.

Space and equipment requirements for the test are minimal. Marking tape, measuring tape and blindfold are the only supplies needed.

The test measures the deviation from a straight line following a series of steps and 360 degree turns while blindfolded. The score is simply the total perpendicular distance deviated from the straight line. One problem with the test is that the score provides little information about the exact nature of the errors made by the examinee. Large scores (i.e., large deviations from the line) could occur for a variety of reasons, such as the failure to walk a straight line and the failure to turn 360 degrees accurately. Although the different types of performance errors might be indicative of specific problems, the recorded score could not be used for diagnostic purposes. Also, small deviations may be recorded following the total series of steps and turns because deviations from one component of the series may negate those from another component. Thus, a small score would be obtained when, in fact, errors occurred in each component of the trial.

Conceptually, the test fails to provide information that would be useful for assessing motor abilities in physical activity or sport situations. Seldom, if ever, are individuals asked to perform while blindfolded. Vision is a powerful source of information in most movement environments. Thus, the measurement of blindfolded examinees on a spatial orientation task seems of limited value for sport or physical education settings.

SUMMARY

Major Strengths:

1. Walking a Straight Line with Turns is a test that requires minimal space and equipment for administration.

2. The test can be administered by one individual.

Major Weaknesses:

1. The test has little scientific merit.

2. The test does not show a relation between the test measurement and specific performance errors.

3. The fact that the test requires total body movements of blindfolded examinees dissociates the test from sports and physical activities.

Overall, the Walking a Straight Line with Turns test is unacceptable and has little to offer in sport research.

Chapter 8

MUSCULAR ENDURANCE

DYNAMIC MUSCULAR ENDURANCE TESTS OF THE ARMS

ABSOLUTE ENDURANCE OF UPPER BODY TEST

Reference.
Baumgartner, T. A., & Jackson, A. S. (1987). *Measurement for evaluation in physical education.* Dubuque: Wm. C. Brown, pp 186, 188-190.

Additional Source.
Safrit (1990, pp. 482-486).

Purpose.
To measure the absolute endurance of an examinee's muscles of the upper body.

Objectivity.
Not reported.

Reliability.
Not reported.

Validity.
Construct validity was established.

Age and Sex.
Not reported, but suitable for children through adult.

Equipment.
A stopwatch and a Universal Gym or similar weight training machine.

Space Requirements and Design.
A clear, level area large enough to position the Universal Gym in the center.

Directions.
The three lifts Baumgartner and Jackson recommend for measuring absolute muscular endurance of the upper body are the bench press, curl and latissimus dorsi pull (more commonly known as the lat. pull). The recommended procedures for executing these lifts are described in the test "One Repetition Maximum (1-RM) Upper Body Strength Tests." The tester needs to select a weight which is appropriate for the lift to be performed for the age group being measured. The weight selected must be such that everyone in the group can do at least one repetition. Baumgartner and Jackson recommend the following weights for a group of male college freshmen: bench press = 110 pounds, curl = 50 pounds and lat. pull = 100 pounds.

After the lift to be used has been decided upon and the appropriate weight has been selected, the examinee performs as many repetitions as possible. Each repetition must be completed within a three second interval and no new repetition may be initiated before the next new three second interval. The examinee must initiate each new repetition in the original starting position, and he/she cannot drop the weight, after lifting the weight upward, in order to stay within the three second interval. Each test is stopped whenever the examinee fails to complete a repetition correctly, or he/she fails to maintain the three second cadence.

Scoring.
The score for each test is the number of repetitions completed.

Norms.
Baumgartner & Jackson (1987, p. 189) men; Hoeger (1989, p. 48) men and women.

REVIEW

LARRY W. TITLOW, Ph.D

Professor of Physical Education
University of Central Arkansas
Conway, AR 72032

Tests of muscular endurance have been a part of the testing continuum in physical education as long as muscles have been tested. There are two common means of measuring muscular endurance - relative and absolute. To rule out strength as a factor, relative tests use percent of either maximal strength or body weight to establish the weight to be used for testing. Absolute tests utilize the same resistance for all, regardless of the examinee's strength or weight. There is no established relationship between relative endurance and strength. Correlations of r = .75 to r = .97 between absolute endurance and strength are reported by deVries (1986). It should be obvious that if a load of 100 pounds were used for examinees of widely varying strength, a weak examinee would be working near maximum while a strong examinee would be working at considerably less than maximum.

Reliability of the Baumgartner and Jackson procedure is not reported; however, other tests of muscular endurance using the same procedure have reported intraclass correlations from r = .88 to r = .94 (Titlow, Unpublished master's thesis, U of Houston, 1970). Construct validity for the procedure is reported by Baumgartner and Jackson. Objectivity is not reported but should not be a problem. The only exception could be determining when an examinee fails to complete a lift within the allotted three seconds. Examinees are required to initiate a new repetition at the beginning of each three second interval; a problem could develop if the tester does not carefully observe the examinee to guarantee full compliance.

The test requires either a Universal Gym or similar weight training device and a stopwatch. The equipment should be readily available in most schools and fitness settings. Free weights could be substituted so long as adequate safety precautions are followed. The stopwatch is required to set the three second cadence. An improvement would be to use a tape recorder and a prerecorded tape with a three second cadence. This would ensure that the cadence is precise and that all examinees have the same cadence. This also allows the tester to observe the examinee more carefully. Failure of the tester to maintain the cadence while using the stopwatch would invalidate the procedure. The procedure could be adapted for simultaneous testing of several examinees if more than one tester is available and a tape is used. Testers would only be required to count and record repetitions. Since 40 repetitions can be performed in two minutes

using the three second cadence, examinees can be tested quickly. Since this is a test of muscular endurance, the involved area of the body will become fatigued. The procedure may also be used as a training method for the development of muscular endurance.

Baumgartner and Jackson report the procedure was tested using college males. The procedure would probably have validity for both sexes, and a wide age range, so long as the weights selected were light enough so that the weakest examinee could perform at least one repetition. Zero scores cannot be adequately interpreted in tests of muscular endurance and must be avoided. With adequate motivation, discrimination among examinees should be good.

Examinee risk is minimal using the Universal or similar equipment. Free weights increase the risk, but proper spotting and adequate safeguards reduce the risk to an acceptable level. Examinees should be warned that there is a possibility of delayed onset soreness following the testing. Examinees experiencing unusual difficulty, pain, or discomfort should discontinue the test.

Norms are provided for college males. Residual score norms based on body weight are provided for both college females and males. Other age group norms are currently unavailable.

SUMMARY

Major Strengths:

1. Requires little time to administer and can be used for groups if additional testers and equipment are available and a tape recorder is used.

2. Norms are provided for college females and males.

3. Adaptable for all age groups as the weight load can be modified.

4. Eliminates strength as a factor in testing muscular endurance.

Major Weaknesses:

1. Lack of norms for age groups other than college.

2. Guidelines for weight selection for other age groups not provided.

Muscular endurance is a component of physical fitness that is generally measured using tests of one or two specified muscle groups, usually sit ups or pull ups. The procedures recommended by Baumgartner and Jackson provide acceptable tests of muscular endurance, although only tests of the upper body and arms are described. This procedure allows one to measure any muscle group in the body by modifying the test procedures to a specific movement that can be performed with a Universal Gym or other similar weight training devices. Studies that employ these procedures have reported good reliability for other muscle groups and construct validity is established. Objectivity is high unless the tester allows examinees to proceed after failing to maintain the cadence. There is minimal danger in the procedure and normal safeguards for weight training are adequate. The procedure is not only useful for testing but is also a good training method for the development of muscular endurance.

CHIN UP (SUPINATED GRIP) TEST

Reference.

Fleishman, E. A. (1964B). *The structure and measurement of physical fitness*. Englewood Cliffs: Prentice Hall, pp 51, 59, 114.

Additional Source.

Baumgartner & Jackson (1982, p. 208).

Purpose.

To measure the muscular endurance of an examinee's elbow flexor and shoulder extensor muscles.

Objectivity.

Not reported.

Reliability.

r = .93 with no time limit and r = .95 with 20 second time limit (Fleishman, 1964B, p. 59).

Validity.

Construct validity was established.

Age and Sex.

Suitable for females and males, age 12 - adult.

Equipment.

An adjustable horizontal bar.

Space Requirements and Design.

A clear, level area approximately 2m (6') square with the bar and the examinee in the center.

Directions.

The examinee assumes a vertical hanging position with the arms fully extended and the feet above the floor. The hands should be approximately shoulder width apart with the palms facing the body (i.e., forearms supinated). On command, the examinee pulls upward until the chin is above the level of the bar and then returns to the starting position. During the movement, the legs should remain straight and the body should not swing. If the examinee does start to swing, the tester may place an arm across the front of the examinee's thighs. The examinee repeats the up and down movement as many times as possible. One trial is adequate unless, for some reason, the examinee did not receive a fair chance.

Scoring.

The score is the number of properly completed chins.

Norms.

Baumgartner & Jackson (1982, p. 209) youth but sex not given; Corbin & Lindsey (1985, p. 58) men and women; Fleishman (1964A, p. 55) boys and girls; Fleishman (1964B, p. 114) boys and girls; Maryland (1986, p. 19) boys and girls;

McCaughan (1975, p. 15) boys; New York (1958, pp. 53-55) boys; New York (1966, pp. 48-53) boys; Ross et al. (1985, p. 65) boys and girls; Safrit (1986, Appendix A-40) boys and girls; Safrit (1990, pp. 378, Appendix A-41) boys and girls.

NOTE: Fleishman (1964B, p. 51) scored one for a regular chin up and one-half when the arms were not fully extended in the down position or the chin did not reach the bar in the up position.

REVIEW

NANCY STUBBS, Ed.D.

Assistant Professor
Physical Education
Wichita State University
Wichita, KS 67208

The Chin Up Test has been used for a number of years to estimate the muscular endurance of the elbow flexors and the shoulder extensors. However, most chin up or pull up type tests have used the overhand grip (palms away) instead of the supinated grip. This particular test correlates well with other tests of endurance or dynamic strength. These tests include Flexed Arm Hang, Dips, and Rope Climb. All these tests require examinees to either support, or repeatedly move their body weight. The validity of this test was established by construct. The reliability was established in a study conducted at the United States Naval Training Center on male Navy recruits with an average age of 18 years, 3 months and is given as r = .93. Trained testers were used in the study. If directions are followed by each tester, the test should be objective. However, some factors which could vary with each tester are the time allowed for stopping in a single position by the examinee and the amount of kicking and twisting allowed.

The test does not require a lot of expensive equipment or much space. However, bars should be consistent in size and should be higher than the tallest examinee to be tested. The test requires one tester per examinee, but could be performed in partners or groups of three. The time required to administer the test for one examinee is short, but the total time for group testing would be dependent upon the number of bars available and the size of the group. The test is also a conditioning exercise for arm and shoulder endurance. The major problem with this test, as with any test which involves supporting or moving body weight, is the weight of the examinee. The heavier examinee may have the same absolute strength, but must move a heavier weight and, therefore, would not score as well. Fleishman (1964) does recommend a score of one-half when a full chin is not made. However, many females of adolescent age and older may not have the strength to lift their body weight even to score one-half. This test is more of a screening test for arm and shoulder endurance and probably should not be used for more precise measurement.

SUMMARY
Major Strengths:

1. It can be used for large group screening.

2. It is a test as well as a conditioning drill.

3. It does not take skill by the examinee to perform the test.

Major Weaknesses:

1. It discriminates against heavier examinees.

2. It may be difficult to ensure that all examinees in a group are tested alike if more than one tester administers the test, as in a group testing.

3. Females may not be able to do one chin up.

This test would be an acceptable screening test for groups, but would not be acceptable for precise measurement of absolute muscular endurance. The greatest problem would be consistent administration in group settings and weight and sex of the examinees.

DIPS TEST

Reference.
Johnson, B. L., & Nelson, J. K. (1986). *Practical measurements for evaluation in physical education.* Edina, MN: Burgess, pp 141-143.

Additional Sources.
Jensen & Hirst (1980, pp. 88, 90); Miller (1988, pp. 181-182).

Purpose.
To measure the muscular endurance of an examinee's elbow extensor and shoulder flexor muscles.

Objectivity.
r = .99 by Recio cited in Johnson and Nelson (1986, p. 141).

Reliability.
r = .90.

Validity.
Face validity.

Age and Sex.
Suitable for females and males, age 8 - adult.

Equipment.
A set of gymnastic parallel bars, or dip bars, mounted on a wall high enough so the examinee's feet will not touch the floor when he/she assumes a lowered bent arm position. The bars should be approximately shoulder width apart.

Space Requirements and Design.
A clear, level area approximately 2m (6') square with dip bars mounted to the wall or an area approximately 2m x 4m (6' x 12') with a set of parallel bars positioned in the center.

Directions.
The parallel bars should be set to a minimum height of, approximately the examinee's shoulders. The examinee grasps the bars and jumps up to a straight arm support position. On command, the examinee lowers the body until the arms form an angle less than 90 degrees at the elbows. To complete the movement, the examinee returns to the straight arm support position. During the movement, the examinee should not be permitted to swing, and the legs should remain straight. The movement is continued for as many repetitions as possible.

Scoring.
The score is the number of properly completed movements accomplished during one trial. A second trial is normally not needed unless the examinee failed to receive a fair chance on the first trial.

Norms.
Evans (1973, p. 386) rugby players; Johnson & Nelson (1986, p. 143) men; Stokes et al. (1986, p. 172) men; Texas (separate pamphlet, no page numbers) boys.

REVIEW

DOUGLAS J. GOAR, Ph.D.
Chair and Associate Professor
Health, Physical Education and
Recreation
Kentucky State University
Frankfort, KY 40601

The parallel bar Dips Test has had a long history of use as a test to measure arm and shoulder girdle muscular endurance and as a component of muscular strength. Sargent (1897) first incorporated the dip test in the Intercollegiate Strength Tests for men. Dips were included in the boy's portion of the Rogers Strength Inventory and Physical Fitness Inventory (Rogers, 1926). Dips were also used in McCloy's Strength Index (1931), Anderson's Weight Strength Tests for girls (1936), Cozen's Muscular Strength Test for boys (1940), Larson's Muscular Strength Test for boys (1940), the WAC (Women's Army Corps) Physical Fitness Rating (1944), and the Illinois Motor Fitness Inventory for college men developed by Cureton (1947). Since that time however, the Dips Test has seen little use and generated limited interest either as a single test or as a component of a test battery for muscular endurance.

Muscular endurance is generally defined as the capacity for a muscle, or muscle group, to resist fatigue while continuing to function at some prescribed work or weight load. In the case of the Dips Test, this load is relative, instead of absolute, since it is dependent on the weight of the examinee. Based on its past use and acceptance as an indicator of muscular endurance by many of the founding fathers of the physical education profession, the Dips Test is considered to have face validity.

Reliability has been reported at r = .90 or higher. Objectivity has been reported between r = .89 to .99 for test batteries which included the Dips Test and was deemed dependent on the training and experience of the tester.

A quick review of the professional literature and measurement textbooks in physical education or exercise science indicates that the Dips Test has been replaced by other measures of both relative and absolute arm and shoulder girdle muscular endurance. The equipment needed to administer the test (i.e., parallel bars or a dip station) are not always readily available. Further, the nature of the equipment limits the number of examination stations most generally to two, one station at each end of a set of parallel bars, making the amount of time needed to administer the test excessive. There is also some risk involved with the test as examinees reach the point of fatigue and could fall onto the bars or to the floor.

Most references to the test indicate that it was principally used for male examinees who were older and more physically mature. It has been noted that most females lack the upper body strength to achieve even one complete dip. Normative data is so out of date or incomplete that it is of no current practical value. The fact that

the Dips Test relies on the relative weight of the examinee makes it statistically cumbersome to use for most research purposes.

The dip is still useful as a conditioning and self evaluation procedure as evidenced by the incorporation of dip stations into most brands of modern weight training equipment. Examinees can easily score themselves and should be able to "feel" if they have dipped down far enough to reach the 90 degree elbow joint angle criteria. Once an individual has developed the muscular endurance to easily handle her/his relative weight, the principle of overload can be applied by suspending additional weight at the waist with a belt or strap.

SUMMARY

In summary, it appears that the Dips Test is generally inadequate for research or teaching except for use as a self evaluation and conditioning activity. The lack of effort on the part of physical education professionals to maintain any normative data, or include the Dips Test into professionally recognized evaluation procedures which measure arm and shoulder girdle muscular endurance, is a strong indication of its shortcomings. Procedures which have achieved greater popularity than the Dips Test include push ups, modified push ups, and squat thrusts. The dependence of the Dips Test on relative instead of absolute weight makes it difficult to use for comparisons between examinees. The demonstrated inappropriateness of the test for females limits the use to the male gender only. The availability of weight training equipment which has absolute workload increments that may readily be applied to both females and males and which has the capability to isolate major muscle groups for examination, has made the Dips Test obsolete.

MODIFIED PULL UP TEST

Reference.

The State Department of Education (1958). *The New York State physical fitness test* (experimental ed.). Albany: State Department of Education, pp 23-27, 57-60.

Additional Sources.

Clarke & Clarke (1987, p. 121); Jensen & Hirst (1980, pp. 95-96); Miller (1988, p. 178).

Purpose.

To measure the muscular strength (endurance) of an examinee's elbow flexor and shoulder extensor muscles.

Objectivity.

Not reported.

Reliability.

Not reported.

Validity.

Not reported.

Age and Sex.

Females, age 12 - 18.

Equipment.

A mat and an adjustable horizontal bar.

Space Requirements and Design.

A clear, level area approximately 3m (10') square with the horizontal bar in the center and the mat positioned under the bar.

Directions.

The examinee stands erect in front of the horizontal bar while the tester adjusts the height of the bar even with the bottom of the examinee's sternum. The examinee then grips the bar with the palms up (i.e., forearms supinated) and slides her feet under the bar until the straight arms form a 90 degree angle with the chest. The body must be kept straight and form an approximate 45 degree angle with the floor. The examinee's body weight rests on the heels which are braced by the tester placing her/his foot sidewise under the examinee's insteps. Once in this ready position, the examinee pulls upward until her chest touches the bar and then returns to the ready position. This sequence is scored as one complete pull up. The sequence is repeated as many times as possible without rest. Throughout the test, the body must remain straight; the arms must be straight in the down position, and the chest must touch the bar in the up position. If the examinee commits any of these faults during the execution of one pull up, the tester should not count that particular pull up.

Scoring.

The score is the number of properly executed pull ups.

Norms.

American Alliance (1975, p. 59) college women; Hoeger (1986, p. 37) women; Johnson & Nelson (1986, p. 382) girls (variation); Metheny et al. (1945, p. 309) girls (variation); National Marine (no date, p. 13) girls; New York (1958, pp. 57-60) girls; New York (1966, pp. 57-62) girls; President's Council (1987, pp. 1-3) USSR girls.

REVIEW

JAMES A. RICHARDSON, Ed.D.

Assistant Professor
Exercise Science and Wellness
The University of South Dakota
Vermillion, SD 57069

As with many tests of this nature, the New York State Physical Fitness Test: Modified Pull Up suggests that strength and endurance are identical, which is not completely accurate. Therefore, the "purpose" of the test is not consistent with the definitions of strength and endurance.

With the lack of objectivity, reliability, and validity measures, it is difficult to support this test when dealing with junior high and senior high school teachers who would be applying this test.

The space required is reasonable and can be found in most any school. The design of the apparatus seems to be less than complete. There are some questions that come to mind. How high must the bar be off the mat? How is the bar secured? How is the support mechanism secured? How is the 45 degree angle measured? These questions should be answered to insure a safe administration of the test.

In the directions, if the bar is at the sternum, how can the arms be at 90 degrees to the chest when the examinee is prone? The directions should read ". . . the straight arms form a 135 degree to the chest. . . ." This would provide a 45 degree angle at the heels, and the superior side of the shoulder.

In addition, the tester placing her/his foot in a way to support the feet of the examinee suggests that the tester is restricted in her/his movement. This situation causes an unsafe situation in relation to assisting the examinee if she starts having difficulty.

Further, in relation to scoring, there is no definition of a "rest." Does this mean that this test requires continuous action?

SUMMARY

Major Strengths:

1. It is easy to administer.

2. It requires a small amount of space.

3. It requires little equipment.

4. It requires little formal training.

Major Weaknesses:

1. It is limited in the specificity of the purpose.

2. There is no differentiation between "strength and endurance."

3. It has no stated objectivity, reliability, or validity.

4. It has no description of the support standard for the horizontal bar.

5. It has no definition of time between the beginning and the end of one pull up.

6. During the entire test, the body and hands are in a state of static contraction which will cause the examinee to experience an artificial increase in systolic and diastolic blood pressure.

The New York State Physical Fitness Test's Modified Pull Up is not an acceptable test of strength or endurance. This test places the body of the examinee in danger from the standpoint of blood pressure. With the general condition of today's youth, it would be advisable to choose some other test of shoulder girdle strength. It would be a difficult test to recommend to teachers who are evaluating the general, or shoulder specific, physical condition of their classes.

MODIFIED PULL UP TEST (BAUMGARTNER)

References.

Baumgartner, T. A. (1978). Modified pull up test. *Research Quarterly,* 49(1):80-84.

Baumgartner, T. A. et al. (1984). Equipment improvements and additional norms for the modified pull up test. *Research Quarterly for Exercise and Sport,* 55:64-68.

Baumgartner, T. A., & Jackson, A. S. (1987). *Measurement for evaluation in physical education and exercise science.* Dubuque, IA: Wm. C. Brown, pp 200-201.

Additional Sources.

Baumgartner & Jackson (1982, pp. 209-210); Baumgartner & Jackson (1991, pp. 239-241); Hastad & Lacy (1989, pp. 200-202); Johnson & Nelson (1986, pp. 135, 137); Miller (1988, p. 179); Safrit (1986, pp. 271-272); Safrit (1990, pp. 403-404).

Purpose.

To measure the muscular strength and/or endurance of an examinee's arms and shoulders.

Objectivity.

Not reported.

Reliability.

Estimates have been reported exceeding r = .90.

Validity.

Face validity was obtained measuring muscular strength and/or endurance of the arms and shoulders.

Age and Sex.

Females and males, grades 1 - college.

Equipment.

A pull up bar mounted on one end of a 2.44m (8') long incline board and a scooter board .46m x .91m (1.5' x 3') (see Baumgartner & Jackson (1990, p. 240).

Space Requirements and Design.

A clear, level area approximately 3m (10') square with the pull up board mounted to a wall or in a doorway so that it forms a 30 degree angle with the floor. The scooter board is placed on the incline board.

Directions.

The examinee assumes a prone position on the scooter board with the bottom of the sternum aligned with the top edge of the scooter board. The examinee then grips the pull up board and assumes a diagonal hanging position with the arms fully extended. The hands should be placed on the pull up bar approximately shoulder width apart with the palms of the hands facing the incline board (i.e., forearms pronated). The examinee pulls her/himself upward until the chin is over the bar and then returns to the diagonal hanging position. The examinee repeats this movement as many times as possible.

Scoring.

The score is the total number of repetitions completed.

Norms.

Baumgartner (1978, p. 83) women; Baumgartner et al. (1984, pp. 64-68) boys, girls men and women; Hastad & Lacy (1989, p. 202) boys and girls; Jackson et al. (1982, p. 164) boys and girls; Johnson & Nelson (1986, p. 137) boys and girls; Miller (1988, p. 180) boys, girls, men and women; Stokes et al. (1986, p. 171) women.

REVIEW

SHARON SHIELDS, Ph.D.

Associate Professor
Teaching and Learning
Peabody College of Vanderbilt
University
Nashville, TN 37232-8285
and
TERESA SHARP, M.Ed.

Research Assistant
Clinical Nutrition
Vanderbilt University Medical Center
Nashville, TN 37232-8285

The Modified Pull Up Test has been validated in the literature. Face validity was obtained measuring muscular strength and/or endurance of the arms and shoulders. Reliability estimates have been reported exceeding r = .90. The test is reproducible by various investigators thus substantiating its' objectivity. The test does not require the active participation of another individual which makes the scoring more objective. The tester, however, is put in the role of motivator to the examinee in order to elicit optimal performance on the test.

Facility and equipment requirements are minimal and inexpensive making the test practical for most settings. Equipment mounting may pose some problems which would make the test prohibitive as a field based measure. The test is not time consuming and this would make it practical for large group testing. The test can be utilized as a drill for aspects of conditioning and training. Precautions should be taken to screen for any shoulder or back injuries or hypertension in the examinees prior to testing. The test, administered under the required conditions, should pose no undue orthopedic or cardiovascular risk to the examinee. This test is validated for females and males in grades one through college, which make it suitable for use as an evaluation tool in educational settings. The test

scoring is objective and can be easily utilized by the examinee for self evaluation. Norms are available, but have not been updated since 1984.

SUMMARY

Major Strengths:

1. A valid and reliable test.

2. Easily administered.

3. Can be used for self evaluation.

4. Norms are available.

5. Excellent test for school settings due to low cost equipment.

Major Weaknesses:

1. Not suitable for field based testing.

2. All age groups have not been validated.

3. Has some dependency on personal motivation.

4. Health screening information needs to be acquired before test administration.

The test is acceptable as an assessment of muscular strength. The test lends itself as an easy self evaluation tool, however examinee motivation may bias the test results.

MODIFIED PULL UP (NCYFSII) TEST

References.
Pate, R. R. et al. (1987). The modified pull up test. *Journal of Physical Education, Recreation and Dance,* 58(9):71-73.

Ross, J. G. et al. (1987). New health related fitness norms. *Journal of Physical Education, Recreation and Dance,* 58(9):66-70.

Additional Sources.
Clarke & Clarke (1987, pp. 163-165); Hastad & Lacy (1989, p. 294); Johnson & Nelson (1986, p. 381); Safrit (1990, pp. 405-406).

Purpose.
To measure the muscular strength/endurance of an examinee's elbow flexor and shoulder extensor muscles.

Objectivity.
Not reported.

Reliability.
Not reported.

Validity.
Not reported.

Age and Sex.
Females and males, age 6 - 18.

Equipment.
A special pull up apparatus with an adjustable bar (see the first reference) and a small mat.

Space Requirements and Design.
A clear, level area approximately 3m (10') square with the pull up apparatus in the center. The small mat should be placed directly under the pull up bar.

Directions.
The examinee assumes a supine position with her/his arms extended vertically directly below the bar. The bar's height is adjusted so that it is 2.5cm - 5.0cm (1" - 2") above the examinee's fingertips. An elastic band is then stretched across the uprights holding the pull up bar, at a height of 18cm - 20cm (7" - 8") below the bar. Once the apparatus is properly adjusted, the examinee grips the bar with the palms facing away (i.e., forearms pronated). The examinee then assumes a straight body position with only the heels touching the floor. Beginning with the arms completely straight, the examinee pulls upward until the chin is hooked over the elastic band and then returns to the down position. This sequence is scored as one pull up. The examinee executes as many pull ups as possible. Throughout the test, the examinee's body must remain straight, the arms must be straight in the down position and the chin must be hooked over the elastic band in the up position. If the examinee commits any of these faults during the execution of one pull up, the tester should not count that particular pull up.

Scoring.
The score is the number of properly executed pull ups.

Norms.
Franks (1989, pp. 42-47) boys and girls; Hastad & Lacy (1989, p. 290) boys and girls; Johnson & Nelson (1986, p. 382) girls; Ross et al. (1987, p. 69) boys and girls; Vermont (1982, pp. 14-15) boys and girls.

REVIEW

BLANCHE W. EVANS, Ed.D.

Exercise Physiologist
Indiana State University
Terre Haute, IN 47809

The validity, objectivity and reliability of the test are not cited and limit its research value. However, other muscular strength and endurance tests, such as the Modified Pull Up (Baumgartner, 1978), report an intraclass reliability of .90. Because the pull up movement is performed until arm and shoulder fatigue, it is logical to assume that some element of muscular strength and endurance is involved. The test has local norms for girls and boys ages 6 to 9 with additional norms expected for ages 6 to 18. Additional data needs to be obtained to make the test more nationally appealing. The directions, as written, are somewhat confusing and may result in some problems with consistency during testing. The review articles were excellent and are highly recommended reading prior to apparatus construction or test administration.

Some advantages of the test include minimal space requirements for equipment, simplicity in equipment design, and economy in equipment construction. The time required to administer the test is minimal and will vary with the number of pull ups completed. Because the actual exercise is not complicated and the rules of test administration are not involved, the exercise may be used as part of other class activities for development of muscular strength and endurance. During testing situations, a trained tester is required to assure body alignment is maintained fo each repetition and to check that the chin clears the elastic band. However, the body alignment and test procedures involve only straight body position, overhand grip with thumb wrap, and chin over the band, so examinees may be taught to self administer the test or work in teams. Though the body position is new for most examinees, it is not difficult to perform and may be mastered with a few trials. The height of the bar for the beginning position is such that an examinee can assume the starting position with little difficulty. One major advantage of the test is that it results in very few zero scores, providing positive feedback to examinees. Therefore, this pull up test discriminates muscular strength and endurance at the lower end of the scale better than the traditional pull up and flexed arm hang tests.

Though the need for specially designed equipment is a disadvantage, the apparatus may be made at minimal cost. It may even be made by adapting existing equipment. The test is not dangerous, but caution should be used when supervising the test area. A protective pad should be placed under the exercise area to prevent or minimize the chance of injury should

an examinee's grip fail as a result of fatigue or perspiration. In addition, caution should be used in the selection of the material for the elastic band. An examinee could receive cuts or burns from inappropriately selected material used for the pull up elastic band. The use of a small board, or foot stop, might keep an examinee from slipping out of position and releasing the grip. Whether such a board would alter the test outcome is not known.

SUMMARY

Major Strengths:

1. Simplicity of design.

2. Ease of administration.

3. Low cost of the modified pull up test.

4. Its positive feedback about muscular strength and endurance make it an attractive exercise and test choice.

5. The test may be used for self evaluation or assessment of progress.

6. The positive presentation of the test with virtually no zero scores is quite appealing and should prove satisfying to both examinees and teachers.

Major Weaknesses:

1. Even though local norms are provided for ages 6 to 8, national norms would enhance the appeal of the test to teachers.

2. The lack of objectivity, reliability and validity measures is a negative.

This is an excellent test that takes into account the weaknesses of other upper body muscular strength and endurance tests. Further research should be conducted to provide additional norms for national appeal. The test is an excellent educational tool for use in teaching, testing, and demonstrations of muscular strength and endurance.

MODIFIED PUSH UP TEST

Reference.
Johnson, B. L., & Nelson, J. K. (1986). *Practical measurements for evaluation in physical education*. Edina, MN: Burgess, pp 139-140, 142, 379, 382.

Additional Sources.
Clarke & Clarke (1987, p. 122); Jensen & Hirst (1980, pp. 91, 93-95); Kirkendall et al. (1980, p. 325); Miller (1988, pp. 182-183).

Purpose.
To measure the muscular endurance of an examinee's elbow extensor and shoulder flexor muscles.

Objectivity.
Not reported.

Reliability.
As high as r = .93, Johnson and Nelson (1986, p. 139).

Validity.
As high as r = .72 with Roger's Short Index by Stumiller and Johnson (1976) cited in Johnson and Nelson (1986, p. 139).

Age and Sex.
Suitable for females and males, age 6 - adult.

Equipment. None.
Space Requirements and Design.
A clear, level area approximately 3m (10') square with the examinee in the center.

Directions.
The examinee assumes a prone position on the floor. The knees are bent 90 degrees so that the lower legs stick up in the air. The hands, fingers pointed forward, are positioned directly beneath the shoulders. The body is raised from the floor until the arms are straight and then lowered until the chest touches the floor. This sequence is scored as one complete push up. The sequence is repeated as many times as possible without rest. Throughout the test, the body must remain straight with the knees bent 90 degrees, the arms must be straight in the up position and the chest must touch the floor in the down position. If the examinee commits any of these faults during the execution of one push up, the tester should not count that particular push up.

Scoring.
The score is the number of properly executed push ups.

Norms.
Alexander et al. (1985, p. 9) girls and women on 30 second speed push up test; Chrysler/AAU (1990, p. 6) girls; Fitness Institute (1981, no page) girls and women; Hoeger (1989, p. 50) women;

Johnson and Nelson (1986, p. 142, 382) girls and college women; Kirkendall et al. (1980, pp. 328-330) boys and girls (variation); Lindsey et al. (1989, p. 9) women; Metheny et al. (1945, p. 309) girls;

National Marine (no date, p. 9) girls; New York (1958, pp. 51-52, 56-57) boys and girls; New York (1966, pp. 45-47, 54-56) boys and girls; O'Connor & Cureton (1945, p. 314) girls; Pyke (1986, p. 9) boys and girls (variation); Van Gelder & Marks (1987, p. 189) women.

REVIEW

E. R. BUSKIRK, Ph.D.
Professor of Applied Physiology
The Pennsylvania State University
University Park, PA 16802

This test measures shoulder girdle and arm strength, particularly that of the elbow extensors. With the arms extended, the body weight is supported both by the arms and the knees. Support by the latter, rather than the toes, qualifies the test as a modified push up. When performed properly, the test, is indeed, one that tests both shoulder girdle and elbow extension strength and strength endurance. Data on reliability are available with correlation coefficients among repeated measurements of the order of 0.90 or higher. Instructions for proper conduct of the test are relatively simple. There should be no problem teaching testers the proper procedure. Thus, consistency among testers should be easy to achieve. The test requires participation of no more than one tester. In fact, one tester could test two or three examinees at one time after being properly trained.

Facility and space requirements are minimal. The environmental conditions should be non-stressful, and only light weight clothing should be worn. Any shirt should be rather tight fitting in order for the tester to be sure that the chest touches the floor. The equipment requirements are minimal. The floor surface should be non slip and also non abrasive. A padded surface, such as the foam mats used in gymnastics for floor exercises, would be appropriate. Although the test is easy to administer, attention needs to be paid throughout the test to the examinee's body alignment both in the up and down positions. The test sequence may be repeated as many times as possible without rest by a given examinee, but for many fit people, a reasonable limit should be set depending on the population surveyed and the goals of the testing. Push ups can be used to develop arm and shoulder girdle strength and endurance. The test is suitable for most all age levels except, perhaps, for the very young or elderly. The test is not dangerous if the examinee is appropriately instructed and supervised. As indicated previously, use of a padded surface should preclude any facial injuries. Muscular injuries are highly unlikely. Scoring is objective when the testers are properly trained, and only appropriate movements are counted. The test could be used as part of a general fitness or strength testing battery. Norms are available for different age groups for both genders.

SUMMARY
Major Strengths:
1. The test is easy to administer.
2. The test does measure shoulder girdle and particularly elbow extension strength and endurance.

Major Weaknesses:
1. It is limited applicability to the very young and elderly.
2. The fact that very fit and strong examinees can do modified push ups for many minutes, or even hours.
3. Also, the test, if conducted to volitional exhaustion, has a subjective endpoint.

The test is acceptable for classroom demonstrations and field research. Gross differences in strength and strength endurance can be ascertained. As part of a test battery for the appraisal of physical fitness, the Modified Push Up Test could be used in research to test shoulder girdle and elbow extension strength and endurance.

PULL-UP TEST

Reference.

AAHPER (1975). *AAHPER youth fitness manual.* Washington DC: American Alliance for Health, Physical Education and Recreation, p 16.

Additional Sources.

Barrow et al. (1989, pp. 108, 113-115); Baumgartner & Jackson (1987, p. 279); Baumgartner & Jackson (1991, pp. 260, 267); Bosco & Gustafson (1983, pp. 95, 97-98);

Clarke & Clarke (1987, pp. 120-121, 214-215); Hastad & Lacy (1989, pp. 196-197, 233-234, 237-238, 285); Jensen & Hirst (1980, pp. 93-95); Johnson & Nelson (1986, pp. 105, 134-135); Kirkendall et al. (1980, p. 269);

Kirkendall et al. (1987, p. 150); Miller (1988, pp. 177-178); Safrit (1981, p. 239); Safrit (1986, pp. 268-270); Safrit (1990, pp. 400-402); Verducci (1980, pp. 248, 282-287).

Purpose.

To measure the muscular endurance of an examinee's elbow flexor and shoulder extensor muscles.

Objectivity.

r = .99 by Recio, cited in Johnson and Nelson (1986, p. 134).

Reliability.

r = .89 by Klesius, cited in Verducci (1980. p. 287).

Validity.

Not reported.

Age and Sex.

Females and males, age 8 - adult.

Equipment.

An adjustable horizontal bar or doorway gym bar or inclined ladder or a horizontal ladder.

Space Requirements and Design.

A clear, level area approximately 2m (6') square with the horizontal bar and examinee in the center. A clearance height of 1m (3') above the bar.

Directions.

The examinee grips the horizontal bar and assumes a vertical hanging position with the arms fully extended and the feet above the floor. The hands should be approximately shoulder width apart with the palms of the hands facing away from the body (i.e., pronated grip). On command, the examinee pulls upward until the chin is above the level of the bar and then returns to the starting position. During the movement, the legs should remain straight, and the body should not swing. If body swing does start to occur, the tester may place an arm across the front of the examinee's thighs to stop any swinging movement. The examinee repeats the movement as many times as possible.

Scoring.

The score is the number of properly completed movements. One trial is adequate unless, for some reason, the examinee did not receive a fair chance.

Norms.

Alabama (1988, pp. 13-15, 18-19) boys and girls; American Alliance (1975, pp. 34, 49, 54, 60) boys and men; American Alliance (1988, pp. 28-29) boys and girls; American Alliance (1989, pp. 10-11) boys and girls;

American Alliance (1990, pp. 10-11) boys and girls; Chrysler/AAU (1990, p. 6) boys; Barrow et al. (1989, p. 105) boys and girls; Baumgartner & Jackson (1987, pp. 279, 286) boys; Baumgartner & Jackson (1991, pp. 260, 288-289) boys and girls;

Clarke & Clarke (1987, pp. 162, 166) boys; Evans (1973, p. 386) rugby players; Getchell (1983, p. 48) men; Greenberg & Pargman (1989, p. 81) men; Hastad & Lacy (1989, pp. 197, 284) boys and girls; Hoeger (1986, p. 37) men;

Johnson & Nelson (1986, pp. 106, 136, 203-204, 205, 207) boys, men, and army and navy; Kirkendall et al. (1980, pp. 283-284) boys; Kirkendall et al. (1987, p. 157) boys; Lindsey et al. (1989, p. 9) men and women; Miller (1988, pp. 178, 234) boys and girls; National Marine (no date, p. 11) boys; President's Council (1987, pp. 1-7) USSR boys; President's Council (1988, pp. 4, 7) boys and girls; President' Council (1989, p. 8) boys and girls;

Safrit (1986, p. 275) boys; Safrit (1990, pp. 342, 347, 352); Shannon (1989, p. 45) high school football players; Stokes et al. (1986, p. 171) men; Virginia (1988, pp. 15, 19) boys and girls.

REVIEW

STEVEN J. ALBRECHTSEN, Ph.D.
Director
Human Performance Laboratory
University of Wisconsin-Whitewater
Whitewater, WI 53190

The Pull-Up Test is a traditionally recognized and frequently administered test of muscular endurance. Almost all examinees are familiar with the test, and most examinees have previously performed pull ups. The test is not acceptable for measuring muscular strength, as performance is dependent upon a combination of both muscular endurance and muscular strength, including a minimal level of muscular strength which many examinees do not possess. The validity of the test for measuring muscular endurance is limited because of this requirement for a minimal level of muscular strength.

The reliability of the Pull-Up Test is high, but it may be affected if the examinees participate in related exercise prior to the administration of the test. The objectivity of the test is high, and the test does not require the participation of another individual who could affect the performance of the examinees. Norms and standards have been developed for a variety of age groups and other specific populations.

The equipment necessary for the Pull-Up Test is readily available or easily improvised. The instructions specify an overhand grip with the palms of the hands facing away from the body. A similar test can also be administered using an underhand grip with the palms facing toward the body. Wells (1971) maintains that the underhand grip involves greater use of the biceps. With the overhand grip the involvement of the biceps is diminished because the tendon is wrapped around the radius and effective arm leverage is reduced.

The completion of a single pull up requires examinees to possess sufficient muscular strength to be able to lift their body weight. The results of the test for most populations are positively skewed, and the test may not adequately discriminate among a significant percentage of examinees who are unable to lift their body weight and perform a single pull up. Available norms and standards indicate increasing repetitions with increasing age among children and decreasing repetitions with increasing age among adults. Norms for the AAHPERD Youth Fitness Test (1976) indicate that 50 percent of 10 year old boys are able to perform no more than a single pull up. While pull up performance improves with increasing age in children, a substantial percentage of children at all ages are unable to perform a single pull up. The recently developed Physical Best (1988) indicates a health fitness standard of only one pull up for boys ages 5 - 10 increasing to only five pull ups for boys ages 15 - 18. The various norms and standards for adults show similar problems with increasing age.

It is recommended that muscular endurance be assessed using tests that involve a smaller percentage of body weight or muscular strength. The Modified Pull-Up Test by Baumgartner (1978) was developed to reduce the importance of muscular strength and to provide a broader distribution of scores with greater discrimination. Examinees who are unable to perform at least one traditional pull up are usually able to achieve a non zero score using the Modified Pull-Up Test. The Modified Pull-Up Test by Baumgartner is reviewed elsewhere in this publication.

SUMMARY

Major Strengths:

1. The examinees are familiar with the test.

2. The equipment for the test is readily available or easily improvised.

3. The test is simple to administer.

4. Norms and standards are available for evaluating the results of the test.

Major Weaknesses:

1. The test involves a relationship between muscular endurance and muscular strength.

2. The test requires that the examinees possess a minimal level of muscular strength.

3. The results of the test are positively skewed and may not discriminate adequately.

The Pull-Up Test is an acceptable test for teaching when the examinees possess an adequate level of muscular strength and when the limitations of the test are considered in evaluating the results. The Pull-Up Test is an unacceptable test for research because of the relationship between muscular endurance and muscular strength.

REVIEW REFERENCES

AAHPER (1976). *Youth fitness test manual.* Washington, DC: American Alliance for Health, Physical Education and Recreation.

AAHPERD (1988). *Physical best.* Reston, VA: American Alliance for health, Physical Education, Recreation and Dance.

Baumgartner, T. A. (1978). Modified pull up test. *Research Quarterly,* 49:80-84.

Wells, K. R. (1971). *Kinesiology.* Philadelphia: Saunders.

PUSH UP TEST

Reference.
Johnson, B. L., & Nelson, J. K. (1986). *Practical measurements for evaluation in physical education.* Edina, MN: Burgess, pp 137-141, 207.

Additional Sources.
Clarke & Clarke (1987, pp. 121-122, 157); Jensen & Hirst (1980, pp. 90-91); Kirkendall et al. (1980, p. 231); Kirkendall et al. (1987, p. 109); Miller (1988, p. 182).

Purpose.
To measure the muscular endurance of an examinee's elbow extensor and shoulder flexor muscles.

Objectivity.
r = .99 by Recio (1972), cited in Johnson and Nelson (1986, p. 138).

Reliability.
r = .76 with 15 second time limit and r = .88 with unlimited time using test-retest method by Fleishman (1964B, p. 59).

Validity.
Face validity.

Age and Sex.
Suitable for males.

Equipment. None.

Space Requirements and Design.
A clear, level area approximately 3m (10') square with the examinee in the center.

Directions.
The examinee assumes a prone position on the floor with the body straight. The hands, fingers pointed forward, are positioned directly beneath the shoulders. The examinee raises his body from the floor until the arms are straight and then lowers his body until the chest touches the floor. This sequence is scored as one complete push up. The sequence is repeated as many times as possible without rest. Throughout the test the examinee's body must remain straight; the arms must be straight while the examinee is in the up position, and the examinee's chest must touch the floor in the down position. If the examinee commits any of these faults during the execution of one push up, the tester should not count that particular push up.

Scoring.
The score is the number of properly executed push ups.

Norms.
Alexander et al. (1985, p. 9) Canadian women; Canadian Minister (1979, p. 18) men and women; Fitness Canada (1986, p. 37) boys, girls, men and women; Fitness Institute (1981, no page numbers) boys and men; Hoeger (1986, p. 37) men;

Johnson & Nelson (1986, pp. 141, 207) boys and men, army and navy; Kirkendall et al. (1980, pp. 235-240) boys, men and women; Kirkendall et al. (1987, pp. 113-117) boys, men, and women; Miller (1988, p. 182) men and women; Lindsey et al. (1989, p. 9) men and women;

National Marine (no date, p. 8) boys; Pollock & Wilmore (1990, p. 687) men and women; Shannon (1989, p. 45) high school football players; Stephens et al. (1986, p. 15) men and women; Strokes et al. (1986, p. 172) men and women; Van Gelder & Marks (1987, p. 189) men.

REVIEW

JEFFREY C. RUPP, Ph.D.

Associate Professor
Health, Physical Education,
Recreation and Dance
Georgia State University
Atlanta, GA 30303

The test would seem to have some degree of validity. However, the test constructors assume face validity, and no comparisons to other tests are cited. Reliability is acceptable when time is not limited for the test. Use of a 15 second time limit significantly reduced reliability and may be more a measure of muscular power than endurance. Objectivity was excellent as reported by Recio (1972). One problem with this test becomes evident when an examinee cannot perform one push up. Under these circumstances, it is questionable whether the examinee is deficient in muscular strength, endurance, or both. Many times this test is given where a partner counts the number of correctly performed push ups. This may significantly reduce the objectivity estimates cited above.

This test does not require any equipment or a significant amount of space. Large numbers of examinees can be tested in a relatively short time period when partners score the test. The administration of the test is simple, however as stated previously, the tester must be able to identify what constitutes an acceptable push up.

The test is appropriate for the intended age range, however the procedures are not modified for those who may not be able to perform one repetition. This will limit the usefulness of the test. The test can be easily practiced and should be familiar to most examinees. Norms are readily available, however many are outdated.

This test is suitable for research purposes, but it should be noted that there are better tests of muscular endurance for these muscle groups. An example would be a bench press test using a standard percentage of a one repetition maximum lift.

SUMMARY

Major Strengths:

1. Facility and/or space requirements are minimal.

2. No special equipment is required.

3. Test is relatively easy to administer.

4. Test does not require an inordinate amount of time to administer.

Major Weaknesses:

1. No validity coefficient is reported.

2. Test is not modified for lower abilities.

3. Scoring requires knowledge of what constitutes a proper push up.

4. Test does not discriminate as well as some other tests.

This is an acceptable test for teaching purposes. However, if it is used for research purposes, scoring should be done by a qualified tester (not a partner). In addition, the ability of the test to measure muscular endurance is questionable if the examinee cannot perform one repetition.

DYNAMIC MUSCULAR ENDURANCE TESTS
OF THE ABDOMEN AND/OR HIPS

HANGING HALF-LEVER TEST

Reference.
McCloy, C. H., & Young, N. D. (1954). *Tests and measurements in health and physical education.* New York: Appleton-Century-Crofts, p. 174.

Additional Sources.
None.

Purpose.
To measure the muscular endurance of an examinee's abdominal and hip flexor muscles.

Objectivity.
Not reported.

Reliability.
Not reported.

Validity.
Not reported.

Age and Sex.
Not reported, but suitable for females and males, age 8 - adult.

Equipment.
An adjustable horizontal bar, doorway gym bar, inclined ladder, or a horizontal ladder.

Space Requirements and Design.
A clear, level area approximately 2m (6') square with the horizontal bar in the center.

Directions.
The examinee assumes a vertical hanging position with the feet above the floor. On command, the examinee raises the legs until they are parallel to the floor and then returns the legs to the vertical position. The body should not be permitted to swing nor should the knees be allowed to bend during the movement. [The editor assumes that the horizontal bar is grasped with the palms of the hands facing forward.]

Scoring.
The score is the number of movements that can be executed continuously.

Norms.
Not reported.

REVIEW

MICHAEL MANGUM, Ph.D.
Assistant Professor
Physical Education and Leisure Management
Columbus College
Columbus, GA 31993

The original test, as described by McCloy and Young (1954), required examinees to hang from a horizontal bar, to raise the legs until parallel to the floor, and then to return to the vertical position without swinging or allowing the knees to bend.

For this analysis the test was modified in two important ways. First, the hip flexor station of the Universal Gym was utilized in lieu of the horizontal bar. Secondly, hip flexion was performed as described by McCloy and Young and also by raising the knees to the chest (referred to here as a "hip curl"). In addition, sit ups (bent knees with partner stabilizing feet) were also performed. Each test provided for maximal repetitions within one minute.

Twenty-three examinees (20 females and 3 males) performed each of the three tests (sit ups, modified half lever, and hip curl) on two occasions, prior to familiarization and after four weeks of training/familiarization with the tasks. Means, standard deviations, and Pearson correlations were calculated to allow comparison of sit ups and each of the other tests. In addition, the two variations of the half lever were correlated.

Informal biomechanical/kinesiological analysis of all three tasks (sit up, hip curl, and modified half lever) would suggest that each would be of value as a measure of abdominal/hip flexor muscle endurance. These data do not speak directly to the actual validity of these items (in the absence of acceptable criterion) but do raise some interesting questions and observations.

Table 1. Mean one minute repetitions for sit ups, hip curl, and modified half lever

	Pretest			After Familiarization		
	Mean	SD	Range	Mean	SD	Range
Sit Up	23.1	7.3	14-42	31.4	8.4	14-50
Hip Curl	25.9	9.2	0-43	31.8	9.9	14-47
Mod Half Lever	11.7	6.3	0-23	18.5	8.2	0-33

Table 2. Bivariate correlations (r) and coefficients of determination (r^2) for sit up, hip curl, and modified half lever

	Pretest		After Familiarization	
	r	r^2	r	r^2
Sit Up/Hip Curl	-.18	.03	-.01	0
Sit Up/Mod Half Lever	.29	.08	.20	.04
Hip Curl/Mod Half Lever	.45	.20	.74	.55

It is apparent that the modified half lever or the hip curl cannot be used interchangeably with sit ups as a measure of abdominal/hip flexor endurance. Performance in one task is not comparable to performance in another, despite the observation that mean responses on the hip curls were similar to sit ups before and after familiarization/training on each task.

The tests clearly discriminate among performances. However, it appears, subjectively, that anthropometric factors (such as adiposity, distribution of adiposity, etc.) may play a major factor in the discrimination and not muscle endurance per se. An analogy may be made to pull ups, where a large body weight affects pull up performance adversely.

SUMMARY

1. "Validity" of the tests are inherent in the biomechanical/kinesiological requirements of the tasks.

However, test should be utilized to reflect specific training or suitability to a specific task. Interchangeability of tests is not apparent, with possible exception.

2. Correlation between half lever and hip curl was modest after familiarization with the tasks (.74) and suggest that they may possibly be interchanged. The hip curl is recommended as a lead in training tool to the half lever.

LEG LIFTS TEST

Reference.

Fleishman, E. A. (1964B). *The structure and measurement of physical fitness.* Englewood Cliffs: Prentice Hall, pp 59, 128, 168-169.

Additional Source.

Jensen & Hirst (1980, p. 99).

Purpose.

To measure the muscular endurance of an examinee's abdominal and hip flexor muscles.

Objectivity.

Not reported.

Reliability.

r = .84 for 20 second test (Fleishman, 1964B, p. 59) and r = .89 for test-retest (Fleishman, 1964B, p. 128).

Validity.

Construct validity was established.

Age and Sex.

Suitable for females and males, age 8 - adult.

Equipment.

A stopwatch and a mat.

Space Requirements and Design.

A clear, level area approximately 3m (10') square with the mat in the center.

Directions.

The examinee assumes a supine position on the mat with hands clasped behind the neck. A partner holds the examinee's elbows to the mat. On command, "Ready, Go," the examinee raises both legs until they attain a vertical position and then lowers them to the floor. This sequence is repeated as many times as possible in 30 seconds. The knees should remain straight and the legs together during the entire movement.

Scoring.

The score is the number of leg lifts performed during the 30 seconds.

Norms.

Beunen et al. (1988, pp. 33, 83, 95) boys; Evans (1973, p. 386) rugby players; Fleishman (1964A, p. 57) boys and girls; McCaughan (1975, p. 15) boys; Ostyn et al. (1980, pp. 104, 127-140) boys; Simons et al. (1990, p. 101) girls.

REVIEW

JOSEY H. TEMPLETON, Ph.D.

Assistant Professor
Health and Physical Education
The Citadel
Charleston, SC 29409

Reliability for this test has been established, but objectivity has not. Objectivity could easily be established as the test is simple to explain, easy to evaluate, and involves only the examinee, a partner, and the tester.

The equipment and facility required for the test are readily available. The leadership and expertise required to administer this test are easily within the capabilities of any physical educator.

Since the testing period is only 30 seconds, it can be administered easily to an entire class in a short amount of time with one-third of the class performing the test, one-third acting as partners holding the examinee's elbows to the mat, and the other one-third serving as evaluators to determine the vertical lift and lowering of the legs. Younger evaluators should have "until they attain a vertical position and then lowers them to the floor" demonstrated and clarified for them.

The test is a dynamic, repetitive task of 30 seconds duration during which the examinee performs as many identical movements as possible. Because some examinees may be able to continue repetitive movements of this type for a long period, it is necessary to impose a time limit. Whether 30 seconds provides adequate time in which to measure muscular endurance, rather than speed of movement for examinees of varying age and fitness levels, is open to question. The test is a measure for endurance; therefore, one trial is appropriate.

Based on a recent article concerning physical activities that may be damaging to the lower back (Lindsey & Corbin, *JOPERD,* October, 1989, pp. 26-32), this test would not be suitable for use as a drill to promote learning and/or conditioning for the general public. It might be appropriate in some situations, but not for a general physical education class. The test has questionable suitability for the recommended age level and ability level of females and males, ages 8 to adult. The results of numerous research projects indicate that the abdominal muscles are weak in most children and adults; and, that many adults have lower back problems for which this type movement would be contraindicated.

If the information about abdominal muscle weakness is considered, the test discriminates among most of its recommended users. The test could also be potentially dangerous for its recommended users. In their article, Lindsey and Corbin (October, 1989, pp. 26-32) suggested that an injury could occur the first time an activity was performed or after it had been performed numerous times. They specifically referred to the bilateral straight leg raise activity and suggested that a "microtrauma" occurs with each repetition of an exercise that violates physiologic movements or normal joint mechanics. They also emphasized that, according to the law of specificity, individuals should practice the same exercises, using the same muscles on which they would be tested, to score well. If this were the case for the Leg Lifts Test, considerable damage might be done to examinees who had not practiced or not practiced sufficiently to develop the muscles to perform the test for a determination of muscular endurance.

The scoring of the Leg Lifts Test cannot really be considered objective because the tester must determine if the legs are raised to vertical and then lowered to the floor with the legs together and knees straight while counting the number of lifts. It is not just a simple matter of counting the lifts. It would be difficult for an examinee to determine if her/his own legs reached vertical while meeting the other performance criteria, counting and timing himself/herself. Therefore, the test would not be suitable for self evaluation.

The test is of suitable precision for research purposes, but that is about where the line should be drawn. Because of the danger of potential injury, the test should not be considered for research purposes using individuals from the general public. Other considerations which would have to be made when using the test are the differences in leg lengths of examinees of the same sex and age, and the motivational levels of the examinees when performing a test which might be difficult and painful if they do not have good abdominal and hip flexor strength.

SUMMARY

Major Strengths:

1. It is easy to administer when considering facility, equipment, and training of testers.

2. A large number of examinees can be tested at one time.

3. It can measure the abdominal and hip flexor muscular endurance of an examinee who has developed adequate strength to perform the movements of the test.

Major Weaknesses:

1. It could be dangerous and/or painful for most examinees.

2. It might not measure muscular endurance in some untrained/unfit examinees.

3. It is difficult to standardize the movement of the legs (based on leg length) and the level of motivation of the examinees.

The most important reason that the Leg Lifts Test is unacceptable for research and teaching is the potential for injury to the untrained/unfit examinee. This should be sufficient reason to select and/or develop safer tests to measure abdominal and hip flexor muscular endurance.

PARTIAL CURL UP TEST

References.
Faulkner, R. A. et al. (1989). A partial curl up protocol for adults based on an analysis of two procedures. *Canadian Journal of Sport Sciences,* 14:135-141.

Fitness Canada (1986). *Canadian Standardized Test of Fitness (CSTF).* Ottawa, Canada: Government of Canada Fitness and Amateur Sport.

Additional Sources.
None.

Purpose.
To measure the endurance of the abdominal muscles in the adult population.

Objectivity.
Not reported.

Reliability.
Not reported.

Validity.
Not reported.

Age and Sex.
Females and males, age 18 - 69 + .

Equipment.
A mat, goniometer, metronome, marking tape, and two 30cm (12") long measuring sticks.

Space Requirements and Design.
A clear, level area approximately 3m (10') square with the mat positioned in the center. The metronome is placed next to the mat.

Directions.
The metronome is set at 50 beats per minute to produce 25 curl ups per minute. The examinee assumes a supine position (i.e., lying on the back) on the mat with the knees bent 90 degrees. The correct knee angle should be verified by the tester using the goniometer. The examinee's head rests in the tester's hand which in turn rests on the mat. A piece of marking tape is placed on the mat under each heel to mark the spot the heels must remain throughout the test. The examinee's arms are held straight at the sides of the body with the palms of the hands resting on the mat. A measuring stick is positioned under

each hand so that the zero mark is even with the fingertips. The curl up is executed by initially flattening the lower back against the mat, followed by a slow curl up of the trunk and a sliding of the palms of the hands over the measuring sticks until the fingertips reach the 12cm (4.72") mark if the examinee is less than 40 years of age and the 8cm (3.15") mark if the examinee is 40 years of age or older. The examinee then returns to the starting position. Both the curl up and return movements are executed in a slow, controlled manner in cadence with the metronome. The two movements should use the same amount of time. The test is stopped when the examinee cannot maintain the proper cadence (i.e., falls behind two repetitions), cannot reach the 8cm or 12cm mark, or completes a maximum of 75 curl ups. If the examinee fails to reach the 8cm or 12cm mark during the first few attempts, a score of zero is recorded.

Scoring.
The score is the number of properly executed curl ups completed up to a maximum of 75.

Norms.
Fitness Canada (1986).

REVIEW

MYRNA M. SCHILD, Ed.S.

Assistant Professor
Physical Education
Southern Illinois University
Edwardsville, IL 62026

The Partial Curl Up Test has been derived from the standardized Curl Up/Sit Up Test which has been widely used for many years. The Full Curl Up Test has recently been judged by experts in exercise and sports medicine to be unsafe for general populations. Because of its innate design as a time dynamic repetitive test, form becomes secondary to performance. Back injuries, especially those affecting the vertebrae and intervertebral discs of the cervical and lordotic curves, have been a common complaint by Full Curl Up examinees. Also, the primary purpose of the Full Curl Up Test is to measure abdominal strength, but this is often negated by the hip flexors which usually prevail. The recent mobilization toward accountability in exercise technique makes a good, safe measure of abdominal strength a necessity.

Since the objectivity, reliability and validity are not given, it is difficult to project these values for the Partial Curl Up Test. However, since this test is similar to the Full Curl Up Test, it is probable that these scientific aspects could be developed and/or fulfilled. If the tester requires the examinee to perform the Partial Curl Up Test in the manner described, it is surmised that the test should adequately serve as a measure of abdominal strength, and it should also measure this physical component consistently when it is administered by different testers.

The Partial Curl Up Test considers safety and concern for injury. It requires nominal facilities and space. It also encourages learning the proper function of the abdominal muscles and applying this knowledge toward proper conditioning techniques. Because of test design and precise directions for implementation, few demands are made of the tester concerning expertise and time required to administer the test. However, in some cases, obtaining a goniometer and metronome may be difficult. Although the test is recommended for adults only, other age groups could easily participate. Also, if provisions for achievement were stated, anyone could self evaluate using this test for practice purposes. Norms are not provided for this test, but it is conceivable that they could be developed

through research. The success of the test depends on the accuracy of the tester and adherence to the test requirements.

SUMMARY

Major Strengths:

1. A high safety rating (the test uses a rate of speed and a position of extremities which reduces trauma of spinal column).

2. A high rated measure of abdominal strength (similar to abdominal "crunches").

3. The test is quick and easy to administer.

4. The test encourages concurrent learning and proper techniques of physical conditioning.

5. The test could be adapted for almost anyone (except the severely handicapped).

Major Weaknesses:

1. Equipment (goniometer and metronome) required.

2. Recorded repetitions are subject to accuracy of the tester.

3. Scientific aspects need to be included (statement of objectivity, reliability, validity, and norms for confirmation).

4. Test could be administered to younger ages than the recommended 18 years.

The Partial Curl Up Test is an acceptable test (possibly excellent, with revisions).

REVIEW REFERENCE

Schild, M. (1990). *Exercise education - A personal approach to weight control and wellness*. Florissant, MO: Auto-Review Publishers.

SIT UP TEST

Reference.
Scott, M. G., & French, E. (1959). *Measurement and evaluation in physical education.* Dubuque: Wm. C. Brown, pp 299-301.

Additional Sources.
Barrow et al. (1989, pp. 107, 109-110, 117, 131, 141); Baumgartner & Jackson (1982, pp. 211-214, 248, 261-264); Baumgartner & Jackson (1987, pp. 202, 264, 280, 297-299, 304, 312); Baumgartner & Jackson (1991, pp. 241-243, 263, 283-285, 287);

Bosco & Gustafson (1983, pp. 98-99); Clarke & Clarke (1987, pp. 155, 157, 159, 163-165, 213-214); Hastad & Lacy (1989, pp. 193-196, 230-231, 233, 238, 283-285, 287, 293); Jensen & Hirst (1980, p. 98); Johnson & Nelson (1986, pp. 108, 111, 131-134, 379, 384);

Kirkendall et al. (1980, pp. 231, 270-271, 299); Kirkendall et al. (1987, pp. 109, 151-152, 169, 397); Miller (1988, pp. 174-175); Safrit (1981, pp. 240-241); Safrit (1986, pp. 238-241, 275-277, 440); Safrit (1990, pp. 241, 364, 366-367, 370-372); Verducci (1980, pp. 248, 281-282, 284, 287).

Purpose.
To measure the muscular endurance of an examinee's abdominal muscles.

Objectivity.
Not reported.

Reliability.
r = .94 for 140 college women; r = .68 for first graders; and r = .77 for sixth graders as derived by Magnusson; r = .94 for a random sample of first through ninth graders by Buxton cited in Scott and French (1959, p. 299).

Validity.
r = .48 and r = .52 during two successive studies between sit up scores and work output on an ergometer.

Age and Sex.
Females and males, grades 1 - college.

Equipment.
A mat.

Space Requirements and Design.
A clear, level area approximately 2m x 3m (6' x 10') with the mat in the center.

Directions.
The examinee assumes a seated position on the mat with the feet flat, knees bent, and the back straight. The angle of knee flexion is determined by placing the hands on the shoulders with the elbows resting on top of the knees. The examinee then reclines on her/his back while keeping the hands on the shoulders, with an assistant holding the feet firmly in place. On command, the examinee flexes the trunk far enough to touch the elbows to the knees and then returns to the mat with the head not touching. The examinee does as many of the up and down movements as possible in one minute. The examinee may stop and rest during the one minute period.

Scoring.
The score is the number of correctly completed sit ups executed in one minute.

Norms.
Alabama (1988, pp. 13-17) boys and girls; American Alliance (1975, pp. 27, 35, 59-60) boys, girls, college men and women; American Alliance (1980, pp. 11-21, 32-33) boys and girls; American Alliance (1985, pp. 11-13, 16, 20-21) college men and women; American Alliance (1988, pp. 28-29) boys and girls;

American Alliance (1990, pp. 10-11) boys and girls; Alexander et al. (1985, p. 9) Canadian women; Arizonia (1983, pp. 3-28) boys and girls; Barrow et al. (1989, pp. 105, 120, 130, 139-140) boys, girls, men and women; Baumgartner & Jackson (1982, pp. 213, 262, 264) boys and girls; Baumgartner & Jackson (1987, pp. 280, 286, 299, 305, 314) boys and girls;

Baumgartner & Jackson (1991, pp. 243, 261, 267, 284-285, 287-289) boys, girls, men and women; Brown et al. (no date, p. 13) boys and girls; Candian Association (1980, pp. 37-60) boys and girls; Canadian Minister (1979, p. 19) men and women; Chrysler/AAU (1990, p. 6) boys and girls; Clarke & Clarke (1987, pp. 162, 166) boys and girls; Fitness Canada (1986, p. 39) boys, girls, men and women; Fitness Institute (1981, no page numbers) boys, girls, men and women; Franks (1989, pp. 42-47) boys and girls; Getchell (1983, p. 48) men and women; Greenberg & Pargman (1989, pp. 80-81) men and women;

Hastad & Lacy (1989, pp. 194-195, 284, 288) boys and girls; Hawaii (1989, pp. 19-20) boys and girls; Haydon (1986, p. 57) boys and girls; Hoeger (1986, pp. 35, 37) men and women; Hoeger (1989, p. 50) men and women; Jackson & Ross (1986, p. 33) men and women; Johnson & Nelson (1986, pp. 110, 133-134, 203-204, 207, 382) boys, girls, men and women, army and navy;

Kirkendall et al. (1980, pp. 235-240, 276-277, 284-285, 331-332) boys, girls, men and women; Kirkendall et al. (1987, pp. 113-117, 157, 173, 399-401) boys, girls, men, women, boys and girls normal and special populations; Maryland (1986, p. 20) boys and girls; Metheny et al. (1945, p. 309) girls; Miller (1988, pp. 176-177, 234) boys, girls, men and women;

National Marine (no date, p. 7) boys and girls; New York (1977, pp. 34-42) boys and girls; New York (1984, pp. 34-42) boys and girls; O'Connor & Cureton (1945, p. 314) girls; Pollock & Wilmore (1990, pp. 672-683, 686) men and women; President's Council (1987, pp. 4-5) USSR girls; President's Council (1988, pp. 2, 7) boys and girls;

President's Council (1989, p. 8) boys and girls; Pyke (1986, p. 9) boys and girls; Rhode Island (1989, pp. 23-26) boys and girls; Ross et al. (1985, p. 64) boys and girls; Ross et al. (1987, p. 70) boys and girls; Safrit (1986, pp. 240, 277, Appendix A-36) boys and girls; Safrit (1990, pp. 342, 345, 347, 352, 370-372, Appendix A-37) boys and girls; Scott & French (1959, pp. 308-310) women; Shannon (1989, p. 45) high school football players;

Simons et al. (1990, p. 100) girls; South Carolina (1983, pp. 15, 30-38) boys, girls, men and women; Stephens et al. (1986, p. 15) men and women; Stokes et al. (1986, p. 171) men and women; Van Gelder & Marks (1987, p. 186) men and women; Vermont (1982, pp. 14-15) boys and girls; Virginia (1988, pp. 16, 20) boys and girls.

NOTE: Some common variations of the above mentioned sit up movement are as follows:

(1) The hands are held behind the neck with the elbows pointed to the side.

(2) The hands are placed on the opposite shoulders with the elbows remaining against the ribs.

(3) The arms are extended along the sides of the body with the hands remaining on the mat.

(4) The arms are extended with the hands moving along the top of the thighs.

(5) The hands are placed on the shoulders with the legs straight. The examinee bends forward until the elbow touches the opposite knee. This movement is repeated continuously, alternating right and left.

(6) The movement may be performed without the feet being held in place.

REVIEW

CHARLES W. ASH, Ph.D.

Associate Professor
Physical Education
State University of New York,
College at Cortland
Cortland, NY 13045

The Sit Up Test is designed to measure muscular endurance of the abdominal muscles. The validity, when compared to work output on an ergometer, was between $r = .48$ and $r = .52$. It is also classified as having face validity. The test is very reliable ($r = .68$ to $r = .94$) and objective ($r = .98$). The test does require the assistance of another individual, which could affect the test results.

The Sit Up Test can be administered in a relatively small space on a mat with an assistant to hold the feet in place. The scoring procedure is simply the number of "correct" repetitions the examinee executes in one minute. In order to familiarize the examinee with the correct technique, the tester should have the examinee execute the sit up with the correct movement.

The test can be used as an activity in a class setting or in a private setting for the purpose of improving the muscular endurance/strength of the abdominal wall muscles, and for developing the technique of executing the test.

If the test is performed as described, there is little risk of injury. However, if the hands are locked behind the head, there is a chance of injury to the extensor muscles of the cervical region. There is also a danger to the posterior portion of the head if the head is not held above the mat when the trunk is being extended in the return position. For some individuals with chronic (structural) lower vertebral abnormalities, or individuals with acute lower back muscle spasms, this exercise is a contraindicated activity because of the stress to the lumbar area.

Sit up data has been normalized across ages and gender and are reported by many state associations in their fitness test manuals.

SUMMARY

Major Strengths:

1. The test requires very little equipment and/or space.

2. The test can be administered easily to a large group in a short period of time.

3. It is a measure of abdominal endurance without the use of expensive modern isokinetic or isotonic equipment.

4. It can be used by any individual almost anywhere for the purpose of improving abdominal endurance/strength.

Major Weaknesses:

1. The safety precautions need to be emphasized in order to avoid injury.

2. Many repetitions can be scored as correct when, in fact, the repetitions were performed incorrectly.

The Sit Up Test is an acceptable test for teaching and for limited research use for the purpose of determining the endurance of the abdominal muscles as long as the precautions are followed. It has been, and will continue to be, a criterion measure test because of its ease of administration to large groups and its cost effectiveness.

DYNAMIC MUSCULAR ENDURANCE TEST OF THE BACK

BACK LIFT OR WING LIFT TEST

Reference.
McCloy, C. H., & Young, N. D. (1954). *Tests and measurements in health and physical education.* New York: Appleton-Century-Crofts, pp 175-176.

Additional Sources.
Jensen & Hirst (1980, p. 99); Kirkendall et al. (1980, p. 232); Kirkendall et al. (1987, p. 112).

Purpose.
To measure the muscular endurance of an examinee's trunk extensor muscles.

Objectivity.
Not reported.

Reliability.
Not reported.

Validity.
Test has face validity.

Age and Sex.
Suitable for females and males, age 8 - adult.

Equipment.
A stopwatch.

Space Requirements and Design.
A clear, level area approximately 3m (10') square with the examinee positioned in the center.

Directions.
The examinee assumes a prone position with the hands clasped behind the head. On command, "Ready, Go," the examinee raises the head and trunk until only the lowest portion of the rib cage is still in contact with the floor. The examinee quickly returns the upper body to the floor and then repeats the raising and lowering movements as fast as possible for one minute. The head and arms do not have to touch the floor during the lowering movement.

To help standardize procedures, an assistant who is about the same body height as the examinee assumes a prone position on the floor with her/his head opposite the examinee's head.

The assistant places her/his right elbow on the floor and looks over her/his clenched fist. The examinee then raises her/his upper body until her/his eyes are on the same level as the assistant's eyes.

Scoring.
The score is the number of upward movements executed in one minute.

Norms.
Kirkendall et al. (1980, pp. 235-240) boys, men and women; Kirkendall et al. (1987, pp. 113-117) boys, men and women; McCloy & Young (1954, pp. 175, 179) girls and women.

REVIEW

DON HARDIN, Ph.D.
Professor of Kinesiology
University of Texas at El Paso
El Paso, TX 79968

This test measures the endurance of spine and neck extensors and shoulder retractors, groups of muscles not tested often.

The test may require that the group being tested be divided into two groups, one group taking the test and the other acting as test assistants as described by McCloy and Young (1954). Also, obese examinees or those with large abdomens, may rock while doing the test, requiring someone to hold their legs.

The test, if done as designed, would yield data accurate enough for research.

The test is easily scored, and good norms are available. The norms scatter the population well. This is helpful if the test is to be used in a test battery.

SUMMARY

Major Strengths:

1. Measures muscle groups not often tested.

2. Good norms.

3. Fast; taking one minute.

4. No special equipment needed.

Major Weaknesses:

1. Should be given as designed to keep students working equally.

2. No validity or reliability data.

3. Little demand for test data.

This test is an acceptable test to measure the muscle groups it was developed to measure. Its best use would be as a test included in a test battery to measure overall muscular endurance. The test is seldom given alone, except maybe, in a research study where the spinal extensors and shoulder retractors were being assessed.

DYNAMIC MUSCULAR ENDURANCE TESTS OF THE LEGS

BENCH JUMPS TEST

References.
Hockey, R. V. (1981). *Physical fitness: The pathway to healthful living.* St. Louis: Mosby, pp 63, 65.
Hoeger, W. W. (1986). *Lifetime physical fitness and wellness.* Englewood, CO: Morton Publishing, pp 36-37.

Additional Sources.
None.

Purpose.
To measure the muscular endurance of an examinee's leg extensor muscles.

Objectivity.
Not reported.

Reliability.
Not reported.

Validity.
Not reported.

Age and Sex.
Suitable for females and males, age 14 - adult.

Equipment.
A sturdy bench 41cm (16") high and a stopwatch.

Space Requirements and Design.
A clear, level area approximately 2m (6') square with the examinee and bench in the center.

Directions.
The examinee assumes a standing position facing the bench. On command, "Ready, Go," the examinee is given a one minute period to jump up on the bench and down from the bench as many times as possible. If examinees become fatigued, they may step up and down for the remainder of the minute.

Scoring.
The score is the number of times both feet touch the floor after the bench jump.

Norms.
Hockey (1981, p. 65) men and women; Hoeger (1986, p. 37) men and women; Hoeger (1989, p. 50) men and women; Shannon (1989, p. 45) high school football players.

REVIEW

PHILLIP BISHOP, Ed.D.

Associate Professor
Health and Human Performance
University of Alabama
Tuscaloosa, AL 35487

As presented, the Bench Jumps Test is not a valid measure of leg extensor endurance because of the time limit involved, the skill component, and the variability in the examinees' body weights. Because of the time limit involved, performance on this test is at least partially a power assessment, which is dependent upon cardiovascular fitness as well as leg muscle endurance. Since the speed at which the examinee jumps or steps is partially determinant of the score, technique is probably also a key factor. Examinees with creativity or prior experience may be able to adopt strategies for improving their scores without improving their leg muscle endurance. A third complicating factor is body weight. An examinee who must move large amounts of body fat up and down will undoubtedly score much lower than a very lean examinee who has equivalent absolute leg muscle endurance. The inclusion of separate female/male norms suggests this is the case, since body composition is the major gender difference involved in performance on this test. The instructions are not clear or detailed enough, which detracts from objectivity. The tester should be advised to allow adequate practice. The lack of validity and reliability information is a serious flaw.

What this test appears to be is a very simple, straightforward means of assessing an examinee's ability to transport their own body weight vertically. This test reflects one operational definition of muscular endurance. Other people conceptualize muscular endurance as the ability to exert a given force repeatedly. This force may be an absolute value or a fraction of an examinee's maximal force. Depending upon the user's definition of muscular endurance and measurement objective, the test might be favorably modified by making it a step test and extending its duration to 3 to 5 minutes to help reduce the influence of cardiovascular endurance incumbent in fast paced stepping. Substituting stepping for the jumping/stepping mix prescribed by the test constructor should also reduce the influence of skill or strategies. Specifying what constitutes a jump, or preferably, a step would also be helpful. Replacing jumping with stepping, extending the time frame, and emphasizing steady pacing should also improve the safety of the test. As for all physical performance tests, allowing the examinees to practice the test several times on days preceding the actual test date should improve both the validity and reliability of the results. The modifications obviously render existing norms useless.

SUMMARY

Major Strengths:

1. The test is very simple to administer and score.
2. With modification, the test may be useful in some applications.

Major Weaknesses:

1. Cardiovascular fitness is a key factor in the test.

2. This test attempts to measure examinees' ability to move their body weight vertically, which may not correspond with the concept of muscular endurance.

3. The time period of measurement may be too short.

4. The speed required and the jumping motion may be a safety risk.

5. The directions are sketchy, and the lack of validity and reliability information makes evaluation difficult.

As written, this test is an inadequate test of leg extensor muscle endurance. Lengthening the test time and restricting examinees to stepping rather than jumping may permit better determination of examinees' ability to move their body weight vertically.

CALF RAISE TEST

Reference.
Arnot, R., & Gaines, C. (1986). *Sports Talent.* New York: Penguin Books, p 234.

Additional Sources.
None.

Purpose.
To measure the endurance of an examinee's ankle extensor muscles.

Objectivity.
Not reported.

Reliability.
Not reported.

Validity.
Not reported.

Age and Sex.
Not reported, but suitable for females and males, age 6 - adult.

Equipment.
A block of wood approximately 10cm x 10cm x 60cm (4" x 4" x 24") and a stopwatch. A staircase could be substituted for the block of wood.

Space Requirements and Design.
A clear, level area approximately 3m (10') square near a wall. The block of wood is positioned on the floor near the wall.

Directions.
The examinee stands barefooted with the ball of the dominant foot on the wooden block facing the wall. The examinee places the hands on the nearby wall to assist with balance. On the signal, "Ready, Go," the examinee fully extends the ankles raising up on the tiptoes and then lets the heels fall below the level of the toes. Each sequence of raising and lowering of the heels counts as one repetition. The examinee tries to do as many repetitions as possible in 30 seconds.

Scoring.
The score is the number of correctly executed repetitions performed in 30 seconds.

Norms.
Arnot & Gaines (1986, p. 234) age and sex are not stated.

REVIEW

DONALD R. CASADY, Ph.D.
Professor of Exercise Science
University of Iowa
Iowa City, IA 52241

The Calf Raise Test is undoubtedly derived from a similar movement (frequently called heel raises or rise on toes) done with the balls of both feet on a raised object for the purpose of developing the strength, endurance, or size of the muscular portion of the lower leg. Muscular endurance tests are often classified as falling into three or four different categories. The Calf Raise Test is a timed, dynamic, repetitive test of 30 seconds duration during which the examinee performs as many identical movements as possible. Because some examinees may be able to continue repetitive movements of this type for a long period of time, it is necessary to impose a time limit. Whether 30 seconds is an adequate span of time during which to measure muscular endurance rather than speed of movement for examinees of varying ages and fitness levels is open to question.

The Calf Raise Test suffers from the fact that it is not included as a muscular endurance test in any of the 15 or so measurement and evaluation books in physical education and exercise science that have been published during the past decade. Several reasons undoubtedly account for this omission. The fact that validity and reliability estimates are unavailable may render this test suspect to some. However, few would argue that logical validity is inherent in the test. The lack of norm tables, or any criterion referenced standards, also weakens its appeal. Although this test involves the endurance of muscle groups used extensively every day, this possible asset cannot make up for its several deficiencies.

On the positive side, the Calf Raise Test requires little training of the examinees to prepare them for a test that involves everyday movements. The test directions are uncomplicated; hence, it is simple to administer. Other advantages are that only simple, inexpensive equipment is required, one-half of a group may be tested at a time, and for most examinees the scorers can be classmates. The space needed for conducting this test should pose few, if any, problems.

On the negative side, a number of weaknesses severely limits the use of the test for testing muscular endurance. Because the calf muscles are repeatedly exercised each day, a test of their endurance may give an unrepresentative sample of overall muscular endurance. The 4" x 4" block on which the test is performed can be unstable and cause an examinee to fall off while performing the test. Stair steps or a board only 1.5" or 2" high provide a safer surface. Some examinees find that placing their hands on a wall in front of them to be somewhat awkward while performing an up and down motion. Younger examinees may have difficulty identifying their dominant leg. Counters frequently report counts that do not agree with other counters for an examinee; thus calling the objectivity of the scoring into question. However, it is a simple test to self score. This difficulty of scoring accurately is exacerbated by the range of motion specified for the test. The directions call for lowering the heel until it is level with the ball of the foot; however, most examinees tend to depress their heel markedly lower than this. On the other hand, examinees with equal foot size vary in the height of the heel raise. Johnson and Nelson (1986) emphasize that definite guidelines must be observed when scoring such tests since small deviations can significantly influence final scores. Similarly, the end score of muscular endurance tests depends on the motivational level of the examinee. It may be difficult to hold motivation factors constant while testing. Johnson and Nelson (1986) also state that timed and untimed muscular endurance test items may correlate poorly with one another. For many examinees,

30 seconds of performing this test may be a better measure of speed of movement than endurance. On the other hand, the use of unlimited repetition of a leg or foot movement is not practical because of the amount of testing time that may be required for a few high scoring examinees. Revision of this test, such as using a timed cadence as is done with step tests, or having each examinee perform with both feet while holding a weight equal to bodyweight, probably would not sufficiently improve it to render it satisfactory as a test of muscular endurance, especially when compared to other more satisfactory tests of muscular endurance that are frequently used.

SUMMARY

Major Strengths:

None.

Major Weaknesses:

1. A possible poor sample of muscular endurance.

2. It may not measure muscular endurance for some examinees.

3. The block of wood on which the test is performed may rotate during the testing session creating the possibility of an injury.

4. An accurate count of the number of repetitions performed is subject to disagreement.

5. It is difficult to standardize the range of movement of the foot and the level of motivation of the examinees.

The weaknesses of the Calf Raise Test of Muscular Endurance far outweigh its strengths and make it an unacceptable test. Better tests of muscular endurance are available and should be used in teaching and/or research.

SQUAT JUMPS TEST

References.

McCloy, C. H., & Young, N. D. (1954). *Tests and measurements in health and physical education.* New York: Appleton-Century-Crofts, p 176.

Johnson, B. L., & Nelson, J. K. (1986). *Practical measurements for evaluation in physical education.* Edina, MN: Burgess, pp 137, 139, 207.

Additional Source.

Jensen & Hirst (1980, p. 98).

Purpose.

To measure the muscular endurance of an examinee's legs.

Objectivity.

Not reported.

Reliability.

Not reported.

Validity.

Not reported.

Age and Sex.

Not reported, but suitable for females and males, age 8 - adult.

Equipment. None.
Space Requirements and Design.

A clear, level area approximately 2m (6') square with examinee in the center.

Directions.

The examinee clasps the hands together on the top of the head and stands with the right foot approximately 30 cm (12") in front of the left foot. The examinee squats down until the left buttock makes contact with the left heel. The examinee then jumps vertically so the legs are fully extended and the feet leave the floor. The examinee returns to a squat position with the left foot in front of the right foot and the right buttock touching the right heel. The placement of the feet should be alternated throughout the test. The movements should be continuous. Once the movements are not continuous, the test is stopped.

Scoring.

The score is the number of squat jumps properly performed.

Norms.

McCloy & Young (1954, p. 176) boys; Johnson & Nelson (1986, p. 139) men and women, army and navy standards.

NOTE: Johnson and Nelson (1986) recommend that an adjustable bench or a stack of mats, as high as the lower edge of the examinee's patella, be placed behind the examinee. The score is the number of times the examinee's buttocks touch the bench top or the mat. They report an objectivity coefficient of r = .99 and a reliability coefficient of r = .82 for their version of the test.

REVIEW

SYNE ALTENA, Ed.D.
Professor of Physical Education
Dordt College
Sioux Center, IA 51250

The Squat Jump Test proposes to measure the muscular endurance of the legs. Attempts have been made to establish the reliability (Prestidge, 1972) and objectivity of the test (Recio, 1972). Face validity was accepted as the criterion for validation.

The test seemed to pose two problems when administered to a group of high school subjects.

The first problem centers on the lack of clarity as to what age group the test is intended. McCloy and Young (1954) suggest that the test be administered to examinees age 8 to adult. Johnson and Nelson (1979) suggest the age level intended be from 10 to college. Anyone using this test would be confused as to what age level is appropriate for this test.

The second problem relates to the jump whereby the examinee jumps upward from a squat position extending the legs and switching the position of the feet while in the air. The examinees tested often have trouble with coordination and balance. The squat jumps were not done smoothly and various rhythms and body positions were observed.

SUMMARY

Major Strength:

1. The criterion measure of face validity seemed to be justified. The major muscles of the legs were taxed as to muscular endurance.

Major Weaknesses:

1. The squat jumps require motor skills such as coordination and balance.

2. There are no published norms for younger examinees.

3. The examinees can use the adjustable bench as a springboard to the next jump.

4. It would be difficult to test a large group because each examinee would need a bench adjusted to the height of the patella.

Based on the above weaknesses, the reviewer concludes that the Squat Jump Test is not practical as a test to measure the muscular endurance of the legs.

STATIC MUSCULAR ENDURANCE TESTS

ARM HANG OR FLEXED ARM HANG TEST

Reference.
Scott, M. G., & French, E. (1959). *Measurement and evaluation in physical education.* Dubuque: Wm. C. Brown, pp 297-298.

Additional Sources.
Barrow et al. (1989, p. 115); Baumgartner & Jackson (1982, pp. 208-209); Baumgartner & Jackson (1987, pp. 279-280); Baumgartner & Jackson (1991, pp. 260, 263); Bosco & Gustafson (1983, pp. 99-100);

Clarke & Clarke (1987, pp. 157, 159); Hastad & Lacy (1989, pp. 198-200, 234); Jensen & Hirst (1980, pp. 98-99); Johnson & Nelson (1986, pp. 132-134); Kirkendall et al. (1980, pp. 269-270); Kirkendall et al. (1987, pp. 150-151, 401);

Miller (1988, pp. 179, 181); Safrit (1981, p. 240); Safrit (1986, pp. 268-270, 272-274, 439-440); Safrit (1990, pp. 240-241, 400-402, 406-409); Verducci (1980, pp. 282-284, 287).

Purpose.
To measure the muscular endurance of an examinee's arms and shoulders.

Objectivity.
r = .99 Johnson and Nelson (1986, p. 132).

Reliability.
r = .83 on first graders and r = .90 on sixth graders were obtained by Magnusson cited in Scott and French (1959, p. 297); r = .67 on children, grades one to three, was obtained by Morris cited in Scott and French (1954, p. 297).

Validity.
Test has face validity.

Age and Sex.
Suitable for females and males, age 6 - adult.

Equipment.
An adjustable horizontal bar, doorway gym bar, inclined ladder, or horizontal ladder, and a stopwatch.

Space Requirements and Design.
A clear, level area approximately 2m (6') square with the horizontal bar in the center. A height clearance of approximately 1m (3') above the bar.

Directions.
The examinee grasps the bar with the hands approximately shoulder width apart and the palms facing the body. On command, the examinee should spring upward or have assistance in order to place the chin above the level of the bar. The upper arms should be aligned against the sides of the body. The examinee should hang straight with the weight being held by only the hands. The examinee should attempt to hold this position as long as possible. The editor notes that the overhand grip (i.e., palms facing away from the body) is more commonly used for this test.

Scoring.
The score is the length of time the chin is held above the bar, or until it is lowered to the same level as the bar.

Norms.
Alabama (1988, pp. 41-42) boys and girls; Alexander et al. (1985, p. 9) Canadian women; American Alliance (1975, pp. 26, 44) girls; Baumgartner & Jackson (1982, p. 210) girls; Baumgartner & Jackson (1987, p. 279) girls; Baumgartner & Jackson (1991, pp. 260, 289) girls;

Beunen et al. (1988, pp. 33, 82, 94) boys; Brown et al. (no date, p. 12) boys and girls; Canadian Association (1980, pp. 36-60) boys and girls; Chrysler/AAU (1990, p. 6) girls; Clarke & Clarke (1987, pp. 162, 166) girls; Getchell (1983, p. 48) women;

Greenberg & Pargman (1989, p. 81) women; Hastad & Lacy (1989, p. 199) girls; Hawaii (1989, pp. 19-20) boys and girls; Haydon (1986, p. 56) boys and girls; Johnson & Lavay (1988, pp. 25-29) boys and girls (handicapped); Johnson & Nelson (1986, pp. 135, 203-205) girls and women;

Kirkendall et al. (1980, pp. 275-276, 331) boys and girls; Kirkendall et al. (1987, pp. 157, 404-405) boys and girls, normal and special populations; Miller (1988, p. 181) girls; Ostyn et al. (1980, pp. 105-106, 127-140) boys;

President's Council (1988, pp. 5, 7) boys and girls; President's Council (1989, p. 8) boys and girls; Rhode Island (1989, pp. 25-26) boys and girls; Safrit (1986, p. 275) girls; Safrit (1990, p. 347) boys and girls; Simons et al. (1990, p. 101) girls; Virginia (1988, pp. 48-49) boys and girls.

NOTE: A variation of this test is to maintain a static position with the bar at eye level and to stop the test when the head falls below the level of the bar (e.g., see Canadian Association 1980).

REVIEW

MARK J. MEKA, M.S.
Assistant Professor
Health and Physical Education
Lake Tahoe Community College
South Lake Tahoe, CA 95702

The Flexed Arm Hang Test measures the muscular endurance of the arms and shoulders in a consistent and reliable manner.

Only one individual is needed to administer the test with the directions being fairly simple and easy to follow. Facility and/or space requirements are minimal, with an extended wall bar, or a hallway bar, being all that is required. The height of the bar will determine whether a ladder or stool is necessary for ease of starting. Multiple bars could be used to save time for testing large groups, and selected students could serve as testers. The time needed to administer the test is also minimal, with most examinees completing it in less than one minute.

All ages can be tested; however, the two extremes of young children and older adults may have some difficulty. This test seems to be best suited for the teen to middle age ranges. Safety is a consideration when first starting. Hitting the chin on the bar could occur.

Scoring is basic, with total time recorded before the examinee's chin touches the bar. This method of scoring is very objective, as long as the examinee does not raise her/his chin to avoid contact with the bar. Scoring and evaluating oneself could be done with a clock in view for recording time.

Performed correctly, the test is suitably precise and could be used for research purposes.

SUMMARY

Major Strengths:

1. Ease of administration.

2. Simple objective scoring.

3. Space and equipment needs are minimal.

4. Short time requirements for each examinee.

5. Selected students could administer the test to assist the examiner when large numbers are to be tested.

Major Weaknesses:

1. The test may be too difficult for younger and older age groups.

2. The test may have some limiting factors relative to body weight and/or obesity.

The Flexed Arm Hang Test, as described, is an acceptable test and adequate for research and/or teaching. Research correlations could be attempted with other traditional upper body endurance tests. Likewise, data could be gathered relative to different races, body types and conditioning levels.

A consideration might be made regarding isolation of the examinee being tested. Some examinees experience embarrassment when they are watched because of the "shaking" that occurs when they are tiring.

ISOMETRIC LEG SQUAT (WALL SIT) TEST

Reference.
Chrysler Fund-AAU Physical Fitness Program (1990). *1989-90 test manual.* Bloomington, IN: Amateur Athletic Union, pp 5-6.

Additional Source.
Jensen & Hirst (1980, p. 99).

Purpose.
To measure the muscular endurance and strength of an examinee's leg muscles, primarily the quadriceps group.

Objectivity.
Not reported.

Reliability.
Not reported.

Validity.
Not reported.

Age and Sex.
Not reported, but suitable for females and males, age 6 - adult.

Equipment.
A stopwatch.

Space Requirements and Design.
A clear, level area approximately 1m (3') square next to a smooth wall.

Directions.
The examinee assumes a sitting position against a wall without the aid of a chair. The knees are bent at a 90 degree angle so that the thighs are parallel to the floor and the lower legs are perpendicular to the floor. The feet are flat on the floor, pointed straight ahead and hip width apart. The examinee's head and shoulders are positioned against the wall. Once in the above position, the tester starts the stopwatch and stops it when the examinee can no longer hold the stationary position.

Scoring.
The score is the maximum time, measured in minutes and seconds, the proper position is held.

Norms.
Chrysler/AAU (1990, p. 6) boys and girls.

NOTE: The test can also be administered with the examinee using one leg at a time for support. Arnot and Gaines (1986, p. 150), *Sports Talent,* New York: Penguin Books, presents norms for such a test for both men and women.

REVIEW

JOHN B. GRATTON, Ph.D.
Chair
Kinesiology and Health Science
Bee County College
Beeville, TX 78102

The Isometric Leg Squat is a valid test of muscular endurance. The test should be a reliable and consistent measurement instrument. There would be no problems caused by inconsistency among different testers. The only situation which must be monitored closely is the body position of the examinee (i.e., the 90 degree angle of the legs). The participation of other individuals is not necessary. The test could be administered to a small or large group with no interference occurring.

Space requirements are not a problem. Each examinee requires a three foot space. There are no equipment requirements other than a stopwatch. The test is easy to administer, and little expertise is needed on the part of the tester. However, each examinee would need a partner to observe the proper position of the examinee and note when the position could no longer be held, thereby terminating the test. With younger aged populations, adult supervision of this process might prove more reliable.

The time requirement could be excessive when testing high school or college aged examinees. A fit examinee could hold the prescribed position for an extended period of time. Using the one leg version of the test should alleviate that situation.

This test is not recommended as a drill to promote conditioning. The test is suitable for the intended age groups. There is no discrimination among different ability levels.

There is one aspect of the test that could prove dangerous. An examinee could hold the position until extreme quadriceps fatigue sets in and then be unable to regain an upright position. This examinee could slide down the wall and suffer abrasions. The observer of each examinee should be cautioned to assist the examinee in regaining an upright stance. The test scoring is extremely objective. A younger aged examinee would have trouble self administering the test. The norms cited in the test description are very appropriate.

SUMMARY

Major Strengths:

1. The test is appropriate for a wide range of examinees.
2. The test can be easily administered by testers without a great deal of expertise required.
3. The test is easily scored and should provide consistent results.

Major Weaknesses:

1. The time required to administer the test could be excessive.

2. The test could be dangerous to certain examinees, especially those who are obese.

3. Particular attention must be paid to the beginning body position of each examinee.

The Isometric Leg Squat is an excellent test of muscular endurance. The results should be very consistent, and the norms available should provide a sound basis for research purposes. The test is appropriate for a wide range of ages and requires little expertise by the tester. The test should be of great benefit to elementary and secondary school teachers.

STATIC GRIP ENDURANCE TEST

References.

Nagle, F. J. et al. (1988). Time to fatigue during isometric exercise using different muscle masses. *International Journal of Sports Medicine,* 9:313-315.

Maughan, R. J. et al. (1986). Endurance capacity of untrained females and males in isometric and dynamic muscular contractions. *European Journal of Applied Physiology,* 55:395-400.

Additional Sources.
None.

Purpose.
To measure an examinee's ability to maintain a static muscle contraction for as long as possible.

Objectivity.
Not reported.

Reliability.
Not reported.

Validity.
Not reported.

Age and Sex.
Not reported, but suitable for females and males, age 6 - adult.

Equipment.
A grip dynamometer and a stopwatch.

Space Requirements and Design.
A clear, level, area approximately 3m (10') square with the examinee standing in the center.

Directions.
After adjusting the dynamometer to fit the hand, the examinee exerts maximum force following standard grip strength testing procedures. Once the examinee's maximum grip strength is known, the tester then calculates a specified percent of this maximum to use in measuring the static muscular endurance of the finger flexors. For example, Nagle et al. (1988) used 30 percent of the maximum, with the test being terminated when the examinee could not maintain a grip force within 10 percent of the score representing 30 percent of maximum strength. Nagle et al. (1988), found a mean time of 3.39 minutes with a range of 2.2 to 5.0 minutes for 10 men whose average age was 24 years. Using a higher percent

of an examinee's maximum strength, results in reduced endurance time. For example, Buck et al. (Nagle et al., 1988, p. 315) used 40 percent of maximum and derived a mean time of 2.1 minutes in the handgrip.

Scoring.
The score is the length of time, measured to the nearest tenth of a second, that the examinee maintains her/his grip force at the required level.

Norms.
Nagle et al. (1988, p. 313) men; Maughan et al. (1986, p. 396), men and women for 20, 50, and 80 percent of maximum in knee extension.

NOTE (1): The above testing procedures can also be modified so that the test is terminated whenever the force drops below the specified percent of maximum being used (e.g., 30 percent) or whenever the force drops below the specified maximum and remains below the specified maximum for a given time (e.g., three or five seconds).

NOTE (2): The above procedure can be used to measure the static endurance of most muscle groups in the body.

REVIEW

WALTER R. THOMPSON, Ph.D.

Director
Laboratory of Applied Physiology
School of Human Performance and
Recreation
The University of Southern Mississippi
Hattiesburg, MS 39406-5142

The word isometric is from the Greek term "isosmetrikus" which has a literal translation of "equality of measure" (Fardy, 1981). Isometric work or tests that measure isometric strength (or endurance) require the development of tension without a subsequent shortening of muscle fibers. Tests of isometric strength were first developed by Clarke (1948) and later used as a training method.

One of the earliest studies utilizing isometric contractions in the development of strength was that of Hettinger and Muller (1953). These researchers demonstrated that a muscle contraction of only six seconds at a given percentage of maximum produces an increase in strength. This hypothesis has been tested subsequently with the same result. Tests of endurance, however, using the technique of isometric (or static) contractions are lacking in the scientific literature.

An early concern of scientists and clinicians in the use of isometric contractions, whether for the study of strength or endurance was that of the pressor response. The most often cited physiological reactions measured were blood pressure and heart rate, although changes in cardiac output were later raised as an issue. Fardy (1981) has indicated that research supports the use of repeated isometric contractions to realize gains in both strength and endurance because the pressor responses are not of the magnitude originally thought.

The Static Grip Endurance Test cited in Nagle et al. (1988) required 10 healthy, male subjects to participate in three tests of isometric endurance. Subjects were required to maintain a sustained isometric contraction at 30 percent of maximal voluntary contraction (MVC) of three major muscle groups. The hand grip, leg extension, and dead lift were the exercises of choice in the study. Time to fatigue was not different between the three exercises (hand grip = 3.39 +/- 0.92 min; leg extension = 3.61 +/- 1.67 min; dead lift = 3.68 +/- 1.34 min; p >0.05). Although these researchers were most interested in the pressor responses, they reveal means and standard deviations that can serve as a guide to other researchers interested in developing normative data. Maughan et al. (1986) offer similar data at different intensities of effort.

While validity for isometric strength tests is available (Baumgartner & Jackson, 1987), none has been developed for isometric (or static) endurance tests. Reliability coefficients are estimated to be 0.90 or greater (Hastad & Lacy, 1989) for hand grip strength tests, but none are available for endurance tests. However, reliability correlation coefficients of between 0.74 and 0.90 have been reported for the flexed arm hang, a test that is similar in design to that

which is reported here (Johnson & Nelson, 1986). Because a dynamometer is used for the hand grip (i.e., a measure that is consistent), objectivity is assumed to be high.

SUMMARY

Major Strengths:

1. This test requires the use of a hand grip dynamometer and stopwatch (both of which are available commercially). It has an advantage over the other tests of endurance because of its relative low cost.

2. The test's assumed acceptable objectivity.

3. Although no reliability or validity data are available for this particular test, it can be assumed to be acceptable.

4. The small space requirement.

5. Although most facilities have only one dynamometer, the time commitment allows for mass testing.

Major Weaknesses:

1. Since no normative data are available, the test application has limited use.

2. While validity and reliability data are available for hand grip strength tests, none have been developed for hand grip endurance.

3. If the examiner is interested in demonstrating increases in endurance subsequent to a training program, this test can be a valuable instrument if it is specific to the type of training.

4. While some research has indicated that pressor responses to repeated or sustained isometric contractions are not exaggerated, caution still must be exercised for those subjects who have a history of cardiovascular or cerebrovascular disease (e.g., hypertension).

The Static Grip Endurance Test has not yet been fully evaluated. Certainly, the concept seems valid yet more research needs to be accomplished before it can be an acceptable measure of endurance. Second, this test will only measure endurance of the finger flexors (i.e., grip) making it a very specific test. However, other devices are available to measure other joints in both extension and flexion, strength and endurance. Modifications of the Nagle et al. (1988) hand grip test can be used once normative data are developed. To become an acceptable test, many more subjects of varying ages, heights and weights will need to be tested so adequate comparisons can be made (Safrit, 1990).

REVIEW REFERENCES

Baumgartner, T., & Jackson, A. (1987). *Measurement for evaluation in physical education and exercise science.* Dubuque, IA: Wm. C. Brown.

Clarke, H. H. (1948). Objective strength tests of affected muscle groups involved in orthopedic disabilities. *Research Quarterly,* 19:118-147.

Fardy, P. S. (1981). Isometric exercise and the cardiovascular system. *The Physician and Sportsmedicine,* 9(9):43-56.

Hastad, D. N., & Lacy, A. C. (1989). *Measurement and evaluation in contemporary physical education.* Scottsdale, AZ: Gorsuch Scarisbrick.

Hettinger, T. L., & Muller, E. A. (1953). Muscular performance and training. *Arbeitsphysiologie,* 15:111-126.

Johnson, B. L., & Nelson, J. K. (1986). *Practical measurements for evaluation in physical education.* Edina, MN: Burgess.

Maughn, R. J. et al. (1986). Endurance capacity of untrained males and females in isometric and dynamic muscular contractions. *European Journal of Applied Physiology,* 55:395-400.

Nagle, F. J. et al. (1988). Time to fatigue during isometric exercise using different muscle masses. *International Journal of Sportsmedicine,* 9:313-315.

Safrit, M. J. (1990). *Introduction to measurement in physical education and exercise science.* St. Louis: Times Mirror/Mosby.

STATIC PUSH UP (HOLD HALF PUSH UP) TEST

References.
Fleishman, E. A. (1964B). *The structure and measurement of physical fitness.* Englewood Cliffs: Prentice Hall, pp 52-53, 59.
Hoeger, W. W. (1986). *Lifetime physical fitness and wellness.* Englewood, CO: Morton Publishing, pp 36-37.

Additional Source.
Bosco & Gustafson (1983, pp. 100-101).

Purpose.
To measure the muscular endurance of the elbow extensor and shoulder flexor muscles.

Objectivity.
r = .85 Fleishman (1964B, p. 59).

Reliability.
Not reported.

Validity.
Not reported.

Age and Sex.
Females and males.

Equipment.
A stopwatch.

Space Requirements and Design.
A clear, level area approximately 3m (10') square with the examinee in the center.

Directions.
The examinee assumes a prone horizontal position on the floor with the hands at the sides of the body about chest level. The examinee raises to a position where the elbows are flexed at a 90 degree angle or less. The chest of the examinee should be two to three inches off the floor. The stopwatch is started when the examinee is stable and is stopped when the elbow angle changes and/or the examinee's body no longer remains straight. Except for the feet and hands, the examinee's body cannot touch the floor. The examinee's head, neck, back and legs must remain straight.

Scoring.
The score is the total number of seconds that the static position can be maintained.

Norms.
Chrysler/AAU (1990, p. 6) boys and girls; Fleishman (1964B, p. 59) men; Hoeger (1986, p. 37) men and women.

REVIEW

DEBRA A. BALLINGER, Ph.D.

Assistant Professor
Health, Physical Education and Recreation
Old Dominion University
Norfolk, VA 23529-0196

Muscular endurance, the ability of a muscle group to exert submaximal force for extended periods, can be measured for both static and dynamic contractions. As described, the Static Push Up specifically measures the time, in seconds, that the push up position can be maintained, and this has face or content validity. Reliability is moderately high at .85. However, since no objectivity references are presented, the tester must interpret the results with caution. Such data should be gathered and compared with other established tests measuring dynamic and static strength and endurance in the upper arm and shoulder muscle group (e.g., dips, dynamic push ups, pull ups and flexed arm hang). The purpose of measuring muscular strength and endurance is presumably to predict the ability of individuals to perform various tasks requiring endurance. Most arm strength and endurance tasks involve dynamic movements. Therefore, the usefulness of this static test for predictive ability has yet to be established.

The test directions are clear and concise. While the objectivity of the test is not reported, the scoring by the use of a stopwatch, recorded to the nearest second, is easy to determine. For females and an extremely obese population, variations in the above ground distance might pose a problem considering differences in chest circumference. The body position could vary significantly with respect to distance from the floor. Furthermore, explicit direction needs to be given with respect to allowance of movement once in the static position.

Another real concern is the requirement that examinees raise from the floor into the starting position. Examinees lacking strength to overcome the combined forces of gravity and inertia will not be able to utilize the test. While the lack of strength may disqualify an examinee, there is no mention of the test being one of strength, as well as endurance. The principle of specifity in training and testing needs to coincide, there needs to be assistance allowed into the position, or an alternative means of measuring the force being applied throughout the resistance test. Body weight is not constant across examinees. No reference is given to adapting the muscular endurance score relative to the examinee's weight. A modified or submaximal endurance test should be developed, with corresponding normative data presented, as an alternative to the norms given (i.e., provide norms for the same test using the "modified push up" position of knees on the floor). One possibility is to allow the tester the option of assisting the examinee into the starting position and beginning the timed test upon release.

Within the test directions, mention should be made of the need for standardizing such testing conditions as time of day, sleep, medications, and motivation. Tests of strength and endurance require a maximum effort by the examinee being tested, and such factors can conceivably alter the reliability of the test's results. Other reliability considerations include the fact that the test allows only one trial. Possibility of previous practice or learning effects are ignored. The tester should be provided guidelines for type and length of warm up exercises.

SUMMARY

Major Strengths:

1. Its ease of administration.

2. Its economy in terms of equipment, facilities and personnel.

3. A conduciveness to self testing and practice by the examinee.

4. The little time required to complete the test.

5. Ease of training and high objectivity of testers.

Major Weaknesses:

1. A concern for sex bias.

2. The lack of objectivity and validity scores.

3. Lack of consideration for body weight or maximum strength of the examinee when comparing test scores.

4. Lack of safety guidelines for warm up, time of day, motivation, etc.

The Static Push Up Test has promise for use if validity and objectivity criterion are established. The test could be useful for physical education teachers in school settings without extensive equipment or facilities. The test is easy to administer, economically feasible and fast. Students could be trained to help partners complete testing with relatively high objectivity. Without established criterion references, however, tests such as the flexed arm hang or dynamic push ups are recommended for their predictive validity in arm and shoulder strength and endurance. This reviewer encourages further collection of data, revision of directions, and creation of modified versions of the test to account for variations in sex, lean body mass, and relative strength of examinees.

Chapter 9

POWER

POWER TESTS OF THE ARMS/UPPER BODY
MISCELLANEOUS TESTS

TIMED BENCH PRESS TEST

Reference.
Baumgarter, T. A., & Jackson, A. S. (1975). *Measurement for evaluation in physical education.* Boston: Houghton Mifflin, p 151.

Additional Sources.
None.

Purpose.
To measure the ability of an examinee to exert power with the arms.

Objectivity.
Not reported.

Reliability.
Not reported.

Validity.
Not reported.

Age and Sex.
Not reported, but suitable for females and males, age 14 - college.

Equipment.
Appropriate weights, preferably a bench press weight machine (e.g., a Universal Gym) and a timing device accurate to a hundredth of a second with a special starting and stopping device (e.g., the Dekan Automatic Performance Analyzer).

Space Requirements and Design.
A clear, level area approximately 5m (15') square with the weight machine positioned in the center. The special start switch is positioned on the weight machine so that the timer is stopped when the weight is in its resting position and is started when the weight is lifted. The special stop switch must be positioned on the weight machine so that the timer will be turned off when the weight is lifted a given distance (e.g., .61m or 2').

Directions.
The examinee assumes a supine position on the bench and places the hands on the bench press handle ready to move the weight. When ready and without a set signal, the examinee presses the weight up as fast as possible. The examinee must keep her/his back flat on the bench throughout the lift. The amount of weight to be lifted can be specified either as a set amount for all examinees (e.g., 100 lbs.) or as a percentage (e.g., 50 percent) of the maximum each examinee can lift in one repetition.

Scoring.
The score is calculated from the following equations:

(1) Work = (F x D) where F (force) is the amount of weight lifted in kilograms or pounds and D is the distance the weight was moved in meters or feet.

(2) Power = W/T where W is the amount of work calculated above and T is the time it took to perform the work.

Norms.
Not reported.

REVIEW

HARRY BEAMON, Ed.D.
Professor
Health, Physical Education, and
Recreation
Tennessee State University
Nashville, TN 27209-1561

The purpose of the Timed Bench Press is to measure the ability to exert power with the arms. This test does not address objectivity, reliability, and validity. Therefore, many researchers will question the use of a test that does not have any reportings on these criteria. The test can be administered without the aid of another individual.

The facilities and space are readily available in most teaching settings and should not present a problem in the administration of the test. However, the equipment needed for the test could cause considerable problems in some programs. The timer with the special start and stop switches and the Universal Gym could be too expensive. The test does not require much time to administer, nor does it require additional personnel to assist in administration. The test is suitable for various age levels, however, it does discriminate if not used in homogeneous groupings of age and sex. The test has no apparent dangerous aspects to it. It can be scored objectively even though no objectivity coefficient was reported, and it can be used for self evaluation. The test needs more refinement to be considered for research purposes.

SUMMARY

Major Strengths:

1. The test is easily administered, and the scoring is simple.

2. The facilities and space are usually available in a school setting.

3. The test is suitable for a variety of age levels.

4. The test can be scored objectively and used for self evaluation.

Major Weaknesses:

1. Objectivity, reliability, and validity were not reported.

2. Equipment for test could be too expensive.

The Timed Bench Press would be acceptable for measuring the ability to exert power with the arms. However, test reliability and validity must be established for research purposes.

VERTICAL ARM PULL TEST (DISTANCE)

Reference.
Johnson, B. L., & Nelson, J. K. (1986). *Practical measurements for evaluation in physical education*. Edina, MN: Burgess Publishing, pp 212, 214-216.

Additional Sources.
Bosco & Gustafson (1983, pp. 93-94).

Purpose.
To measure the ability of an examinee to exert power with the arms.

Objectivity.
r = .99.

Reliability.
r = .97.

Validity.
r = .80 with vertical power pull test (work/time).

Age and Sex.
Males, age 14 - college.

Equipment.
A thick rope approximately 3m (10') long securely attached to a ceiling beam so it hangs vertically, marking tape, a tape measure, and a chair.

Space Requirements and Design.
A clear, level area approximately 3m (10') square with the rope in the center hanging vertically and touching the front edge of the chair.

Directions.
The examinee is required to be dressed in shorts, light shirt, and no shoes. The examinee takes a sitting position in a chair in which the seat is at least .38m (15") above the floor. The examinee grasps the rope as high as possible while still keeping the buttocks on the chair. The preferred hand is placed the higher of the two. A piece of marking tape is placed just above the top hand. The examinee then lifts the legs up assuming a piked position and pulls as hard as possible moving the lower hand as high as possible. The examinee must hold this position until the tester again places a piece of marking tape just above the top hand. After the examinee has grasped the rope, it is permissable to close the legs around

the rope to assist in holding the position. During the pull, the examinee must not let the feet touch the floor - if the feet do touch the floor, the trial is disregarded. Three legal trials are given. Just prior to the last trial, the tester should say, "This is your last pull. Try to beat your last two pulls." The distance is measured vertically between the lower edges of the two pieces of tape.

Scoring.
The score is the best distance of the three trials measured to the nearest cm (1/4").

Norms.
Johnson & Nelson (1986, p. 216) high school athletes, boys and college men.

REVIEW

CRAIG J. CISAR, Ph.D.

Associate Professor
Human Performance
San Jose State University
San Jose, CA 95192-0054

The Vertical Arm Pull Test does appear to have face validity in measuring the power generated by the muscles of the arms and shoulder girdle as they pull the body upward, even though the time required to complete the task is not measured. In addition, acceptable concurrent validity was demonstrated when the test was correlated (r = .80) with the vertical power pull test (work/time). The Vertical Arm Pull Test has also been reported to have high reliability (r = .97). The high reliability of the test may be due to the fact that the test required the performance of a relatively basic movement pattern, which, in the absence of muscle fatigue, should be capable of being consistently repeated. The test has been reported to have high objectivity (r = .99), which, in part, would appear to be due to the simplistic method of scoring. An additional factor which enhances the reliability and validity of the test is that the active participation of another individual is not required or involved in the test, and hence, an examinee's performance is independently measured.

The Vertical Arm Pull Test has minimal facility and equipment requirements. Furthermore, the test is relatively easy to administer, generally requiring only one tester. In fact, the test could be self administered with only slight modification of the recommended testing protocol. Thus, an examinee could use the test for self evaluation. The test can be quickly administered as it requires only three trials of a relatively basic movement pattern. Also, since the task is primarily dependent upon the phosphagen energy system, the rest period required between trials in order to obtain reliable and valid results is minimal. The high reliability of the test suggests that the three trials are adequate in order to obtain valid test results. Thus, in terms of the time required to administer the test, the test would appear to be suited for both individual and group assessment of upper body muscular power. Since the test involves a fairly basic, but specific movement pattern, the usefulness of the test in the promotion of learning and conditioning is limited to sports and activities which involve that specific movement pattern, such as pole vaulting, gymnastics, and rock climbing.

As indicated in the test description, the test was developed on adolescent and college aged males. Hence, its use in the assessment of upper body muscular power should be limited to this population. Within the age and gender limitations, the test does appear to discriminate among its intended users. The test constructor suggested that the test may be useful in indicating potential in pole vaulting and gymnastics. The test may also be useful in evaluating performance potential in other sports which require upper body muscular power such as rock climbing, swimming, and wheelchair sports. Generally, the dangerous aspects of the test appear to be minimal. However, if the test were used to evaluate muscular power in paraplegic populations, additional testers should be involved in order to assist examinees in returning to the sitting position. Test norms have been developed for high school and college pole vaulters and gymnasts, college men, high school boys, and junior high school boys. However, the norms may need reevalua-

tion and updating, since they were developed in the early 1970's. Although the Vertical Arm Pull Test is a practical field test, the test is not of suitable precision for research purposes for several reasons. First, the test does not directly take into account movement time or force production in its calculation of power. The results of the test are based solely on the power component of distance. Second, interexaminee variability in arm length is not taken into account in the determination of the test results. Third, the test results are expressed in distance units of measurement (cm or in) rather than in the preferred power units of measurement (Kgm/s or watts).

SUMMARY

Major Strengths:

1. The test has acceptable validity.

2. The test has high test-retest reliability.

3. The test has high objectivity and assesses an examinee's performance independently.

4. The test is relatively easy to administer requiring minimal facilities and equipment.

5. The test is a suitable method of field testing for individual and group assessment of upper body muscular power.

6. The test is generally safe to administer and can be self administered.

Major Weaknesses:

1. The use of the test is limited to adolescent and college aged males.

2. The use of the test in learning and conditioning is generally limited to sports and activities that involve the same specific movement pattern required in the test.

3. The test is not of suitable precision and quality for research purposes.

In conclusion, the Vertical Arm Pull Test is an acceptable field test for assessing upper body muscular power in adolescent and college aged males but is inadequate for research purposes and has limited application in the promotion of learning and conditioning.

POWER TESTS OF THE ARMS/UPPER BODY
PUT/THROW TESTS

MEDICINE BALL PUT (SITTING IN CHAIR) TEST

Reference.
Johnson, B. L., & Nelson, J. K. (1986). *Practical measurements for evaluation in physical education.* Edina, MN: Burgess, pp 214, 217.

Additional Sources.
None.

Purpose.
To measure the ability of an examinee to exert power with the arms.

Objectivity.
r = .99 by Ford (1969) cited in Johnson and Nelson (1986, p. 214).

Reliability.
r = .81 college females and r = .84 college males.

Validity.
r = .77 with scores computed from power formula.

Age and Sex.
Suitable for females and males, age 12 - college.

Equipment.
A 2.72 kilogram (6 pound) medicine ball, sturdy folding chair, marking tape, tape measure, and a strap approximately 1.5m (5') long.

Space Requirements and Design.
A clear, level area approximately 3m x 11m (10' x 35') with a chair positioned behind a "scratch" line near one end of the 11m (35') length.

Directions.
The examinee sits in the chair with the strap placed around the chest and under the armpits. A partner stands behind the chair and holds the strap tight to prevent any trunk movement by the examinee. The examinee grasps the ball with one hand on each side of the ball. The ball is held about chest high. When ready, the examinee draws the ball back against the chest just under the chin and then forcefully pushes the ball forward and upward. Three trials are given in suc-

cession. A practice trial may be taken before scoring to serve as warm up and to acquaint the examinee with the test.

Scoring.
The score is the best of the three trials measured to the nearest .30m (foot). The distance is measured from the "scratch" line just in front of the chair to the spot where the back of the ball first touched the surface.

Norms.
Johnson & Nelson (1986, p. 217) college men and women.

NOTE (1): Medicine balls of other weights are frequently used to adapt the test to the ability of the examinees.

NOTE (2): To prevent splitting the seams of the medicine ball, mats may be placed in the landing zone.

REVIEW

SAMUEL CASE, Ph.D.

Professor of Physical Education
Western Maryland College
Westminster, MD 21157

The underlying reasoning behind the concept of this test is valid if all examinees throw a medicine ball at the same trajectory. Examinees who are capable of producing more power with their arms should be able to throw a medicine ball farther than examinees who are not as powerful. The fact that the examinee is seated and restrained by a strap around the chest insures that the arms alone are used to generate the power. Unfortunately, the validity of this test may be compromised by the fact that examinees may throw the medicine ball at an angle greater than or less than the optimum angle of release. For example, a powerful examinee who releases the medicine ball at an angle of 25 degrees may not exhibit as much arm power as an examinee who releases it between 40 degrees and 45 degrees. This may account for the marginal validity coefficient of 0.77.

According to the information describing the test, the reliability coefficient is 0.81 and the objectivity coefficient is 0.99. Usually, the objectivity coefficient is somewhat lower than the reliability coefficient. However, no references are cited reporting the circumstances under which the reliability and objectivity coefficients were obtained. At any rate, the reliability coefficient is, at best, borderline acceptable for a test of this type.

The requirements for administering the test are reasonable. Nothing extraordinary is required in terms of equipment, facilities, or space. Furthermore, one tester could easily organize a class so that this test could be administered efficiently. Since the motions used in this test are probably unfamiliar to most students, and only three trials are given, it might be better if an opportunity were given for the students to practice.

This test, although suitable for its intended age group, is not suitable for drill or conditioning purposes. The skill learned has little carry over value and there are better, more efficient exercises for improving power in the arms. For safety reasons, it is important that the area in which the medicine ball lands be kept clear. The assistants responsible for marking the spot where the ball lands should be instructed not only in the proper techniques for marking the distance the ball is put, but they should also be cautioned about not getting hit by the ball. Getting hit by a six pound medicine ball could be an unpleasant experience.

Since the scoring simply involves measuring the distance that the ball travels, the test is objective, easily scored, and can be used for self evaluation. This test is unsuitable for research purposes because of the low reliability and validity coefficients. Furthermore, better tests are available even though they require expensive equipment, such as arm ergometers or isokinetic dynamometers.

The available norms for females and males are questionable since they were based on a limited sample using only one age group at only one institution. However, if a physical educator were to use this test, it would not be difficult to establish norms for a specific population.

SUMMARY

Major Strengths:

1. It can be administered with ease.
2. It uses readily available equipment.

Major Weaknesses:

1. Its low reliability.
2. Its low validity.

This test is unacceptable for research purposes because of its inherent weaknesses and the fact that other tests are available. However, it is acceptable for its intended purpose in the classroom situation because of its ease of administration and the fact that normative data could be made available. Additionally, there are very few tests that perform the intended function of this test.

MEDICINE BALL PUT (SITTING ON FLOOR) TEST

Reference.

Fleishman, E. A. (1964B). *The structure and measurement of physical fitness.* Englewood Cliffs: Prentice Hall, pp 52, 59, 134.

Additional Sources.

None.

Purpose.

To measure the ability of an examinee to exert power with the arms.

Objectivity.

Not reported.

Reliability.

r = .73 for test-retest.

Validity.

Construct validity was established.

Age and Sex.

Suitable for females and males, age 15 - college.

Equipment.

A 4.08 kilogram (9 pound) medicine ball, with a 1.27 cm (1/2") wide strip of tape around its circumference, marking tape, and a tape measure.

Space Requirements and Design.

A clear, level area approximately 3m x 10m (10' x 30') with a "scratch" line placed near one end of the 10m (30') length.

Directions.

The examinee sits on the floor with arms outstretched and fingertips directly above the "scratch" line. The examinee grips the ball so that the strip of tape around it is perpendicular to the floor and parallel to the front of the examinee's chest. The examinee must place the palms of the hands on the sides of the ball forward of the tape. It is not permissable to place the hands behind the ball or to "cock" (i.e., extend) the wrists or to move from the sitting position. When ready, the examinee draws the ball back against the chest and then forcefully pushes the ball forward and upward. Three trials are given.

Scoring.

The score is the best distance (the editor assumes it is measured to the nearest .30m or foot) of the three trials.

Norms.

Fleishman (1964B, p. 59) men.

NOTE (1): Medicine balls of other weights are frequently used to adapt the test to the ability of the examinees.

NOTE (2): To prevent splitting the seams of the medicine ball, mats should be placed where the balls land.

REVIEW

THOMAS E. BALL, Ph.D.

Professor of Physical Education
Northern Illinois University
DeKalb, IL 60115

The Medicine Ball Put and various modifications of this test have been used for a number of years to assess the muscular power of the arms and shoulder girdle. While construct validity for the seated medicine ball has been claimed to have been established, research looking at the validity of similar tests does not bear this out. Logically, we might expect an examinee with greater power in the musculature of the arms and shoulders to be able to put an object further than an examinee with less power. Gillespie and Keenum (1987) investigated the validity of the Seated Shot Put Test as a test of muscular power. They found validity coefficients of 0.58 and 0.48 when comparing the Seated Shot Put Test to power calculated from a Bench Press Test. They found validity coefficients of .90 between the two measures. However, when the effect of lean body mass was accounted for statistically, the coefficients dropped to .20. They concluded that, in young wrestlers, the Seated Shot Put reflects differences in muscle mass and not upper body power. Johnson and Nelson (1986) report a validity coefficient of .77 between the distance a six pound medicine ball was put from a seated position and power calculated by a power formula. They did not report the formula used.

The reliability of the various put tests is very good. Reliability coefficients ranging from .77 to .99 have been reported for puts using medicine balls, shots and softballs, and for both seated and standing puts. It would appear that the put test is more reliable when the put is done from a sitting position and when the angle of release is controlled (Gillespie and Keenum, 1987). It is also important to allow the examinees to have several practice trials prior to testing. In addition to having high reliability, the Seated Medicine Ball Put has been reported to have an objectivity coefficient as high as .99 (Johnson & Nelson, 1986).

The administration of the Medicine Ball Put Test does have some moderate drawbacks. The space requirement is for an area of approximately 10 feet by 30 feet, and for some groups, a larger space may be needed. In all likelihood, only one examinee at a time could be tested. With proper warm up and practice, it would be difficult to test a class of 30 students in one 50 minute class period. In addition, at least two people are required to administer the test. Other drawbacks to the use of the test include the limited norms available (Johnson & Nelson, 1986) and the fact that the test is not accurate enough to be used in research.

The test is attractive in that it is easy to administer, can be done either indoors or outdoors, does not require much equipment, the equipment that is required is inexpensive, and the test can be easily modified to test a variety of groups. It is also possible that the test can be self administered after moderate instruction.

SUMMARY

The test is attractive in that it is easily administered and inexpensive. The major drawbacks to the test include the time required to test a large class, the lack of precision and the relative lack of available norms. The test appears to be acceptable for fitness evaluations or teaching, but due to it's imprecision, it is inadequate for use as a research tool.

REVIEW REFERENCES

Gillespie, J., & Keenum, S. (1987). A validity and reliability analysis of the seated shot put as a test of power. *Journal of Human Movement Studies,* 13:97-105.

Johnson, B. L., & Nelson, J. K. (1986). *Practical measurements for evaluation in physical education.* Edina, MN: Burgess.

Mayhew, J. L. et al. (1989). The seated shot put as a measure of upper body power in young wrestlers. Paper presented at the Missouri Academy of Sciences, Jefferson City, MO.

MEDICINE BALL PUT (STANDING) TEST

References.
Barrow, H. M., & McGee, R. (1979). *A practical approach to measurement in physical education.* Philadelphia: Lea and Febiger, pp 142-144.

Fleishman, E. A. (1964B). *The structure and measurement of physical fitness.* Englewood Cliffs: Prentice Hall, p 51, 59.

Additional Sources.
Baumgartner & Jackson (1982, pp. 203-204); Baumgartner & Jackson (1987, pp. 197-198); Baumgartner & Jackson (1991, p. 237); Hastad & Lacy (1989, pp. 281-283); Johnson & Nelson (1986, p. 366); Mood (1980, pp. 237-238); Safrit (1986, pp. 354-356); Safrit (1990, pp. 526-530).

Purpose.
To measure the ability of an examinee to exert power with the arms.

Objectivity.
Not reported.

Reliability.
r = .70 (Fleishman, 1954B, p. 59).

Validity.
Construct validity was established.

Age and Sex.
Suitable for females and males, age 14 - college.

Equipment.
A 2.72 kilogram (6 pound) medicine ball, marking tape, and a tape measure.

Space Requirements and Design.
A clear, level area approximately 8m x 30m (25' x 100'), a 4.57m (15') putting area marked on one end of the 30m (100') length.

Directions.
The examinee takes a standing position in the 4.57m (15') putting area with the ball against the side of the head. The ball is held with the dominant hand under the ball while the other hand is placed on the front of the ball to help with control. The examinee may use the 4.57m (15') putting area in any manner to gain momentum but the projection must be a put and not a throw. The examinee must push the ball forward and upward being sure to keep the putting hand medial to the elbow. If the examinee steps on or over the "scratch" line, it is called a foul and recorded as a trial. Three trials are given in succession. If the examinee commits a foul(s) and/or uses an illegal putting motion on all three trials, additional trials are given until one fair put is made.

Scoring.
The score is the best distance of the three trials measured to the nearest .30m (foot).

Norms.
Barrow & McGee (1979, pp. 143-144) boys and college men with a six pound ball; Fleishman (1964B, p. 59) men with a nine pound ball; Hastad & Lacy (1989, p. 281) boys; Johnson & Nelson (1986, pp. 363, 365-366) boys and men; Mood (1980, pp. 238, 240) boys and men; Safrit (1986, pp. 356, 358) boys and men; Safrit (1990, pp. 528-529) boys and men.

NOTE (1): Fleishman (1954B, p. 51) recommends that the examinee execute the put from a stationary position (i.e., no run up permitted) utilizing trunk rotation and a strong arm shoulder action.

NOTE (2): Medicine balls of other weights are frequently used to adapt the test to the ability of the examinees being tested.

NOTE (3): To prevent splitting the seams of the medicine ball, mats should be placed where the balls land.

REVIEW
WILLIAM F. CLIPSON, Ed.D.

Emeritus Professor
Physical Education
University of Alabama
Tuscaloosa, AL 35486

The Medicine Ball Put (MBP) is scientifically sound since construct validity was established for measuring arm power. Test-retest reliability is reported as 0.893 and objectivity for two scorers as 0.997. In addition, as an indication of motor ability, a validity coefficient of 0.736 was found when compared with a composite of 29 tests measuring eight different components of motor ability (Safrit, 1986).

The MBP requires very little equipment and space, can be easily administered, is easily scored, and requires little expertise to administer. It lends itself to self testing and can be used for both sexes from the upper elementary grades through college by using medicine balls of differing weights.

Norms are available only for boys, grades 7 through 11, and for college men. However, these norms have not been updated in the last 25 years (Johnson & Nelson, 1979).

The danger of someone being hit with the medicine ball is the one hazard that must receive attention. Careful supervision is required. Proper warm up and proper form will protect against arm strain.

If a researcher's purpose is to measure power of the dominant arm, this test may be used. However, if the test is to be administered several times over a considerable period of time, examinees may perfect their form and coordination through practice. The researcher will need to control practice if such is not compatible with her/his research. Also, previous instruction in shot putting form may be a factor for researchers to consider.

SUMMARY
Major Strengths:
1. Objectivity, reliability, and validity.

2. Ease of administration.

3. Potential use in a teaching situation.

Major Weakness:

1. The only major weakness in the test is that practice is necessary for the examinees to feel comfortable with the required putting motion. Practice may be no problem in a teaching situation but may not be desirable for research.

The MBP is acceptable for research when previous experience with the putting motion is not a factor and practice can be controlled. The MBP is an excellent test for teaching situations. It can be used to promote physical fitness and skill in shot putting. It is challenging and interesting since scores improve as power and/or form improve. In teaching, the test has a variety of uses. At one extreme, it can be introduced merely to stimulate interest and to give a program variety. At the other extreme, the test scores can be a part of each examinee's permanent physical development record over a period of years.

REVIEW REFERENCES

Johnson, B. L., & Nelson, J. K. (1979). *Practical measurements for evaluation in physical education*. Minneapolis: Burgess, pp. 358-359.

Safrit, M. J. (1986). *Introduction to measurement in physical education and exercise science*. St. Louis: C. V. Mosby, pp. 354-355.

SHOT PUT TEST

References.

Baumgartner, T., & Jackson, A. (1991). *Measurement for evaluation in physical education and exercise science.* Dubuque: Wm. C. Brown, p 237.

Johnson, B. L., & Nelson, J. K. (1986). *Practical measurements for evaluation in physical education.* Edina, MN, Burgess, pp 214, 217-218.

Additional Sources.

Baumgartner & Jackson (1982, pp. 203-204); Baumgartner & Jackson (1987, pp. 197-198); Jensen & Hirst (1980, pp. 140-142).

Purpose.

To measure the ability of an examinee to exert power with the arms.

Objectivity.

r = .97 reported by Adkison and Martinez cited in Johnson and Nelson (1986, p. 217).

Reliability.

r = .83 reported by Martinez (1982), cited in Johnson and Nelson (1986, pp. 214, 216).

Validity.

Face validity (Johnson & Nelson, 1986, p. 217).

Age and Sex.

Suitable for females and males, age 10 - college.

Space Requirements and Design.

A clear, level, grassy area approximately 8m x 23m (25' X 75') with a restraining ("scratch") line at one end of the 23m length.

Equipment.

A shot of appropriate weight, 2.72kg to 5.44kg (6.1 lbs. 12 lbs.) for the age group being tested, a tape measure, and three sets of small sticks (e.g., tongue depressors) numbered 1 to 5 to be placed in the ground as markers. Johnson and Nelson (1986, p. 217) recommend using a softball.

Directions.

The examinee takes a standing position behind the "scratch" line with the shoulders (i.e., a line through the shoulders) perpendicular to it. The examinee holds the shot or softball in the fingers with the thumb grasping it near the top. The shot is held on the side of the neck just below the ear. The examinee then flexes the hip, knee and ankle joints and simultaneously rotates the trunk backward (i.e., clockwise for a right hander and counterclockwise for a left hander) without moving the feet. After rotating the shot backwards as far as possible, the examinee forcefully rotates the trunk forward and extends the hip, knee and ankle joints. The shot is pushed forward as the examinee straightens the arm (i.e., shoulder flexion and elbow extension). The shot or softball must be put; it cannot be thrown. The feet cannot be moved throughout the put. In Johnson and Nelson's test directions, the examinee is permitted to move across a 2.75m (7') ring. Three trials are given and measured to the nearest foot.

Scoring.

The score is the distance from the inside edge of the "scratch" line to the point of landing measured to the last half-foot. Johnson and Nelson recommend measuring to the nearest foot.

Norms.

Johnson and Nelson (1986, p. 218) young men and women for the softball shot put.

REVIEW

DOUGLAS L. WEEKS, Ph.D.

Assistant Professor
Exercise Science
Ball State University
Muncie, IN 47306

The Shot Put Test was developed as an indicator of muscular power exerted by the arm(s) against a constant weight load. The initial question with regard to the test as an accurate indicator of muscular power is how well test scores correspond to the construct purportedly measured by the test [muscular power]. The test seems to have satisfactory face validity when compared to the traditional definition of muscular power as the ability of a muscle group to deliver maximum force to an object in minimum time. However, studies have not been performed to determine whether the test correlates with more formal mechanical measures of power as indicated by work output (i.e., force x distance) per unit time measurements. Thus, the construct validity of the test has not been established. Reliability estimates have been obtained and indicate that the test delivers consistent scores across multiple administrations to the same examinees. In addition, the measurement procedure seems to afford a high degree of objectivity as indicated by the coefficient of objectivity; thus, one can be assured that any two testers scoring any one performance would arrive at similar scores. It should be cautioned, though, that a standardized measurement procedure be used for each put (e.g., by measuring distance from a common anchor point at the restraining line to the back edge of the impact impression left by the shot). Increased accuracy of measurement, therefore test reliability, will be obtained if measurement is to the nearest inch instead of to the nearest foot, as described.

Administration of the test is straight forward as long as an area is available which can withstand multiple impacts from the shot, and a shot is available which may be handled safely by all examinees. However, a major change in the described procedure of putting while standing is recommended to one in which examinees perform the put while seated in a chair to reduce extraneous body movement. The chair should be aligned with its leading edge perpendicular to the intended direction of the put, thus placing the examinee in a position facing the direction of the put. The rationale for this variation in the standard procedure is based on several studies which show a low correlation between tests of arm power and tests of leg power. Putting from a standing position allows entire body movement so that leg musculature becomes substantially involved, thereby confounding assessment of arm power.

Putting while standing (and to the extreme, allowing movement across a shot put ring as suggested by Johnson and Nelson) may allow examinees of identical arm power to have vastly different scores based on technique differences in putting the shot. The net effect of allowing involvement of extraneous musculature is a decrease in the test's ability to measure what it is

intended to measure, arm power. Therefore, the expected benefit of this change in standard procedure would be an increase in the reliability and validity of the test as an indicator of arm power. Putting from a seated position would also allow the test to be used as an indicator of arm power for wheelchair bound examinees.

An additional recommended change in the standard procedure is the use of a twohanded put, using a pushing motion from beneath the chin, as opposed to the one handed put as described. Not only would a two handed put enable assessment of power in both arms simultaneously, it would also allow easier control of the shot by younger examinees. Allowing examinees practice with the putting technique is also recommended with examinees informed that the greatest distance will be obtained from a release angle of about 30 degrees (based on an average release height of 3 to 4 feet while seated). Even if practice is not possible, examinees should be informed of this optimal release angle, as the angle of release will affect put distance and therefore, the reliability and validity of the test. If practice is allowed, it should not be scheduled on the same day as testing since fatigue has been shown to have a negative effect on power output. Because of fatigue effects, the examinee's best performances should be expected within the recommended three trials administered in succession. Several trials should be administered rapidly to each examinee.

The test seems to have minimal risk to examinees, other than the chance of unexpectedly dropping the shot. This risk may be decreased by employing a two handed put procedure. Keeping the putting area clear of examinees, and making the examinees aware that the shot may roll after impact will additionally increase the safety of the test. Due to minimal safety risks, the test is suitable for age 10 and above if they are physically able to handle the shot. The size and weight of the shot should be adapted to accommodate the physical ability of the examinees. However, a shot of the same weight should be used for all examinees within a grade or age group. It is recommended that the use of a softball in lieu of a shot be reserved for younger examinees. Unfortunately, available norms are based on the softball put; therefore, assessment of performance using a shot will be solely criterion referenced.

SUMMARY

Major Strengths:

1. The test has face validity, is highly reliable, and objective as a traditional field test of arm power.

2. The test is easy to administer and score.

3. The test is applicable to a wide range of ages and either gender.

Major Weaknesses:

1. Statistical criteria for the construct validity of the test has not been established.

2. Norm referenced standards are not available for the shot put, thus eliminating inclusion of the test in norm based studies of motor abilities.

3. The allowance of extraneous body movements will confound measurement of upper body power unless the test is performed from a seated position.

Overall, the test is recommended as acceptable for field testing situations in which devices for direct measurement of work per unit time are not available. The test is adequate as an indicator of potential for varsity athletics, or as an indicator of the ability of a strength training program to increase upper body power. However, it is not recommended that the test be used for student grading since power output is related to rate of muscle contraction which is primarily genetically determined and resistant to modification. The test is also not acceptable for research purposes since a direct measure of work per unit time is not obtained, and construct validity of the test has not been established with other formal measures of mechanical power.

UNDERHAND, BACKWARD SHOT THROW TEST

Reference.
Myers, B. (1986). Testing for field and multi events athletes. *Athletic Journal*, 66:10-12, May.

Additional Sources.
None.

Purpose.
To measure the ability of an examinee to exert power with the body.

Objectivity.
Not reported.

Reliability.
Not reported.

Validity.
Not reported.

Age and Sex.
College track and field athletes.

Equipment.
A stopwatch, tape measure, and various shots: 4kg (8 lbs.) for females, and 7.27kg (16 lbs.) for college age males and older.

Space Requirements and Design.
A shot put circle with an open area approximately 5m x 25m (16' x 82') in front of it.

Directions.
The examinee stands on the toe board facing the back of the circle with the feet shoulder width apart. The shot is grasped in both hands. The examinee then squats, extends the legs, and throws the shot over the head. The examinee may leave the toe board during the follow through and land in the throwing sector. The distance is measured from the inside edge of the toe board to the closest mark made by the shot. The editor assumes three trials are adequate.

Scoring.
The score is the greatest distance measured for the best of three trials.

Norms.
Not reported.

NOTE: (1) For safety reasons, it may be better if the examinee stands in front of the board with her/his toes touching rather than on the toe board.

NOTE: (2) A variation of the above is the two hand overhead forward shot throw. The examinee assumes an upright position facing the landing area. The overhead throw is executed by using the technique similar to the soccer throw in.

REVIEW

EDGAR W. SHIELDS, JR., Ph.D.
Associate Professor
Physical Education, Exercise and
Sport Science
University of North Carolina at
Chapel Hill
Chapel Hill, NC 27599-8605

It should be noted that this item, as developed by Myers (1986), is one of ten items in what he labels a "hybrid" table. Apparently, following years of using multiple tables (e.g., jumps decathlon, throws decathlon, power pentathlon, and IAAF tables) for men or women (often referred to as the Portuguese Tables), Myers developed the "hybrid" table for the purpose of evaluating the talent of jumpers, throwers, and multi eventers in track and field, as well as determining the training and conditioning levels of these athletes. Although somewhat difficult to evaluate from Myer's (1986) presentation of his table, it does not appear that the issues of validity, reliability, or objectivity were ever scientifically addressed, either for the 10 items administered collectively as a battery or for any individual item. One fails to find even a straightforward claim of "face" or "logical" validity. Upon examination of the description of the item, it seems reasonable to suggest that the test may have acceptable objectivity. It is not possible to conclude the same for either validity or reliability.

Assuming that, regardless of the lack of evidence for the test being valid, reliable, and/or objective, one wishes to utilize the underhand, backward shot throw, the following should be considered. The nature of the test is such that active participation of another individual, other than to mark the distance of the throw, is not required and would have no effect on the performance of the examinee. Facility and equipment requirements are not unusual and are normally already in place, assuming track and field is a component of the athletic program. Time requirements should be minimal, and the item could be administered easily by one tester, although two would probably be more efficient if several examinees are to be tested successively. The number of trials, three, is fairly standard and acceptable for power items.

Use of the item to promote conditioning and/or learning is, at best, an equivocal consideration. It would seem very presumptuous to suggest that any conditioning attained by the use of this item as a drill would be as suitable as the task specific conditioning gained by simply practicing the event in which one will participate, which would also promote learning. In that this item, as executed, does not appear to approximate any event in which one would participate, it is not suitable as a learning drill. Disregarding previous statements, it would appear that the item would present no general or specific problems for the age ability levels for which it is intended. While his presentation may weakly suggest that the test can discriminate among the examinees, Myers (1986) does not directly address this issue, and it must be concluded that no evidence exists to verify this characteristic for the item.

A significant concern in administering this test would be the safety of the examinee as well as that of the testers and/or other individuals who may be in the area. Myer's (1986) does, in the interest of safety, note a possible modification in the execution of the item, which would likely reduce the possibility of injury to the examinee, tester, and others, but would certainly not be sufficient to reduce a concern for or precautions relative to, safety. The item is not suitable for self administration or evaluation. Scientifically derived norms are not evident, and the test appears to have been developed for a rather broad category of "college track and field athletes" with no breakdown by age or gender. The item could be administered and scored with sufficient precision to be utilized in research, although initial efforts would need to address the questions of validity, reliability, and objectivity.

SUMMARY

Major Strengths:

1. Easily administered.

2. A minimum of time, personnel, and equipment required.

Major Weaknesses:

1. Safety concerns.

2. Lack of established validity, reliability, objectivity, and discrimination capability.

3. Lack of scientifically established norms.

Any one of these weaknesses and certainly all of them collectively, could be cause to conclude that this test is generally unacceptable for research and/or teaching purposes. As only one item in a battery of 10, Myers (1986) may have an instrument which functions well for him as a part of a whole. The battery of items does appear to have been useful to him in evaluating jumpers, throwers, and multi event collegiate track and field athletes; however, the underhand, backward shot throw as a "stand alone" item for the measurement "power of the body" is judged inadequate at this time, primarily due to the three key test characteristics of validity, reliability, and objectivity being unknown. The systematic evaluation of these issues, along with the ability of the item to discriminate, must be done before the suitability question of use of the item for research and/or teaching can be addressed adequately.

POWER TESTS OF THE LEGS/LOWER BODY
ANAEROBIC CAPACITY/POWER TESTS

MARGARIA ANAEROBIC POWER TEST

Reference.
Margaria, R. et al. (1966). Measurement of muscular power (anaerobic) in man. *Journal of Applied Physiology,* 21:1662-1664, September.

Additional Source.
Johnson & Nelson (1986, pp. 219-222).

Purpose.
To measure the maximum anaerobic power of an examinee by use of a stair climbing exercise.

Objectivity.
Not reported.

Reliability.
+/- 4 percent on values when test was repeated during the same session. Approximately the same values for each subject when the test was repeated every few days with untrained subjects.

Validity.
Values for athletes were significantly higher than the values for untrained subjects.

Age and Sex.
Not reported, but suitable for females and males, high school through adult.

Equipment.
A body weight scale and an electric timer, accurate to at least one-hundredth of a second, with switch mats for starting and stopping the timer.

Space Requirements and Design.
A staircase of 12 to 16 steps, each step 15cm - 20cm (6" - 8") in height. The switch mats are placed on steps 8 (start mat) and 12 (stop mat).

Directions.
The examinee stands in front of the stairs and when ready, runs the stairs, two steps at a time, as fast as possible. The timer is started when the examinee lands on the switch mat on step 8 and is stopped when the examinee lands on the switch mat on step 12. The test may be repeated after a few minutes of recovery. (Note: The exact number of trials to be given is not stated.) The vertical distance the examinee ran is determined by measuring the vertical height directly from the top of step 8 to the top of step 12 or by measuring the height of one step and multiplying by four.

Scoring.
The score is derived by multiplying the examinee's body weight (in kilograms) by the vertical distance of the four steps (in meters) and then dividing by the time required to run the four steps.

> Power = Work/Time = (Body Weight) (Vertical Distance)/Time

Norms.
Not reported.

REVIEW

LINUS J. DOWELL, Ed.D.
Chair, Graduate Programs
Health and Physical Education
Texas A & M University
College Station, TX 77843

The Margaria Power Test was a landmark measurement in its time. Its use was very short lived. Shortly after its inception it was modified by Kalamen in his doctoral dissertation at Ohio University (1968). Validity and reliability for this test are both high and considered to be accurate. Though norms for the Margaria Test are not available, there are guidelines set up for the Margaria-Kalamen Test.

Kalamen also found a correlation of .974 between the Margaria-Kalamen Test and a 50 yard dash with a 15 yard running start. This suggests one might substitute this test with the Margaria-Kalamen Test if cost of timing equipment was a factor. The Margaria-Kalamen Test shows greater power output than the Margaria test probably due to the six meter running start and taking three steps instead of two.

One of the problems with this test is that some examinees have difficulty taking two steps at a time and express doubts and fears about their ability to perform the test safely and successfully. When looking at the data collected on this test it appears that some subjects who showed great anaerobic power on other tests did not do so on the Margaria-Kalamen Power Test. This may validate the idea that the Margaria-Kalamen Power Test may not measure anaerobic power for people who have difficulty in running stairs in a confident manner.

SUMMARY

Major Strengths:

1. Ease in setting up.
2. Scoring is objective.
3. Ease in administration.
4. Reliability of the test.
5. Validity of the test.

Major Weaknesses:

1. Lack of safety in taking two steps at a time.

2. Fear of some examinees lacking the ability to perform this test.

3. The expense of equipment needed.

This is an excellent test for measuring anaerobic power if the equipment needed to perform the test is available. For examinees who have difficulty in running the stairs, the tester might consider the 50 yard dash with a running start as an alternative.

Testing using the Margaria Anaerobic Power Test has been done at Texas A & M University with the women's basketball team, and comparisons were made with a control group. The average score for the women's basketball team was 1175 watts and for the control group 733.6 watts. These measurements were converted to watts to facilitate correlation calculations between this and other tests.

MARGARIA - CHALOUPKA ANAEROBIC POWER TEST

References.

Margaria, R. et al. (1966). Measurement of muscular power (anaerobic) in man. *Journal of Applied Physiology,* 21:1662-1664, September.

Mathews, D. K. (1978). *Measurement in physical education.* Philadelphia: W. B. Saunders, pp 169-170.

Additional Source.

Johnson & Nelson (1986, pp. 219-222).

Purpose.

To measure the maximum anaerobic power of an examinee by use of a stair climbing exercise.

Objectivity.

Not reported.

Reliability.

r = .94 when first five trials were correlated with second five trials.

Validity.

Not reported.

Age and Sex.

Grades 2 - 6, but sex not reported.

Equipment.

A body weight scale and an electric timer accurate to at least one-hundredth of a second with switch mats for starting and stopping the timer.

Space Requirements and Design.

A staircase with 6 to 10 steps, each step 15 to 20cm (6" - 8") in height, with a run up area in front of the first step 6m (19.68') in length. The switch mats are placed on steps two and six.

Directions.

The examinee stands 6m in front of the first step and when ready, runs as fast as possible to the steps, takes and, them two at a time. The timer is started when the examinee lands on the switch mat on step two and is stopped when the examinee lands on the switch mat on step six. Both body weight and the vertical height of the steps are determined in the same manner as in the original Margaria power test.

Scoring.

The score is derived by multiplying the examinee's body weight (in kilograms) by the vertical distance (in meters) of the four steps and then dividing by the time required to run the four steps.

Power = Work/Time = (Body Weight) (Vertical Distance)/Time

Norms.

Mathews (1978, p. 170) boys.

REVIEW

RICHARD LITWHILER, Ed.D.

Associate Professor
Physical Education
Georgia Southwestern College
Americus, GA 31709

This test of anaerobic power has become a standard in research application, basically because very few tests of "anaerobic" power have been developed. If one compounds this fact with a general confusion of the concept of "power," one can understand the difficulty in accurately defining the component as well as accurately measuring it. With terms such as "power," "aerobic power," "anaerobic power," "explosive power," "explosive strength," "athletic power," "muscular power," and "mechanical power" being using to describe this trait, it is easy to understand the general confusion. "Power," as defined in this review, is the "product of force (body weight) times distance (vertical height between step two and step six) divided by time (from step two to step six)." Because of this definition, many of the traditional field tests of power, which do not factor in the weight moved or the time of movement (such as the Vertical Jump or Standing Long Jump) would be considered inappropriate, even though some work has been done in an attempt to include body weight in such calculations (e.g., the Lewis Nomogram).

The reliability of this instrument is well within the accepted limits for performance tests. This result is consistent with the reliability correlations of other "anaerobic" power tests, as well as the more traditional "athletic" power tests, such as the Standing Long Jump and Vertical Jump.

Very little information can be found on the objectivity of the test. If the test directions are strictly followed, the objectivity of the test should be excellent, so long as the timing equipment accurately measures from the starting switch mat to the stopping switch mat to at least one-hundredth of a second. Use of a hand held stopwatch (even a digital watch) would be unacceptable, given the probable timer error over such a short distance and time span.

The space and facility requirements may create a problem. If each of the steps used is not the suggested 174mm high, the norms should not be used. A special stairway may need to be built. The equipment needed includes switch plates and an accurate clock. There are many excellent instruments available, but the majority are beyond the budget of most schools. The test can be administered to only one examinee at a time, but it is neither difficult, nor too time consuming, to do so. Usually three trials are permitted with the best trial recorded as the examinee's score.

It may be important to remember that this test is a revision of the Margaria-Kalamen Power Test (circa 1968) designed for high school and college males, which is in turn an adaptation of the original leg power test of Margaria and associates (circa 1966). The major change made was to shorten the total distance from 1.05 meters to .7 meters for boys grade two through six. Norms are available for elementary school boys (based on only N = 136). Guideline classifications (i.e., five categories, poor to excellent) for men and women ages 15 to over 50 can be found in Mathews and Fox (1976). The test seems suitable for both sexes and most age groups. More current norms should be developed.

There may be some safety concern in any all out effort on a stairway, particularly with the younger examinees. Some short legged examinees may also have trouble negotiating the three step jumps. This test is probably best suited for research, so long as the proper equipment and facilities are available.

SUMMARY

Major Strengths:

1. Easy to set up, administer and score.

2. Highly reliable and should be highly objective.

3. Does not take a great deal of time to administer and directions are not difficult to understand.

4. Could be used for both sexes and most age groups.

5. One of the only true anaerobic power tests suggested.

Major Weaknesses:

1. Electronic equipment needed to insure objectivity and accuracy can be expensive.

2. No current norms; not in general use.

3. Can only test one examinee at a time.

4. Possible safety problem, particularly with younger, motor immature examinees.

5. Measures only leg power.

This test is adequate for research, although current norms should be sought or developed. Precaution should be taken to avoid injury during the test. This test is probably unacceptable for teaching because it is not feasible administratively to test a large number of examinees. Interestingly, it was reported by Fox and Mathews (1981) in *The Physiological Basis of Physical Education and Athletics,* Philadelphia: W. B. Saunders, that a correlation of .974 was found when the results of a 50 yard dash (with 15 yard running start) were compared with the Margaria-Kalamen Power Test. An option to the power test, should the equipment not be available, may thus be considered.

MARGARIA - DEVRIES ANAEROBIC POWER TEST

References.
Margaria, R. et al. (1966). Measurement of muscular power (anaerobic) in man. *Journal of Applied Physiology*, 21:1662-1664, September.

deVries, H. A. (1971). *Laboratory experiments in physiology of exercise*. Dubuque: Wm. C. Brown, pp 101-104.

Additional Source.
Johnson & Nelson (1986, pp. 219-222).

Purpose.
To measure the maximum anaerobic power of an examinee by use of a stair climbing exercise.

Objectivity.
Not reported.

Reliability.
Not reported.

Validity.
Not reported.

Age and Sex.
Not reported, but suitable for females and males, high school through adult.

Equipment.
A body weight scale and an electric timer accurate to at least one-hundredth of a second with switch mats for starting and stopping the timer. A stopwatch may be substituted for the electric timer.

Space Requirements and Design.
A staircase with 12 to 16 steps, each step 15cm to 20cm (6" - 8") in height, with a run up area in front of the first step 2m (6') in length. The switch mats are placed on steps 4 and 12.

Directions.
The examinee stands 6' in front of the first step and, when ready, approaches and runs the stairs as fast as possible, taking two steps at a time. The timer is started when the examinee lands on the switch mat on step 4 and is stopped when the examinee lands on the switch mat on step 12. The average time of three trials is used to calculate power. Both body weight and the vertical distance are determined in the same manner as in the original Margaria power test.

Scoring.
The score is derived by multiplying the examinee's body weight (in pounds) by the vertical distance (in feet) of the eight steps and then dividing by the average time required to run the eight steps.

Power = Work/Time = (Body Weight) (Vertical Distance)/Time

Norms.
Johnson & Nelson (1986, p. 222) boys and men.

REVIEW

JAMES R. MORROW, JR., Ph.D.
Professor
Health and Human Performance
University of Houston
Houston, TX 77204-5331

The Margaria-deVries Anaerobic Power Test is a modification of the original Margaria Power Test. The test, a measure of leg (anaerobic) power with results expressed as a time rate of performing work, indicates the maximum force exerted in the shortest possible time. Various modifications of the test protocol have been developed. Essentially, the time to elevate the body weight a given distance is recorded. Body weight is elevated a specific height by having the examinee run up stairs as quickly as possible while the time to do so is recorded. Variations in the height of stairs and the number of stairs taken with each step have been made. Work is calculated as the examinee's weight times the height traveled (from the step where timing begins to the step where timing ends). Work is divided by the time to complete the elevation.

Reliability coefficients for this form of the test are not reported, nor are objectivity coefficients. Assuming variability among examinees, reliability and objectivity should be quite good when using electronic timing devices. However, the use of hand held watches will reduce these values. Content validity has been reported. Concurrent validity coefficients for particular muscle groups assessed with isokinetic devices have not been reported. Johnson and Nelson (1986) report construct validity has been provided when sprinters scored higher than distance runners and athletes scored higher than nonathletes on this version of the test. While the item reflects content validity, a major consideration is the relatively high correlation expected between test scores and body weights since the work accomplished is a function of the examinee's body weight.

Johnson and Nelson (1986) report this test is "suitable" for college men and women. They provide norms based on the work of Carter (1979) for high school boys and college men. Given the characteristics of the test, the measures obtained, and the limitation related to body weight, the test could probably be administered to subjects of any age. Mathews (1973) reports a modification by Chaloupka for use with elementary age children. Descriptive statistics are provided by Mathews. Given the stairs and climbing nature of the test, reasonable precautions should be taken to ensure a valid measurement (e.g., practice trials and clearly marking which steps start and stop the timing device).

REVIEW REFERENCES

Carter, D. R. (1979). Measurement of anaerobic power in high school and colleges. Unpublished study, Louisiana State University.

Johnson, B. L., & Nelson, J. K. (1986). *Practical measurements for evaluation in physical education.* Edina, MN: Burgess Publishing.

Mathews, D. L. (1978). *Measurement in physical education.* Philadelphia: W. B. Saunders.

MARGARIA - KALAMEN ANAEROBIC POWER TEST

References.

Margaria, R. et al. (1966). Measurement of muscular power (anaerobic) in man. *Journal of Applied Physiology,* 21:1662-1664, September.

Kalamen, J. L. (1968). Measurement of maximum muscular power in man. Unpublished doctoral dissertation, Ohio State University. In Fox, E. L. and Mathews, D. K. (1981). *The physiological basis for physical education and athletics.* Philadelphia: Saunders College Publishing, pp 621-622.

Lamb, D. R. (1984). *Physiology of exercise: Responses and applications.* New York: Macmillan, pp 294-296.

McArdle, W. D. et al. (1986). *Exercise physiology: Energy, nutrition, and human performance.* Philadelphia: Lea and Febiger, pp 167-171.

Additional Sources.

Baumgartner & Jackson (1982, pp. 204-206); Jensen & Hirst (1980, p. 138); Johnson & Nelson (1986, pp. 219-222); Kirkendall et al. (1980, pp. 241, 243); Kirkendall et al. (1987, pp. 119-120).

Purpose.

To measure the maximum anaerobic power of an examinee by use of a stair climbing exercise.

Objectivity.

Not reported.

Reliability.

Not reported.

Validity.

r = .97 using a criterion of a 50 yard dash with a 15 yard running start (Fox & Mathews, 1981, p. 622).

Age and Sex.

Suitable for females and males, high school through college.

Equipment.

A body weight scale and an electric timer accurate to at least one-hundredth of a second with switch mats for starting and stopping the timer.

Space Requirements and Design.

A staircase with 9 to 12 steps, each step 15 - 20cm (6" - 8") in height, with a run up area in front of the first step 6m (19.68') in length. The switch mats are placed on the third step (start mat) and the ninth step (stop mat).

Directions.

The examinee stands 6m (19.68') in front of the first step and when ready, approaches and runs the stairs as fast as possible taking three steps at a time. The timer is started when the examinee lands on the switch mat on step three and is stopped when the examinee lands on the switch mat on step nine. Both body weight and the vertical distance are determined in the same manner as in the original Margaria power test.

Scoring.

The score is derived by multiplying the examinee's body weight (in pounds) by the vertical distance (in feet) of the six steps and then dividing by the time required to run the six steps.

Power = Work/Time = (Body Weight) (Vertical Distance)/Time

Norms.

Fox & Mathews (1981, p. 622) men and women; Kirkendall et al. (1980, p. 244) men and women; Kirkendall et al. (1987, p. 120) boys, girls, men and women.

REVIEW

JOSEPH J. GRUBER, Ph.D.
Professor of Physical Education
University of Kentucky
Lexington, KY 40506-0219

The purpose of this field test is to estimate indirectly the anaerobic power of examinees. Power is work performed per unit of time; usually an all out maximum intensity of big muscle work (e.g., cycling, sprinting, and rowing) for periods of two minutes or less. Any power test is dependent on a specific movement pattern, metabolic pathways (energy system) to support the short duration, high intensity work and motivation of the examinee being tested. Anaerobic power is dependent on the short term anaerobic energy system involving splitting of ATP, CP and a breakdown of glycogen without a supply of oxygen needed to replenish the system. It usually takes two minutes to involve the entire ATP-CO-glycolysis anaerobic metabolic chain. One would expect that appropriate criteria for the validation of a power test would include such things as oxygen debt and blood lactic acid buildup after a power test lasting for several minutes. These criteria have not been utilized in laboratory validation studies of the Margaria-Kalamen Power Test because the test lasts less than two seconds. Instead, other field tests have been utilized in concurrent validity studies. Fox and Mathews (1981) report a correlation of .974 with a 50 yard dash time after a 15 yard running start. McArdle et al. (1986) also report correlations of .56 with the Sargent Jump Test and .67 with a power bicycle test. These same investigators also report correlations ranging from .31 to -.88 between various leg power tests, indicating that leg power performance is highly task specific. Thus, the Margaria-Kalamen Power Test taps the short term energy system of splitting ATP required to sprint up an incline or run a short dash. One must not infer that an examinee who scores high on the Margaria-Kalamen Power Test of the legs will also have high power scores on tests of the arms, etc.

Data on test reliability and objectivity is lacking. However, any professional using the test can do a simple test-retest reliability study across several days. The nature of the test and adherence to directions for test administration should produce reliable data.

The score on the test is not dependent on another individual who might influence the examinee's score.

Space is not a problem as the test can be performed on most staircases. Equipment can be a problem if one does not have a timer that is activated and deactivated by switch mats. However, this reviewer has utilized stopwatches with good accuracy. It is recommended that the average of three trial scores on the test be used. The test is easy to administer and score by one

tester with a minimum of training. The test can be administered to one examinee in less than five seconds.

While the test directions imply only one trial of the test is given, this reviewer recommends three trials in order to take into consideration learning and warm up variables. The test is not suitable as a drill or a conditioning activity due to its extremely short duration and the possibility of tripping while doing repeat trials of the test.

The test is suitable for both sexes of an age range capable of running up a standard flight of stairs. There is no danger to examinees taking the test as long as they are uninjured and warm up prior to the test.

Scores on this test are dependent on body weight. Hence, individual differences in short term energy capacities (two seconds or less) should not be compared across examinees of different body weights having the same time score. The heavier examinee will on the surface, appear to be more powerful. There is no biochemical data to support the level of development of the anaerobic system in this case. Use the test data to compare examinees of the same body weight or among the same examinee before and after training. Examinees can test themselves and monitor their progress over time.

The Margaria-Kalamen Power Test is suitable for use in research if the research involves maximum work done in a very short period of time as this only involves the splitting of ATP. If the power output to be estimated lasts for a minute or two, then CP and glycogen stores are brought into play. This calls for a different duration test. Again, a test is valid for specific purposes. If the Margaria-Kalamen Power Test provides valid data to answer the research question, then use it. Adequate norms from ages 15 through 50 for men and women exist.

SUMMARY

Major Strengths:

1. The test is easy to administer; a large number of people can be tested in a short period of time.

2. The test is inexpensive in terms of time involved, monetary expense, and testing personnel.

3. The test possesses logical and concurrent validity as a measure of leg power lasting for a few seconds.

Major Weaknesses:

1. The test's short duration. An examinee will climb the flight of stairs in .5 to 1.5 seconds at most. This is too short a period of time to challenge the entire anaerobic metabolic pathways, which requires one to two minutes.

2. The Margaria-Kalamen Test should not be used to estimate the power output of other major muscle groups.

This test is acceptable for teaching and research purposes if the test validity provides needed data. It is unacceptable if the aim is to predict times in a 400 meter run. However, if one desires to determine leg power in one second or less, the test is acceptable.

WINGATE ANAEROBIC TEST

References.
Ayalon, A. et al. (1974). Relationships among measurements of explosive strength and anaerobic power. *Biomechanics IV,* Vol. 1, pp 572-577.

Bar-Or, O. (1978). A new anaerobic capacity test -characteristics and applications. Presented at the 21st World Congress in Sports Medicine, Brasilia.

Bar-Or, O. (1987). The wingate anaerobic test: An update on methodology, reliability and validity. *Sports Medicine,* 4:381-394.

Additional Sources.
None.

Purpose.
To measure the peak power, the mean power, and the rate of fatigue of an examinee while pedalling a cycle ergometer.

Objectivity.
Not reported.

Reliability.
$r = .89$ to $r = .98$ (Bar-Or, 1987, p. 386).

Validity.
Numerous r values of 0.75 or more with a variety of anaerobic tasks (Bar-Or, 1987, p. 388).

Age and Sex.
Females and males, children - adult.

Equipment.
An arm or cycle ergometer and a stopwatch.

Space Requirements and Design.
A clear, level area approximately 3m (10') with the ergometer in the center.

Directions.
The examinee assumes a sitting position on the cycle ergometer with the seat height adjusted so that the legs are fully extended at the bottom of the pedalling cycle. Bar-Or (1987) recommends the use of toe stirrups. After an adequate warm up and on the command, "Ready, Go," the examinee pedals as fast as possible against no resistance. Once the initial inertia is overcome, usually two to three seconds after beginning pedalling, a predetermined resistance is then given to the examinee based on her/his body weight. Once this predetermined resistance is set, the tester starts the stopwatch and the examinee continues pedalling at maximum effort for 30 seconds. The tester and several assistants count the number of pedal revolutions and record the number for each three or five second interval of cycling. The resistance each examinee uses was originally based on 0.075 kilopounds (kp) per kilogram (kg) of body weight. This figure has been found to underestimate the highest mean power. Therefore, Bar-Or (1987) recommends that a resistance setting of 0.090 kp/kg of body weight be used with adults and a setting of 0.100 kp/kg of body weight be used with adult athletes.

Scoring.
The peak power, mean power, and fatigue index scores are calculated using the following work formula:

Work (kgm) = (kg resistance) x (number of pedal revolutions x 6).

Peak Power Score
The Peak Power Score (also referred to as the anaerobic power score) is calculated for the three or five second period during which the greatest amount of work was produced.

Mean Power Score
The Mean Power Score (also referred to as the anaerobic capacity or total work score) is calculated for the entire 30 seconds of cycling.

Fatigue Index
The Fatigue Index is determined by plotting and examining the amount of work produced for each three or five second cycling period.

Norms.
Maud, P. J. & Shultz, B. B. (1989, pp. 146-147) men and women.

REVIEW

JAMES M. MANNING, Ph.D.
Associate Professor
Movement Science and Leisure Studies
The William Paterson College of New Jersey
Wayne, NJ 07470

The Wingate Anaerobic Test is an acceptable test to measure power of the arms or legs for either sex of any age. Two major values are obtained from this test. One is peak power or the power which can be generated by the muscles within three to five seconds, and the other is anaerobic capacity, or the mean power generated over 30 seconds. Peak power tests the immediate energy source (stored phosphogens) and involves an intensity of 300 to 375 percent of maximum oxygen consumption. Even though this test is being utilized to examine two energy pathways involving anaerobiosis, care must be used when attempting to evaluate an examinee's specific athletic performance. This test involves skill and the coordination of pedaling. This alternating left and right circular motion could affect the nature of the force application. The use of this test in an attempt to predict performance of a skill which does not specifically mimic the same identical movement may prove to be unsuitable.

The equipment necessary to perform the test is very important, since a calculated workload according to examinee's body weight must be applied at an exact time. The test should be performed on a cycle ergometer modified to permit the instantaneous application of the workload. It is extremely critical that testers follow the directions exactly. Three methods of timing and counting the revolutions are suggested. The least precise would be the use of a stopwatch and counting the number of revolutions in each three or five second interval. Another method would be to attach a microswitch to the cycle frame and magnets to the rim of the flywheel so that the onset of the test and the number of revolutions could be obtained by a computer. A third method would be to video tape the test with a clock in the background so that upon review of the tape, would show the exact number of revolutions and partial revolutions.

The predetermined resistance was originally based on 0.075 kilopounds per kilogram of body weight. Various studies have reported that, in order to obtain the highest power measures, resistances greater than 0.075 kilopounds per kilogram of body weight should be used for adult females and males and for adult athletes. Since those reports were made, different settings have been recommended. Sufficient norms are not available. More research is suggested as the predetermined resistance settings seem to be specific to the population investigated.

The performance of this test may cause an examinee to become light headed and/or nauseous and the exercise should not be performed twice in one day.

SUMMARY
Major Strengths:
1. It is a valid, reliable, objective test for measurement of anaerobic peak power.

2. It is a valid, reliable, objective test for measurement of anaerobic capacity.

3. Power measures can be obtained in a short amount of time.

4. The duration of the test is specific to the anaerobic metabolic process which is being evaluated.

Major Weaknesses:
1. Specific equipment is necessary.

2. Trained testers are necessary.

3. Norms for numerous populations are not available.

4. Well documented workloads which elicit the highest power output have not been established for various populations.

5. The asymmetrical circular pedal motion involves skill and coordination, so some previous experience in performing the test is suggested.

6. Results from this test should not be used to predict specific performance.

The Wingate Anaerobic Test is an acceptable power test, adequate for research and/or teaching because the test protocol meets the physiological metabolic criteria for anaerobic power and anaerobic capacity. As in all research, the test procedures, trained personnel, and the specific equipment needs are extremely important in order to obtain the desired results.

POWER TESTS OF THE LEGS/LOWER BODY
JUMP TESTS

ALTERNATE LEG JUMP FOR DISTANCE TEST

Reference.
President's Council on Physical Fitness and Sports (1987). *USSR youth physical performance test.* Washington, DC: President's Council on Physical Fitness and Sports, pp 1, 10.

Additional Sources.
None.

Purpose.
To measure the explosive power of an examinee's legs in covering the greatest possible horizontal distance.

Objectivity.
Not reported.

Reliability.
Not reported.

Validity.
Not reported.

Age and Sex.
Not reported, but based on the norms provided, it appears intended for females and males, age 8 - 9.

Equipment.
A tape measure and marking tape.

Space Requirements and Design.
A clear, level area approximately 2m x 15m (6' x 50') with a starting line marked off near one end of the 15m length, and the tape measure laid out perpendicular to the starting line for the full 15m length.

Directions.
The examinee stands behind the starting line in a forward stride stance (i.e., one foot just behind the line and the other foot back a comfortable distance). After the signal, "Ready, Go," the examinee jumps as far as possible using a one leg takeoff and lands on the opposite leg. The examinee continues jumping by alternating the leg used to take off with for a total of eight consecu-

tive jumps. The examinee can only have the one foot in contact with the surface throughout the jumping phase of the test.

Scoring.
The score is the distance covered in the eight alternate leg jumps. The editor assumes it is the perpendicular distance from the starting line to the back edge of closest heel at the end of eight jumps that is measured to the nearest cm (half-inch).

Norms.
President's Council (1987, p. 1) boys and girls.

REVIEW

JOHN DAGGER, Ph.D.

Assistant Professor
Physical Education
University of Illinois
Chicago, IL 60680

From a practical stand point, the Alternate Leg Jump For Distance (ALJ) adequately meets most evaluative criteria. It is easy to administer, and requires little training, equipment, time, or space. Although no data are presented, it would appear to provide a fair degree of objectivity, if the tester is positioned appropriately to see and mark the measurement point (with perhaps a piece of tape). Instructions for administration are a bit sparse. For example, there is no indication of how much instruction (or at least demonstration) can be given, how many trials will be given or recorded, nor what age range beyond the limited one noted would be appropriate.

Power is an attribute of motor performance, which is measured in terms of work performed over time (e.g., foot-pounds/second). High performance on a pure measure of muscular power can be conceptualized as the maximum weight moved a standard distance in the shortest time interval and is dependent upon a variety of factors, including the number of muscle groups involved, effective recruitment of contractile units, mechanical efficiency or coordination of the movement pattern, and the nature of the test (e.g., discrete versus continuous and duration of the task). In obtaining such a measure, it is common for empiricists to attempt to control these degrees of freedom limiting their summative effect. For most practical purposes, however, measures of power performance are defined and attributed face validity and are required only to be at least reliably and objectively obtained.

The Alternate Leg Jump For Distance Test (ALJ) is purported to measure "explosive" leg power. It appears to combine elements of short dashes and horizontal (SLJ) or vertical (SVJ) jumping, heretofore the most common measures of leg power in the physical education setting. The ALJ differs from running in that it promotes powerful muscle contraction through a greater range of motion, and produces less horizontal momentum. It would seem to fit the label "explosive" better. The (ALJ) differs from the jumps in that eight repetitions are required in a more sustained performance. All three of the above tests have been criticized on grounds that scores are interpreted without regard for differences in body weight and coordinative status of the examinee. Even at age eight or nine, mechanical differences in these movement patterns exist, yielding a higher score for some lighter or less powerful examinees. By providing a somewhat unique movement task, it is possible that some error attributable to developmental differences will be neutralized. However, a cross validation with some of these measures would be useful in interpreting the test's validity. Also of concern in the matter of practical validity would be the sensitivity of the measure to a general power training program.

Concern over the test's unreported reliability and a hypothesized learning effect led to a brief study, performed on 14 eight and nine year old

males enrolled in an urban recreational day camp. The tester, who held an master's degree in physical education, was a counselor in the camp. Each examinee performed three trials of the test with approximately three minute rest intervals. Then each examinee performed a single retention trial two hours later. Repeated measures ANOVA revealed no learning effect across trials and a test for independence indicated only random variation between trials (T1, T2, and T3) and between T1 and the retention trial (T1 vs. TR). Intraclass correlations (R) were computed at .97 for both the three trial and pretest retention comparisons. This evidence would support administration of a single trial and provide a fair estimate of short term stability of the test.

SUMMARY

Major Strengths:

1. A reliable, and presumed objective, test.

2. Easily and cheaply administered.

3. Can be administered indoors or outdoors.

4. Appears to be a motivating test for children.

Major Weaknesses:

1. Lack of normative data beyond the eight and nine year old range, accompanied by a lack of any report of test standardization procedures.

2. Lack of any validation work.

Due primarily to the unique nature of the task and the focus upon explosive work, this item is, perhaps, better suited to teaching the concept of power to children in a physical education setting than the traditional measures mentioned above. It is currently not known whether this measure would be sensitive to instruction. Lack of appropriate norms on a broad sample of American children would prohibit any norm referenced interpretation. As a pure test of power, this test is not felt to be well enough controlled for empirical analysis.

BOSCO'S MECHANICAL POWER JUMP TEST

Reference.
Bosco, C. et al. (1983). A simple method for measurement of mechanical power in jumping. *European Journal of Applied Physiology*, 50:273-282.

Additional Sources.
None.

Purpose.
To measure the mechanical power of an examinee's legs during a series of vertical jumps.

Objectivity.
Not reported.

Reliability.
r = .95 for test-retest method.

Validity.
r = .87 with modification of Wingate test and r = .84 with 60m dash.

Age and Sex.
Males, age 16 - 30.

Equipment.
A stopwatch and an electrical instrument called the Ergojump. Any electrical timer, accurate to .001 second, with a mat attachment which will start the timer when the examinee leaves the mat and stop the timer when the examinee lands on the mat can be substituted for the Ergojump.

Space Requirements and Design.
A clear, level area approximately 3m (10') square with the Ergojump instrument positioned in the center.

Directions.
The examinee stands on the Ergojump platform and when the signal, "Ready, Go," is given, the examinee begins performing as many maximal vertical jumps as possible in 60 seconds. Throughout the test, the examinee must keep the hands on the hips and bend the knees approximately 90 degrees when in contact with the platform. While the Ergojump instrument keeps the flight time of all the jumps, the tester counts the number of vertical jumps performed during the 60 seconds.

Scoring.
The score is derived by plugging the total flight time, (Tf) and total number of jumps, (n) into the following formula.

$$W = [(g2)(Tf)(60)]/[(4)(n)(60 - Tf)]$$

Where W = the average mechanical power and g = the force of gravity.

Mechanical power per mass unit is then expressed in Watts per kilogram.

Norms.
Bosco et al. (1983, pp. 277-278) basketball players, volleyball players and school boys.

REVIEW

FRANK M. VERDUCCI, Ed.D.

Professor of Physical Education
San Francisco State University
San Francisco, CA 94132

Power is generally defined as the rate at which work is performed. Muscular power measuring instruments usually involve different muscle groups, lengths of time or repetitions, and appropriateness for different populations.

The examinees (16 to 30 years old) were three different groups: 12 regional basketball players from one team (validity), 12 players from an Italian volleyball student team (reliability), and 14 school boys who although physically active did not participate in one specific sport (validity). Limitations appear to be: (1) limited number of examinees, (2) random selection of examinees from a population, and (3) estimating reliability on a different sample from that of validity. A comprehensive validity study expects reliability and validity to be determined on an adequate number of randomly selected subjects from a population.

Concurrent validity was used to validate the test with the criterion scores being a modified Wingate Test for 60 seconds, a Margaria Test and a 30 or 60 meter run.

Table 9-1. Correlation Matrix for the Various Mechanical Parameters Calculated from the Different Tests (Basketball Players)

	1	2	3	4	5
1 Jumping (0-15 s)					
2 Jumping (0-60 s)	.91				
3 Wingate (0-15 s)	.87	.54			
4 Wingate (0-60 s)	.67	.80	.82		
5 Margaria	.12	.03	.18	.19	
6 60m Dash	.84	.58	.73	.50	.20

These tests can be categorized into three groups based on time: (1) less than 5 seconds, (2) 5 to 15 seconds, and (3) 60 seconds. Within each group the correlations tend to be high, while the relationships between different categories tend to be low. The Jumping (0-15), Wingate (0-15) and 60m Dash possess significant relationships of .87, .84, and .73 at the .01 level. A correlation of .80 exists between Jumping (0-60) and Wingate (0-60). The relationships between the different categories tend to be low and not significant. In both Jumping and Wingate tests, the 0-15 second period scores were extracted from the 60 second tests, which resulted in higher correlations between the 15 second and 60 second tests. The length of test time appears to be related to the validity coefficients for basketball players.

The school boy group was administered the Bosco Jumping Test (60 seconds), Wingate (60 seconds), Margaria, and 30m sprint. The only significant relationship occurred between the Wingate (60 seconds) and the 30m sprint, which does not coincide with the results obtained from the basketball players. The Jumping Test correlated .53 with Wingate, .23 with Margaria, and .56 with 30m sprint.

Although the relative reliability coefficients within similar timed tests for basketball players are significant, the Watts per kilograms of body weight are very different between the Jumping and Wingate tests. The mean power output (kgBW-1) calculated in the Jumping Test (0-15s = 24.7, 0-60s = 19.8) was much higher than that computed for the Wingate (0-15s = 8.8, 0-60s = 6.9) Test. This raises a serious validity question

when measuring W x kgBW-1 because the Jumping Test produces mean scores 2.8 times greater than the Wingate Test for the same examinees.

When comparing the mean W x kgBW-1 on the Jumping and Wingate tests, the school boys obtained higher values (22.2, 7.1) than the basketball players (19.8, 6.9). One would expect the basketball players, who jump numerous times in practice, to produce higher scores than the school boys.

Although the test-retest reliability coefficient was .95 for the 0-60 second time, the intraclass correlation coefficient would have been a more appropriate method of estimating reliability. Reliability may be reduced by the examinee not bending the knees to 90 degrees at the beginning of the jump, slight variation in landing and take off positions, a variance in horizontal and lateral displacement, a different knee angle when landing, and a measuring error in flight time.

A total, mechanical power score should be included in the Jumping Test. An individual who has a low mean power score may have a high total power score which should be considered when studying power.

SUMMARY

The subcomponents of the power construct have not been adequately defined and this makes it extremely difficult to evaluate the validity of a general power test.

Major Strengths:

1. Possesses a high degree of validity for estimating power on repeated maximum vertical jumps which continues for 15 or 60 seconds for basketball players.

2. Possesses a high degree of reliability for volleyball players.

3. Appears easy to administer.

Major Weaknesses:

1. Lacks validity as a general power test. (The reviewer suspects that there is no one general power factor.)

2. Limited number and selection of examinees.

3. Reliability not determined on the same subjects as validity.

4. Should add a total power score.

5. Requires special equipment.

6. No adequate norms or standards presented.

7. The large difference in mean power scores between tests.

The Bosco Power Jump Test appears to possess a high degree of logical, or content, validity for estimating power on repeated maximum vertical jumps which continue for 15 or 60 seconds for basketball players. As a general power test, it lacks validity as demonstrated in this study.

NOTE: The reviewer did not have access to an Ergojump instrument during the assessment of this test. When analyzing the reviewer's comments, this must be considered a major limitation of the review.

JUMP WITH WEIGHTS TEST

Reference.

Viitasalo, J. T. (1988). Evaluation of explosive strength for young and adult athletes. *Research quarterly for Exercise and Sport,* 59(1):9-13.

Additional Sources.

None.

Purpose.

To measure the explosive strength of an examinee's legs.

Objectivity.

Not reported.

Reliability.

Examinees below 12 years showed a low reliability on the jump test. As the examinees became older the test became more reliable.

Validity.

r = .66 and r = .69 between the jumping test and the Sargent jump and standing broad jump, respectively.

Age and Sex.

Male athletes, age 10 - 16.

Equipment.

Barbell weights, digital timer, and a platform.

Space Requirements and Design.

A clear, level area approximately 3m (10') square with the platform in the center.

Directions.

The examinee assumes standing position on the platform with barbell weights placed on the shoulders. On command, the examinee jumps as high as possible in sets of three to five trials. The digital timer starts when the examinee's feet leave the platform and stops when the feet return to the platform. The trials were administered at intervals of 5 to 10 seconds. Each set required a different weight with a one to two minute recovery between sets. Examinees who are smaller, lighter, and younger should use barbell loads of 0, 5, 10 and 15 Kg. Loads of 0, 10, 20 and 40 Kg are used for examinees who are older and taller.

Scoring.

The score was the height the body's center of gravity (HCG) was raised. The following equation is used to determine the HCG:

$$HCG = [t^2 \times g]/8$$

Where $g = 9.81 m/s^2$ and t = the flight time

Norms.

None.

REVIEW

THOMAS M. ADAMS, II, Ed.D.

Professor of Physical Education
Arkansas State University
State University, AR 72467

Viitasalo (1988) offers a jumping test designed to measure dynamic, or explosive, leg strength in young male athletes. The test is specifically designed to control non-neuromuscular force producing factors (i.e., the correct timing of the arm swings) that influence the results of traditional jump tests such as the Standing Long Jump and the Vertical Jump.

While the test is designed for young males ages 10 to 16, statistical analysis indicated the test was more reliable on examinees over the age of 12. These findings probably reflect age related development of the neuromuscular characteristics related to force production in prepubescent youth.

The reliability of the Jump With Weights Test tended to show progressively lower values as the barbell loads increased. This would suggest greater variability in force production by the neuromuscular system when explosive strength is generated against increasing loads.

Statistically significant relationships were found when the estimated increase in height of the body's center of gravity for zero load jumps was compared with the more traditional field tests (e.g., Sargent's Jump and the Standing Long Jump).

Statistically significant differences in the reliability of the measurements were found with respect to sport. This would suggest some sports are more conducive to developing the necessary coordination and skill that allow for more reliable vertical jumps. If this is actually the case, a broad application of this test over a variety of sports in which the reliability of the test has not been determined may not be advised.

From a practical standpoint, the test requires a minimal amount of space and could easily be safely administered in 15 minutes or less. The time requirement, however, may limit its use in environments where time restrictions and the number of examinees are factors that influence test selection. Similarly, the equipment required by this test would be more readily available in professional settings and university laboratories. The electronic digital timer and contact mat would not be standard pieces of equipment in most elementary and secondary schools.

One individual is required to administer the test. No influencing effect by the tester on the examinee is expected.

The Jump With Weights Test requires three to five trials at four different weights. Given the nature of the test and the potential for leg fatigue, this requirement is considered reasonable and adequate. The test indicates that "smaller, lighter and younger children" should receive barbell loads of 0, 5, 10, and 15 kg, whereas "older, taller children, and adults" should receive loads of 0, 10, 20, and 40 kg. These generalities require individual tester judgement and expertise. More specific criteria regarding weight selection seem warranted.

Scoring is determined by measuring the average flight time of the best two trials. The height the body's center of gravity is raised is estimated by fitting the determined flight time of the jump into an equation. Normative information specific by age, sex and sport is not available.

The nature of the test procedures and the exactness of the equipment should allow for consistent measurements. However, no direct attempt to determine the test's objectivity was made.

SUMMARY

Major Strengths:

1. The procedures of the test minimize the effects of uncontrollable factors associated with traditional jumping field tests (i.e., impulse from the movement of the arms).

2. The test may be considered reliable for young males, age 12 and older.

3. The test showed significantly high correlations with traditional jumping field tests.

Major Weaknesses:

1. The reliability of the test was positively influenced by age.

2. The inter event reliability would suggest that the test may not be appropriate for all sports.

3. No norms were reported.

4. The test requires some judgement on the part of the tester when selecting barbell weights for the examinees.

5. No attempt to determine the reliability of the test on female athletes was made.

The Jump With Weights explosive strength test can be considered an acceptable test that offers reliable results when applied to males 12 years of age and older. The significant interevent differences would suggest, however, precaution be used before this test is widely applied across differing sports.

LEWIS NOMOGRAM TEST

Reference.

Fox, E. L., & Mathews, D. K. (1981). *The physiological basis of physical education and athletics*. Philadelphia: W. B. Saunders, pp 619-620.

Additional Sources.

Kirkendall et al. (1980, pp. 240-242); Kirkendall et al. (1987, pp. 118-119).

Purpose.

To measure an examinee's ability to exert power with the legs.

Objectivity.

Not reported.

Reliability.

Not reported.

Validity.

Not reported.

Age and Sex.

Not reported, but suitable for females and males, age 8 - adult.

Equipment.

A body weight scale, a yardstick, several pieces of chalk, and the Lewis Nomogram.

Space Requirements and Design.

A clear, level jumping area approximately 2m (6') square next to a smooth wall at least 3.96m (13') high.

Directions.

Body weight is determined in the usual manner to the nearest kilogram (pound) and jumping ability according to the directions written for the vertical jump test.

Scoring.

After the examinee's body weight and vertical jump distance have been determined, a straight edge is laid across the Lewis Nomogram (see Fox & Mathews, 1981, p. 620) connecting the weight and distance scores. The examinee's power output score is then read from the center column expressed in kilogram meters per second (kg-m/sec) or in foot-pounds per second (ft-lb/sec).

Norms.

Not reported.

REVIEW

NOLAN A. THAXTON, D.P.E.

Professor of Physical Education
Medgar Evers College
City University of New York
Brooklyn, NY 11225

The Lewis Nomogram is designed to be used with the Sargent Jump Test. It purports to add the "speed" variable to the body weight and vertical distance jumped aspects of power. Therefore, face validity for this test of power is achieved.

The Lewis Nomogram has possibilities for use from both a practical standpoint and for research purposes. Although the nomogram is purported to add the time element in both metric (kilogram meters per second) and English units (foot pounds per second) to the Vertical Jump Test, no correlation measures are presented for objectivity, reliability or validity. Further, no norms are presented.

The Lewis Nomogram is a safe test that has no dangerous aspects to it. The equipment and space requirements are practical and should be available to most testing situations. The scoring is also easy to understand since it is so straightforward. However, several trials should be allowed. The test would not require an excessive amount of time to administer.

The test is suitable as a drill to promote both learning and conditioning. The test can easily be scored by the examinee and, thus, may be used for self evaluation.

Since no norms are provided, it is questionable whether the test should be used for research purposes, except to be pilot tested to determine its objectivity, reliability and validity. Norms should also be established for the test. A validated test of power, such as the Margaria-Kalamen Anaerobic Power Test, should be used to establish the validity of the Lewis Nomogram Test. Acceptable measurement strategies should be used to establish reliability and objectivity coefficients.

SUMMARY

Major Strengths:

1. It is easy to administer.

2. The test can accomodate large groups of examinees.

3. The equipment needed is relatively inexpensive and readily accessible for testing purposes.

Major Weaknesses:

1. There are no measures of validity, reliability, and objectivity.

2. No norms are available for the test.

The lack of an acceptable validity coefficient is a critical weakness of the Lewis Nomogram. It is essential for the user of this test to establish the fact that it correlates highly with a power test which has already been validated. The test should not be used if such a coefficient of validity cannot be generated.

The Lewis Nomogram Test is an acceptable test with the qualifications and recommendations that are indicated in this review.

SPEED HOP TEST

Reference.
Myers, B. (1986). Testing for field and multi events athletes. *Athletic Journal,* 66:10-12, May.

Additional Sources.
None.

Purpose.
To measure an examinee's leg power, acceleration and coordination.

Objectivity.
Not reported.

Reliability.
Not reported.

Validity.
Not reported.

Age and Sex.
College track and field athletes.

Equipment.
A stopwatch, tape measure, and marking tape or chalk.

Space Requirements and Design.
A clear, level area approximately 2m x 30m (6' x 100') with a starting line and a finish line marked 25m (82') apart.

Directions.
The examinee assumes an upright position behind the starting line. A rocking step is allowed at the start. On command, "Ready, Go," the examinee hops on one leg as fast as possible past the finish line.

The time begins when the examinee's hop foot, usually the dominant leg, comes off the ground behind the starting line. The watch is stopped when the examinee's torso crosses the finish line.

Scoring.
The score is the number of seconds it takes to hop the specified distance.

Norms.
Myers (1986, p. 11) point system for various scores.

REVIEW

DON HARDIN, Ph.D.
Professor
Kinesiology and Sport Studies
University of Texas at El Paso
El Paso, TX 79968

This is a test designed to measure the status of an examinee's leg power prior to, and during, a season of track and field performance. Its initial purpose was to determine what state of training an athlete has achieved, and to see if the athlete's training program is improving leg power. The test was developed primarily for athletes in the field events and is part of a battery of 10 tests used to assess and motivate these athletes during a competitive season and to serve as a "change of pace" in the training regimen.

The validity of the test should be good if procedures are followed carefully and if used with an athlete population.

The norms, however, are for high quality university level athletes and are scored on a decathlon point scale. The times could be converted to a percentile scale, or local norms could be developed to help physical education teachers or coaches at lower competition levels. Probably, some practice attempts would improve performance as balance and coordination are factors in the test as well as the power being measured.

The test does measure leg power well, and performance norms should be established if the test is to be used in settings other than the one which it was designed.

SUMMARY
Major Strengths:

1. Valid test to measure leg power.

2. Administration time is short.

3. Little equipment needed for test.

Major Weaknesses:

1. Norms currently on decathlon scale with female and male athletes same scale.

2. Some practice needed before initial use of test.

This is an excellent test for use in the setting for which it was developed, and its best use would be in a test battery.

The test by itself could be used well in measuring leg power in research studies.

STANDING LONG (BROAD) JUMP TEST

Reference.

AAHPER. *Youth fitness test manual* (1975). Washington, DC: American Alliance for Health, Physical Education and Recreation, pp 20, 29, 37, 46, 51, 56.

Additional Sources.

Barrow et al. (1989, pp. 117-118); Baumgartner & Jackson (1982, pp. 221-222); Baumgartner & Jackson (1987, pp. 282-283); Baumgartner & Jackson (1991, pp. 264-265); Bosco & Gustafson (1983, pp. 91-92);

Clarke & Clarke (1987, pp. 155, 164, 211-213); Hastad & Lacy (1989, pp. 279, 281-282, 293-294, 296-298); Jensen & Hirst (1980, p. 140); Johnson & Nelson (1986, p. 212); Kirkendall et al. (1980, pp. 272, 323-325);

Kirkendall et al. (1987, pp. 153, 397); Miller (1988, pp. 184-185); Mood (1980, p. 237); Safrit (1981, p. 242); Safrit (1986, pp. 279-281, 348-349, 351, 440-441); Safrit (1990, pp. 241-242, 411-414); Verducci (1980, pp. 246-247, 285, 287).

Purpose.

To measure the ability of an examinee to exert power with the legs.

Objectivity.

Not reported, but r = .96 by Clayton (1969) cited in Johnson and Nelson (1986, p. 212).

Reliability.

Not reported, but r's = .88 - .99 reported in a number of studies.

Validity.

Not reported, but r = .61 with a pure power test (Johnson & Nelson, 1986, p. 212).

Age and Sex.

Suitable for females and males, age 6 - college.

Equipment.

Marking tape and a tape measure.

Space Requirements and Design.

A clear, level non slip area approximately 2m x 4m (6' x 12') with a "scratch" line marked .30m (1') in from one end of the 4m (12') length. The tape measure is positioned perpendicular to the "scratch" line with the zero mark above the inside edge of the line.

Directions.

The examinee assumes a standing position with the toes just behind, and the feet perpendicular to, the "scratch" line. The feet are positioned about shoulder width apart. The examinee crouches slightly, swings the arms forward and backward as many times as desired, and then jumps forward and upward. The landing is made on both feet. During the jumping process, the examinee cannot shuffle the feet along the surface. The take off must be made from both feet simultaneously. Three trials are given. If the examinee shuffles the feet or leaves from one foot or steps on or over the "scratch" line, the trial is recorded as a foul. If the examinee fouls all three trials, additional trials are given until one legal jump is made.

Scoring.

The score is the perpendicular distance, measured from the inside edge of the "scratch" line to the closest body part (usually the back heel) contacting the surface, the examinee jumps. The best distance of the three trials is measured to the nearest centimeter/inch.

Norms.

Alabama (1988, pp. 47-48) boys and girls; American Alliance (1975, pp. 29, 37, 46, 51, 56, 59-60) boys, girls, men and women; American Alliance (1990, p. 49) boys and girls; Barrow et al. (1989, p. 122) boys and girls;

Baumgartner & Jackson (1982, p. 222) boys and girls; Baumgartner & Jackson (1987, pp. 283, 286) boys and girls; Baumgartner & Jackson (1991, p. 262) boys and girls; Canadian Association (1980, pp. 37-60) boys and girls;

Chrysler/AAU (1990, p. 6) boys and girls; Corbin & Lindsey (1983, p. 126) men and women; Governor's Commission (no date) boys and girls; Harrison & Bradbeer (1982, pp. 24-25) boy and girl athletes; Hastad & Lacy (1989, pp. 277, 280, 289, 296-297) boys, girls, and women;

Hawaii (1989, pp. 19-20) boys and girls; Johnson & Nelson (1986, pp. 363-364, 370-371, 376-377, 380, 382) boys, girls, men and women; Kirkendall et al. (1980, pp. 278-279, 286-287, 328-330, 333) boys and girls; Kirkendall et al. (1987, pp. 158-159, 397-399) boys, girls, and special populations;

Metheny et al. (1945, p. 309) girls; Miller (1988, p. 184) boys and girls; Mood (1980, pp. 238-239) boys and men; National Marine (no date, p. 10) boys and girls; O'Connor & Cureton (1945, p. 314) girls; President's Council (1987, pp. 2-6) USSR boys and girls;

President's Council (1988, p. 5) boys and girls; Pyke (1986, p. 10) boys and girls; Safrit (1986, pp. 281, 352-353, 356-357) boys, girls, men and women; Safrit (1990, pp. 414, 524-525) boys and girls; Simons et al. (1990, p. 99) girls; Vermont (1982, pp. 14-15) boys and girls.

REVIEW

LEIGH F. KIEFFER, Ph.D.

Professor
Physical Therapy and Exercise Science
S.U.N.Y. at Buffalo
Buffalo, NY 14214

It is important to recognize that tests of this nature (field based evaluations) do not always measure a single factor, such as in this particular instance, power of the legs. Primarily, this is because the factor in question is not a unidimensional entity, but composed of many features that the examinee must possess at the time of testing that are ultimately reflected in the score. For example, developmental maturation, coordination, and amount of practice are factors reflected in the test score, regardless of the number of trials. Undoubtedly, however, there is a general assumption made about these factors when evaluating leg power in this manner.

The test appears to be objective as well as reliable. However, the question of validity might be a concern. This would depend upon how the results were being used. It is conceivable that due to the variability introduced by the factors mentioned above, as well as others, the common variance this test item shares with at least one other test item ($r = .61$ with a pure power test) is low. Therefore, the usefulness of this test from a standpoint of validity is questionable.

The environmental set up and protocol do not appear to detract from objective data gathering. Likewise, it appears that the test can be efficiently administered and scored with a minimum of practice by the testers. Using the item for self testing would be possible under certain circumstances which would have to be built into the protocol beforehand (e.g., having a way to mark the heel when it struck the ground). The only advantage to using this "test" as a drill to promote learning and/or conditioning would be task specific to the goal of improving the skill of the standing long jump.

There are normative data available on the standing long jump other than those identified (e.g., the Special Fitness Test Manual for Mildly Mentally Retarded, the Motor Fitness Test for Moderately Mentally Retarded, and the Adapted AAHPERD Youth Fitness Test for Blind and Partially Sighted Students). Data are available for both age and sex.

SUMMARY

Major Strengths:

1. Easily administered and scored.

2. Objective and reliable based upon investigations using the test.

3. May yield an overall performance of leg power "ability."

4. May be acceptable for specific teaching situations.

Major Weakness:

1. Validity of the instrument.

Acceptable test - in general, the test is adequate for teaching (specific to the task of the standing long jump) and research purposes under certain circumstances. It should be kept in mind that, due to the variables which may potentially influence the results of performance, caution should be taken to explain the circumstances under which the test item is used thoroughly, particularly in research. An operational definition incorporating the use and the implication of scores would be important.

VERTICAL JUMP TEST

References.

Sargent, D. A. (1921). The physical test of a man. *American Physical Education Review,* 26:188, April.

Safrit, M. J. (1990). *Introduction to measurement in physical education and exercise science.* St. Louis: Times Mirror/Mosby: pp 494-495.

Additional Sources.

Baumgartner & Jackson (1982, pp. 220-221); Baumgartner & Jackson (1987, p. 206); Baumgartner & Jackson (1991, p. 246); Bosco & Gustafson 1983, pp. 90-91); Clarke & Clarke (1987, pp. 210-211);

Jensen & Hirst (1980, p. 139); Johnson & Nelson (1986, p. 210); Kirkendall et al. (1980, pp. 240-241); Kirkendall et al. (1987, p. 118); Miller (1988, p. 184); Safrit (1986, pp. 320, 325-326); Verducci (1980, pp. 247-248).

Purpose.

To measure the ability of an examinee to exert power with the legs in jumping vertically.

Objectivity.

r = .90 (Safrit, 1990, p. 495).

Reliability.

r = .93 (Safrit, 1990, p. 495).

Validity.

r = .78 with sum of four power type events in track and field (Safrit, 1990, p. 495).

Age and Sex.

Suitable for females and males, age 6 - college.

Equipment.

A measuring board marked in half-inches and several pieces of chalk.

Space Requirements and Design.

A clear, level jumping area approximately 2m (6') square next to a smooth wall (at least 3.96m or 13' high). The measuring board should be attached vertically to the wall.

Directions.

The examinee stands facing the wall with her/his nose and toes touching the wall. The feet are positioned perpendicular to the wall and touching each other. The examinee then takes a piece of chalk and holds it in the dominant hand so that 2.54cm (1") of its length is exposed. Without moving the feet, the examinee reaches overhead as far as possible and strikes the measuring board with the chalk. The examinee then assumes a new standing position with the feet about shoulder width apart and the side of the body with the chalk in the hand nearest the wall. The examinee crouches slightly, swings the arms forward and backward as many times as desired, and jumps as high as possible striking the measuring board at the peak of the jump. The examinee cannot shuffle the feet across the surface during the take off. If the examinee moves the feet prior to take off, it is counted as a trial, but no score is recorded. Three trials are given.

Scoring.

The score is the perpendicular distance, measured to the nearest half-inch, from the standing reach chalk mark to the jump reach chalk mark. The score is the best distance jumped during the three trials.

Norms.

American Alliance (1966, p. 44) boys and girls; Baumgartner & Jackson (1982, pp. 176, 221) boys and girls, high school and college volleyball players; Baumgartner & Jackson (1987, pp. 180, 207) boys and girls, high school and college volleyball players;

Baumgartner & Jackson (1991, pp. 220, 247) boys and girls, high school and college volleyball players; Beunen et al. (1988, pp. 32, 82, 92) boys; Evans (1973, p. 386) rugby players; Getchell (1983, p. 66) men and women;

Harrison & Bradbeer (1982, pp. 24-25) boy and girl athletes; Hawaii (1989, pp. 19-20) boys and girls; Johnson & Nelson (1986, pp. 211, 376-377) boys, girls, men and women; Miller (1988, p. 184) boys and girls;

Ostyn et al. (1980, pp. 100-101, 127-140) boys; Safrit (1986, p. 326) boys, girls, men and women; Safrit (1990, p. 495) boys, girls, men and women;

Scott & French (1959, pp. 374-375) boys and girls; Simons et al. (1990, p. 100) girls; Texas (no date and no page numbers) boys and girls.

NOTE (1): The standing height is sometimes measured by reaching with both hands to the same maximum height.

NOTE (2): Another variation of the vertical jump involves placement of the nonpreferred hand behind the examinee's back while the preferred hand is held vertically with the arm straight and resting against the side of the head throughout the jumping movement (Clarke & Clarke, 1987, p. 211).

NOTE (3): The vertical jump is also known as the Chalk Jump, Jump and Reach, and the Sargent Jump.

REVIEW

RICHARD MUNROE, Ed.D.

Associate Professor
Exercise and Sport Sciences
University of Arizona
Tucson, AZ 85721

The Vertical Jump has long been accepted (and supported statistically, Sargent 1920's, McCloy 1930's, Fleishman 1960's) as a valid measure of leg power. More recent work by Perrine at UCLA in the development of CYBEX and VERTEC supports the validity of the Vertical Jump as a measure of power. The reliability and objectivity (as well as validity) coefficients reported by Safrit (1990) should be supported by original references. Reliability seems high in view of the problems in achieving an accurate mark at the peak height with the older "chalk" techniques. Development of the VERTEC eliminated this problem and provides extremely consistent measures, as well as making the Vertical Jump a self administering test. Although helpful, another individual is not necessary for the administration of this test when VERTEC is employed.

The only space requirement for this test is a sufficient clear height to allow the maximum jump for the group being tested; 12 feet is usually adequate. The "chalk" test requires literally no equipment but a measuring board and chalk. However, the VERTEC apparatus greatly improves the validity, reliability and practicability of the test, and is reasonable in cost. Three trials are adequate, but should be preceded by appropriate warm up. Three practice trials prior to three measured trials is an appropriate procedure. A great advantage of the Vertical Jump Test is its value as a training system. The VERTEC enhances this capability by providing a "motivating" target (see Scates, A., 1979, "Jumping training at UCLA," *Scholastic Coach,* May/June, p. 24).

This test is suitable for any individual able to execute a standing vertical jump. However, younger children and/or those not well coordinated are extremely difficult to test due to the difficulty of "marking" at the precise peak of the jump. The VERTEC eliminates this problem. The test is highly discriminatory, with scores accurate to one-half inch over a range in excess of three feet. This precision is adequate for research purposes. In addition to those listed, norms are available with the Oregon Motor Fitness Tests, 1962, State Department of Education, Salem, Oregon.

SUMMARY

Major Strength:

1. Its simplicity and accuracy (when administered properly) in measuring perhaps the most important single factor in athletic performance.

Major Weakness:

1. The lack of standardization in test administration; specifically, improper jumping techniques such as run in or crow hop, inaccurate standing reach measurement and errors in securing maximum reach, especially with finger marking techniques.

Overall, this is an excellent test when administered under controlled conditions with reach scores measured by an objective device, not the examinee's own marking. As a wall test with finger marking, the test may be acceptable for non research purposes with the following qualifications:

1. Strict control of jumping action.
2. Maximum standing reach, not just arm above head.

3. Accurate means of recording jump height; no finger held chalk, wet finger on recording surface may be best.

VERTICAL POWER JUMP (WORK) TEST

References.

Glencross, D. J. (1960). The measurement of muscular power; A test of leg power and a modification for general use. Microcarded doctoral dissertation, University of Western Australia).

Johnson, B. L., & Nelson, Jack K. (1986). *Practical measurements for evaluation in physical education.* Edina, MN: Burgess, pp 218-220.

Additional Sources.

Baumgartner & Jackson (1982, p. 206); Bosco & Gustafson (1983, pp. 92-93).

Purpose.

To measure (in terms of work produced) the ability of an examinee to exert power with the legs by jumping vertically.

Objectivity.

r = .99 by Long (1972) cited in Johnson and Nelson (1986, p. 218).

Reliability.

r = .98 (Johnson & Nelson 1986, p. 218).

Validity.

r = .99 with the vertical jump expressed in horse power (Johnson & Nelson 1986, p. 218).

Age and Sex.

Suitable for females and males, age 10 - college.

Equipment.

A body weight scale, chalk dust, a stool or ladder, a hand held calculator, and a jump board approximately .30m x 1.52m (1' x 5') painted black and marked off with horizontal lines one centimeter or .5" apart.

Space Requirements and Design.

A clear, level area approximately 2m (6') square next to a smooth wall (at least 3.96m or 13'high). The jump board should be attached vertically to a wall so that the lower edge is slightly above the standing height of the shortest examinee to be tested.

Directions.

The shoeless examinee's body weight is determined and recorded in pounds. The shoeless examinee stands with the non preferred side nearest the wall and the jump board. The hand nearest the wall is raised overhead perpendicular to the floor while the other hand is used to grasp the waist band in the back of the examinee's trunks. The raised hand is turned outward so that the hand is flat against the jump board. Reach height is taken at the end of the middle finger as the examinee reaches upward as far as possible while standing on the toes. After placing chalk dust on the middle finger, the examinee extends the non preferred arm overhead and grasps the back waist band of the trunks with the other hand. The examinee then crouches to a full squat (buttocks resting on the heels), with the head and trunk held erect and the shoulders square, pauses, and jumps as high as possible (Figure 9-1). The examinee touches the jump board with the non preferred hand at the peak of the jump. The difference between the maximum reach height and the maximum reach on the jump is the Distance Jumped measured in inches. The best Distance Jumped of three trials is recorded. Prior to the final trial, the tester should say, "This is your last jump. Try to beat your last two jumps."

The examinee: (1) cannot shuffle the feet across the floor during the take off, (2) must maintain balance throughout the jump, (3) must keep the head and trunk erect throughout the jump. If the examinee commits any of these faults the trial is recorded as illegal. Adequate practice of the jumping technique will enhance the reliability and validity of the test.

Scoring.

The score is derived by placing the greatest Distance Jumped into the following equation:

Power (Ft.lbs.) = Distance Jumped (inches) x Body Weight (pounds)/12

Norms.

Baumgartner & Jackson (1982, p. 207) boys; Johnson & Nelson (1986, p. 220) girls, men and women.

NOTE: All measurements may be expressed in metric units if preferred.

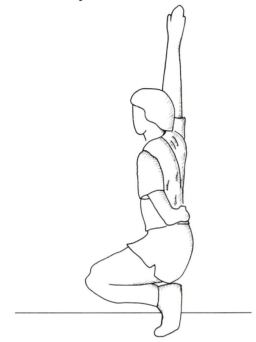

Figure 9-1. Initial position for the Vertical Power Jump.

REVIEW

DOYICE J. COTTEN, Ed.D.
Professor of Physical Education
Georgia SouthernUniversity
Statesboro, GA 30460

The Vertical Power Jump (Work) [VPJ(W)] test is a valid, practical test for measuring leg power. It is a modification of the original Vertical Power Jump (VPJ) test, also devised by Glencross. The VPJ test is an excellent laboratory test which includes all of the components of power (Force x Distance/Time) and yields a score in horsepower.

The VPJ(W) requires the use of the formula, Force x Distance/12, for computation of the power score. This formula includes two of the three elements of power (Force and Distance) and yields a power score in foot pounds. In spite of the fact that the element of time is not directly measured, the validity of the VPJ(W) test when compared to the VPJ test is .989.

Any power test involving jumping must control four factors in order to be valid. These factors are (1) body weight, (2) skill or coordination, (3) height, and (4) stretching or flexibility. The VPJ(W) test controls all four.

First, body weight is multiplied times the distance jumped, so the heavy examinee is not penalized by weight. The 200 pound examinee will receive a higher power score than the 150 pound examinee when each jumps the same distance.

Second, the test eliminates the skill factor by having all examinees jump from a full squat. When directions are followed the examinee goes to a full squat (with buttocks resting on the heels), pauses, and explodes from that stationary position. This simple variation eliminates the advantage held by the examinee who knows how to jump.

Third, the test greatly reduces the advantage of height by measuring the distance between the maximum reach and the maximum jump.

Finally, the test prohibits twisting and stretching during the jump by requiring that the shoulders remain square. This eliminates the advantage held by the flexible examinee.

Since these extraneous factors are eliminated, what factors determine the score? The only remaining factor seems to be the explosive force or power exerted by the legs of the examinee.

Research has yielded validity, reliability, and objectivity coefficients in the high .90's. Lower reliability and objectivity figures should not occur if the tester conscientiously follows test directions.

The tester needs a tall stool or stepladder for administering the test so he/she can be at eye level to the top of the jump. A jump board on the wall is helpful, however tape will do almost as well. A hand held calculator is useful in computing the scores. The test requires little space and can be administered easily and quickly by one tester. Weighing the examinees, testing them, and computing their scores should require less than a minute per examinee.

The VPJ(W) is an objective test that can also be used for both conditioning drills and for self evaluation. It is precise enough for use in research and can be used for ages six and above.

SUMMARY

Major Strengths:

1. The test gives a valid, reliable, and objective measure of leg power.

2. The test can be administered easily and quickly.

Major Weakness:

1. The tester or examinee must make a simple calculation to obtain the score.

The VPJ(W) is an excellent test that is completely acceptable for research and teaching. This is, by far, the best practical measure of leg power available to the teacher. The validity of power scores of most other commonly used power tests is questionable due to the presence of other factors.

POWER TESTS OF THE LEGS/LOWER BODY
RUNNING TESTS

THE PHOSPHATE RECOVERY TEST

Reference.
Dawson, B. et al. (1984). New fitness test for team and individual sports. *Sports Coach*, 8(2):42-44.

Additional Sources.
None.

Purpose.
To measure the ability of an examinee to repeat high intensity, short duration sprints with brief recovery periods similar in nature to what is commonly demanded in a given sport.

Objectivity.
Not reported.

Reliability.
Not reported.

Validity.
Not reported.

Age and Sex.
Not reported.

Equipment.
Fifteen plastic cones, stopwatch, and whistle.

Space Requirements and Design.
A clear, level area approximately 10m (30') wide and 80m (261') long. A starting line should be marked at one end of the 80m length. Another line should be drawn across the width of the field at the 40 meter mark. Beginning at the 40 meter mark, 10 cones are arranged along a sideline with two meters between centers. The cones are numbered 1 to 10 with the numbers all facing the starting line. Four additional cones, preferably of a different size or color, are arranged on the same straight line as the other 10 cones between the 40 meter mark and the starting line. The cones are spaced, four meters apart. These four cones are used to improve the accuracy of the scoring.

Directions.
The examinee takes a position at the starting line, prepared to complete 20 sprints of 7 seconds each with a 23 second recovery time between each sprint. On command, "Ready, Go," the examinee sprints down the field next to the line of cones and stops when the whistle is blown after seven seconds. The tester allows the clock to run while the examinee returns to the starting line. When the stopwatch reaches 25 seconds, the tester warns the examinee that the next sprint is about to begin. At the 30 second mark, the whistle is blown and the examinee begins the next sprint. The examinee continues this procedure until 20 sprints have been completed. The time of the sprint (7 seconds), the recovery period (23 seconds) and the number of sprints (20) should be modified to meet the requirements of the sport of interest. The seven second sprint with 20 repetitions is based on a game analysis of Australian football.

Scoring.
The score is the total number of cones passed during the 20, seven second sprints.

Norms.
Not reported.

REVIEW

JESSE DEMELLO, Ed.D.
Associate Professor
Health and Physical Education
Louisiana State University in
Shreveport
Shreveport, LA 71115

The constructors of this test are correct that there is a tremendous need for a test(s) that measures phosphate energy capacity which is also task specific and relevant. This test appears to have face validity in as much as it does stress the phosphagen energy supplies and it is match specific to Australian football skills and fitness.

There is no available data on the reliability and objectivity of this test, however, the methods by which the examinees are scored appear to be fairly objective in nature.

From a practical stand point, there are no major problems with facilities, if there is a field available. Equipment wise the requirements are reasonable, with perhaps the exception of the unusually high number of plastic cones. However, that could possibly be remedied by painting lines on the field and numbering them. From the tester's standpoint, it is possible to give the test with one stopwatch. However, it requires an unusual amount of concentration. The use of two stopwatches is recommended.

The time (approximately 10 minutes) required to administer the test to each examinee is unreasonable. This means that it would take approximately 500 to 800 minutes to administer the test once, to an average size football squad, or 180 to 250 minutes to administer the test to a typical soccer team. However, it might be possible to reduce the number of repeats by 10 and still maintain validity.

The test could be incorporated into a drill to promote anaerobic conditioning. It is objective and could be used for self evaluation purposes. The test is fairly safe to administer. Due to the maximal intensity running, caution should be taken in adequately warming up to minimize muscle pull type injuries.

From the stand point of appropriateness, the test could be administered to females and males who are older than 12 and younger than 35 and have been found to be free of any disease or condition which may be counter indicative to safe participation. The test does not have suitable precision for research purposes, at least not until further work is done to establish its validity and reliability.

As to this test's ability to discriminate, additional data is necessary before one can comment on that aspect of the test. A possible problem in that regard lies with the procedural step which allows an examinee to rest if and when he/she cannot continue. This not only affects the ratio of exercise to rest (affecting the validity), but also appears to help the examinee in the next sprint, thus affecting the results of the test.

SUMMARY

Major Strengths:

1. The measurement of match specific anaerobic phosphagen capacity.

2. It does not require much equipment, if one does not use cones.

Major Weaknesses:

1. The fact that it takes at least 10 minutes to test one examinee.

2. The procedural step which allows an examinee to take a longer recovery period.

Overall, this test is acceptable for teaching and coaching, and it has the potential to become an excellent test once it is subjected to the appropriate statistical treatment in establishing reliability, validity, and objectivity and some minor procedural changes are made. The test constructors are to be commended for an excellent idea and for addressing a measurement aspect of sport fitness that has long been neglected.

REPEATED 220 YARD SPRINT TEST

Reference.
Semenick, D. (1984). Anaerobic testing - Practical applications. *National Strength and Conditioning Association Journal*, 6(5):45, 72-73.

Additional Sources.
None.

Purpose.
To measure the anaerobic capacity of an examinee through repeated running of the 200 meter (220 yard) sprint test.

Objectivity.
Not reported.

Reliability.
Not reported.

Validity.
Not reported.

Age and Sex.
Female and male college athletes.

Equipment.
Two stopwatches and a tape measure.

Space Requirements and Design.
A 400 meter (440 yard) track or a clear, level surface measuring 200 meters (220 yards) in length.

Directions.
The examinee assumes a standing position at the starting line. On command, "Ready, Go," the examinee sprints 200 meters at maximum speed. Upon completion of the sprint, the examinee is given a rest which is three times as long as it took to run the distance. At the end of the rest, the examinee once again sprints the distance followed by a rest three times as long as the running time. These procedures are repeated until the examinee completes 12, 200 meter (220 yard) sprints.

Scoring.
The score is the average time required to run the 12 sprints.

Norms.
Semenick (1984, p. 73) female and male basketball players.

REVIEW

BARBARA E. AINSWORTH, Ph.D.
Assistant Professor
Physical Education, Exercise and
Sport Science
University of North Carolina
Chapel Hill, NC 27599-8700

This field test is designed to stress the glycolytic lactic acid energy system as a measure of anaerobic work capacity. For a field test to be an accurate estimate of physical work capacity, it should be valid, reliable, and objective. To determine the validity of the Repeated 220 Yard Sprint Test, results should be compared with standard laboratory tests of anaerobic capacity. Standard tests should include the (1) calculation of work, or power output, during 30 to 90 seconds of all out exercise against a fixed resistance on an ergometer (e.g., Wingate Anaerobic Test), and (2) measurement of the blood lactate level following the above type of exercise. There is no indication in the description of the Repeated 220 Yard Sprint Test that it has been validated using standard laboratory tests as the criterion measure, or with other performance outcomes (i.e., basketball player's court performance). Therefore, this test should be validated before it is used to measure or predict anaerobic work capacity.

A test is considered reliable when results are consistent between repeated administrations given by the same tester and objective when multiple testers are used. To determine the reliability and objectivity, examinees should repeat the test two or more times under identical conditions several days apart. There is no indication this has been done for the Sprint Test since reliability and objectivity coefficients are not reported. Therefore, it is not known if this test is a reliable and objective measure of anaerobic capacity.

There are other possible threats to the test's validity. Examinee motivation and maturation, temperature and wind conditions, test familiarity, and possible competition between examinees tested at the same time could affect the results on repeated administrations of the tests. These threats to the test's validity should be examined.

The field test is easy to conduct and requires the use of a flat, oval 200 yard track. The personnel and equipment requirements are simple. However, the testers should be alert, familiar with the use of a stopwatch, and know the testing protocol well. The test is objectively scored (i.e., recording the timed runs in seconds) and easy to administer. It should take about 24 minutes to complete the running and recovery bouts (approximately two minutes per bout); however, additional time should be allotted for appropriate warm up and cool down sessions.

The Repeated 220 Yard Sprint Test seems better suited as a conditioning drill than a test of anaerobic capacity. Three or four thirty second, all out running bouts will probably stress the lactic acid anaerobic energy system sufficiently to measure anaerobic capacity. It appears that the test was developed for collegiate basketball players, and it is unknown if it has been used among athletes in other sports or in other age groups. The test may promote muscle soreness, and possibly injury, due to the repeated nature of the high intensity, short duration, all out running sprints. For this reason, the test seems more appropriate for mature, well conditioned athletes.

Finally, the utility of the Repeated 220 Yard Sprint Test as a test of anaerobic work capacity is questionable. The test lacks a well defined, cumulative scoring method that can be used to quantify and compare the results with standard tests of anaerobic capacity. Further, performance norms are not indicated. This limits its use for comparison of anaerobic capacity against others of a similar age and gender.

SUMMARY

Major Strengths:

1. The test is simple and may be used in most school settings. It does not require knowledge of laboratory testing methods or the use of expensive equipment.

2. It involves only running and does not require one to learn complex motor skills.

Major Weaknesses:

1. The test has not been validated or subjected to reliability and objectivity testing. This limits its utility in measuring and predicting anaerobic capacity.

2. Cumulative scoring methods are not well defined which makes the test results very difficult to interpret.

3. Age and gender specific performance norms are not listed restricting its use in comparing one's performance against a standard or against others.

The Repeated 220 Yard Sprint Test is an unacceptable test of anaerobic capacity for research and teaching purposes. It has not been validated against standard laboratory tests, tested for reliability or objectivity, and does not include a clear overall scoring method to estimate anaerobic capacity. Further, the excessive number of 220 yard repetitions may promote muscle soreness or injury in examinees not conditioned in sprinting. The Repeated 200 Yard Sprint Test seems better suited as a drill to develop rather than test anaerobic capacity.

SUICIDE DRILL TEST

References.

Burke, E. J. (1980). Physiological considerations and suggestions for the training of elite basketball players. In Burke, E. J., ed. (1980). *Toward an understanding of human performance.* Ithaca: Mouvement Publications, pp 293-311.

Semenick, D. (1984). Anaerobic testing - Practical applications. *National Strength and Conditioning Association Journal,* 6(5):45, 72-73.

Additional Sources.

None.

Purpose.

To measure the anaerobic power of an examinee while running a shuttle.

Objectivity.

Not reported.

Reliability.

Not reported.

Validity.

Not reported.

Age and Sex.

Female and male college athletes.

Equipment.

A stopwatch.

Space Requirements and Design.

A regulation basketball court 28.66m (94') long with examinee at one end of the court.

Directions.

The examinee assumes a standing position just behind the baseline (i.e., out of bounds) of a basketball court. On command, "Ready, Go," the examinee sprints four continuous round trips: (1) to the nearest free throw line and back to the baseline, (2) to the midcourt line and back to the baseline, (3) to the farthest free throw line and back to the baseline and (4) to the farthest baseline and back to the baseline/finish. A total of four trials are given with two minutes rest between trials.

Scoring.

The score is the average time required to run the four trials.

Norms.

Burke (1980, p. 310) basketball players; Semenick (1984, p. 73) male basketball players.

REVIEW

JIM L. STILLWELL, P.E.D.
Chair
Human Performance Studies
The University of Alabama
Tuscaloosa, AL 35487

This test is an appropriate measure of anaerobic power. It has face validity, but no level of statistical validity or reliability is given. Although there is no value given for the objectivity of this test, it appears to have consistency.

From a practical standpoint, this test is quite appropriate because it requires no specific equipment for measurement, other than a stopwatch. A regulation basketball court, 94 feet in length, is necessary if the established norms are to be used. The test requires no specific training for the tester. The test is suitable for both females and males of college age.

With regard to danger in administration, there is no need for concern. The test is appropriate for conditioning. Norms are available but only for a select group (i.e., basketball players) and are a bit outdated. Four trials are required for the test with the score being an average of the four trials. The best score of the four trials is recommended, since the variable being measured is power and not endurance. Three or, perhaps, two trials would be sufficient. With the four trials, the two minute rest between trials may not be sufficient for full recovery.

SUMMARY

Major Strengths:

1. It is easy to administer one on one.
2. It requires no specific instrumentation.
3. It is appropriate for a conditioning activity.

Major Weaknesses:

1. It cannot be administered in mass.
2. Test time per examinee is 8 to 10 minutes.
3. Four trials are too many.
4. Recovery time between trials is too short.

5. The name of the test is inappropriate.

The Suicide Drill Test is an appropriate test for measuring anaerobic power. It provides an acceptable measure with limited expense and/or training in its use. It only requires a stopwatch and a regulation basketball court. It is appropriate for females and males and, perhaps, for a wider range of examinees than reported.

THOMSON ANAEROBIC CAPACITY TEST

Reference.

Thomson, J. M. (1981). Prediction of anaerobic capacity: A performance test employing an optimal exercise stress. *Canadian Journal of Applied Sport Sciences,* 6(1):16-20.

Additional Sources.

None.

Purpose.

To provide an accurate prediction of an examinee's anaerobic capacity.

Objectivity.

Not reported.

Reliability.

Not reported.

Validity.

Not reported.

Age and Sex.

College age males.

Equipment.

A red flag, two marker poles 1.5m (4.92') in height, a tape measure, and two stopwatches.

Space Requirements and Design.

A 400 meter track with a marker pole placed on the inner edge of the track at distances of 256m (280 yds) and 329m (360 yds) from the starting line. A timer with a stopwatch is positioned directly across from each marker pole. The tester is at the starting line with the red flag in one hand.

Directions.

The examinee assumes a standing position just behind the starting line. Upon the tester's command, "On your mark ... set ... go," the examinee runs around the track as fast as possible until he passes the 329m mark. The timers start their watches when the tester swings the red flag down simultaneously with the "Go," signal. The first timer stops her/his watch when the examinee crosses the plane of the 256m mark. The second timer stops her/his watch when the examinee crosses the plane of the 329m mark. The ex-aminee should run the entire distance in the inside lane and as fast as possible without pacing himself.

Scoring.

The score is derived by plugging the examinee's running time (T) to the 256 meter mark (measured to the nearest tenth of a second) and the examinee's running speed (S) between the 256m and 329m marks (in meters per minute), into the following formula.

Anaerobic Capacity = 1.72 - [(0.027) x (T) + (0.022) x (S)]

Norms.

Not reported.

NOTE: Running speed (S) is calculated by the following formula:

$$S = (73/t) (60)$$

Where 73 = the number of meters between the 256m and 329m marks, t = the time required to run the 73m which is determined by subtracting the time on the first stopwatch from the time on the second stopwatch, and 60 is the constant used to change the result from meters per second to meters per minute.

REVIEW

DONNA J. TERBIZAN, Ph.D.

Assistant Professor
Health, Physical Education and
Recreation
North Dakota State University
Fargo, ND 58105

It is extremely difficult to determine whether this test is valid, reliable, or objective because no information is given in regard to these aspects. As a test of anaerobic capacity, was it compared to another test that is considered standard? How did the test constructor determine if this test measured anaerobic capacity? The test does appear to measure anaerobic performance, but whether it measures capacity, or power, or whatever is suspect.

The test does require other personnel to be aware of what is going on, as they are timers for this measurement. There must be some error associated with this measurement, as not all timers will begin or stop their stopwatches at the same time. This would affect the test measurement as time is a factor used to measure anaerobic capacity.

This test also appears to have some practical problems. Although it appears to be a quick measurement of anaerobic exercise, the additional timers needed may be a problem. Facility requirements may be a difficulty, as most indoor tracks fall in the 250 to 300 meter distances, not 400 meters. There is only one trial; what happens if the examinee "falls asleep" when the signal to begin is given. It may be a better measure of capacity if the examinee was given a running start, rather than being at a dead stop when the signal to go is given.

This test may or may not be suitable as a drill, as noted above with facility problems. Without the proper distance for measurement, this test becomes suspect.

There are no norms given that would allow for this test to be used as a learning experience. These would need to be included before the test should be considered for this measurement or for teaching. Also, a validity coefficient should be given to show that it was compared to another type of anaerobic capacity test before recommending the test.

SUMMARY

Major Strength:

1. The time involved to administer the test.

Major Weakness:

1. There are no validity, reliability, or objectivity measures given, and these are needed before the test should be considered strong. The use of this test cannot be recommended for this measurement without this additional information.

This test is unacceptable for research or teaching because of the lack of norms and validity.

It may be a test that some researcher would use to do further research, so that validity and reliability measurements could be determined. It is not good for teaching as we attempt to have students look for validity and reliability measurements before using a test of any sort. Until these are available, this test is not recommended.

300 YARD SHUTTLE RUN TEST

References.
National Marine Corps League (no date). *Physical Fitness Program*. Arlington, VA: National Marine Corps League, p 12.

Gillian, G. M., & Marks, M. (1983). 300 yard shuttle run. *National Strength and Conditioning Association Journal*, 5(5):46.

Additional Sources.
None.

Purpose.
To measure the anaerobic power of an examinee through running.

Objectivity.
Not reported.

Reliability.
Not reported.

Validity.
Not reported.

Age and Sex.
Females and males, age 8 - adult.

Equipment.
A stopwatch, a starting pistol for which a whistle may be substituted, two plastic cones, and a tape measure.

Space Requirements and Design.
A clear, level area approximately 3m x 70m (10' x 200') with two cones measured 54.88m (60 yds.) apart.

Directions.
The examinee assumes a standing position behind the starting line. On the command, "Ready, Go," the examinee sprints to the cone 60 yards away and returns to the other cone next to the starting line. The examinee must run around each cone. The test is completed when the examinee has made four and one-half round trips around the two cones. If the examinee knocks over a cone, he/she must return it to its original position before continuing on with the test.

Scoring.
The score is the time measured to the nearest second.

Norms.
National Marine (no date, p. 12) boys and girls; Semenick (1984, p. 73) male basketball and football players.

REVIEW

EUGENE R. ANDERSON, Ph.D.
Associate Professor
Health, Physical Education and Recreation
University of Mississippi
University, MS 38677

The purpose of the 300 Yard Shuttle Run is to determine anaerobic power through running. Since the test does not address such technical standards as objectivity, reliability, and validity, its use for this purpose may be questionable. Norms are available for females and males, ages 8 to 17 +, by the Marine Corps League. The only other active individual besides the examinee is the tester whose responsibilities are limited and should be consistent throughout the testing.

The facilities and space are readily available in most teaching settings and should not be a problem for test administration. The same thing can be said for the equipment to be utilized. Other objects may be substituted for cones if cones are not available. Scoring of the test is relatively simple. Using a stopwatch would be appropriate since the examinee's score is rounded to the nearest second. The amount of time required for each examinee to complete the test may be a problem unless a number of stations are set up. It should take 1.5 minutes per examinee to complete the test. The very nature of the test requires that trials be limited. One trial should be sufficient following an appropriate warm up.

The test is most assuredly suitable to use as a drill or a conditioning technique. Since the test is self paced, it is suitable for a wide range of age groups and for both sexes. Individuals with a high anaerobic tolerance will do well on this test while those who are more suited to aerobic training will score lower. The test should be accident free if the examinees are allowed, and encouraged, to warm up and stretch properly.

Examinees may easily score themselves on this test. It is doubtful that this particular test and scoring procedure could be used for research purposes. The procedure is not precise enough to determine anaerobic power.

SUMMARY

Major Strengths:

1. The test is easily administered and the scoring is simple.

2. The facilities and equipment needed for the test are not uncommon in a school setting.

3. Norms are available for both sexes and a variety of age groups.

Major Weakness:

1. Validity, reliability and objectivity of this test are not provided.

The 300 Yard Shuttle Run would be inadequate for research and/or teaching for the following reasons: (1) since the validity is not given, it is questionable whether or not this test actually assesses anaerobic power, (2) the test is dependent upon the motivation of the examinee. The test is very demanding and requires examinees to call upon their intestinal fortitude.

Chapter 10

REACTION TIME

REACTION TIME TESTS

LATHAM YARDSTICK REACTION TIME TEST

Reference.
Arnot, R., & Gaines, C. (1986). *Sports Talent.*
New York: Penguin Books, pp 163-165.

Additional Sources.
None.

Purpose.
To measure an examinee's choice reaction time.

Objectivity.
Not reported.

Reliability.
Not reported.

Validity.
Not reported.

Age and Sex.
Not reported, but suitable for females and males, age 8 - adult.

Equipment.
A chair and a small table or a student desk chair, and two yardsticks.

Space Requirements and Design.
A clear, level area approximately 3m (10') square with the chair and table positioned in the center.

Directions.
The examinee sits in the chair facing the table with her/his forearms flat on the table. The hands hang over the table's edge with the palms about 15cm (6") apart and facing each other. Each thumb is positioned about 2.5cm (1") from its respective forefinger. The thumbs and forefingers are held parallel to the table's top. The tester stands in front of the examinee and holds a yardstick in each hand at the 36 inch end. The tester holds the yardsticks' zero mark even with the top edge of the examinee's forefingers

and thumbs in the middle of the space between the forefingers and thumbs. The tester then announces, "Ready, Go," and drops one of the two yardsticks within a range of 1 to 10 seconds after saying, "Go." The examinee attempts to close, as quickly as possible, her/his forefinger and thumb catching the yardstick. The distance just above the thumb on the yardstick is recorded. A total of 20 trials are randomly given with 10 for each hand.

Scoring.
The score is the shortest distance the yardstick fell during any of the 20 trials.

Norms.
Arnot & Gaines (1986, p. 165) age and sex are not reported.

REVIEW
JOYCE GRAENING, D.A.

Assistant Professor
Physical Education
University of Arkansas
Fayetteville, AR 72701

Validity of this test is not given, however face validity can be assumed, since catching an object is dependent on an examinee's ability to react to a stimulant. However, the test appears to be testing a very small muscle group - thumb and finger reaction. Reliability of the test is not given, but using 20 trials should allow some consistency. Objectivity is also not given and would appear to be questionable. The directions are not completely clear and there are many dependent variables. The test is dependent on one other individual, the tester, dropping the yardsticks. With 20 random trials, 10 for each hand, it could be very difficult for the tester to keep a count of the number dropped on each side without additional help. The size of the examinee's hands could also be a factor, as could keeping one's finger and thumb 1 inch apart.

This test can be administered using a partner system. Many examinees can be tested within a typical class period. A small testing area is all that is needed. Students can be administered this test while sitting at their own desks in a classroom. Equipment needs are minor. Time requirements are minimal even with 20 trials. However, 20 trials may be excessive. There could be a fatigue or boredom factor. Perhaps reliability should be checked using only 10 trials.

The test appears suitable for examinees ages eight and over as suggested. However, one must remember that reaction time usually decreases with age in older adults. The available norms do not consider age or sex. Scoring this test is relatively simple. It would be impossible for the examinee to score herself/himself. The tester who drops the yardstick would also need scoring help with 20 trials. Recording of the best score is also questionable. Most measurement experts agree that calculating the average score of all trials is the most appropriate scoring procedure rather using than the best trial as this test suggests.

SUMMARY

Major Strengths:

1. Fast to administer.

2. Does not require expensive equipment.

3. Can be administered to both sexes and a wide age range.

Major Weaknesses:

1. Validity, reliability, and objectivity are not given.

2. Test is dependent on another individual.

3. The best of 20 trials may not be the proper way to score.

4. Twenty trials may be excessive - fatigue and boredom may become factors.

5. Norms have not been developed which consider the sex and age of the examinees.

6. Tests only small muscle group reaction time - thumb and forefinger.

Overall, this test is unacceptable for use in research or for teaching purposes. The test has too many grey areas; one should not consider using any test that does not have acceptable validity, reliability, and objectivity. The Nelson Hand Reaction test is recommended instead of this test.

NELSON FOOT REACTION TEST

References.
Nelson, F. B. (1965). The nelson reaction timer. Instruction Leaflet, Lafayette, LA.

Johnson, B. L., & Nelson, J. K. (1986). *Practical measurements for evaluation in physical education*. Edina, MN: Burgess Publishing, pp 256-257.

Additional Source.
Jensen & Hirst (1980, pp. 152-153).

Purpose.
To measure the ability of an examinee to react to a visual stimulus with the foot.

Objectivity.
Not reported.

Reliability.
r = .85 for college men.

Validity.
Face validity.

Age and Sex.
Suitable for females and males, age 8 - college.

Equipment.
A Nelson Reaction Timer and a bench or table.

Space Requirements and Design.
A clear, level, quiet area approximately 3m (10') square with the table or bench positioned 2.54cm (1") from a clear wall.

Directions.
The examinee sits on the table or bench with the ball of her/his bare foot positioned 2.54cm (1") and the heel 7.62cm (3") from the wall. The tester holds the Nelson Reaction Timer between the wall and the examinee's foot so that the Timer's base line is opposite the end of the big toe. The examinee focuses on the concentration zone (i.e., a black shaded area on the timer between the .120 and .130 lines). After the examinee and Nelson Reaction Timer are properly positioned, the tester gives the command, "Ready" and releases the Timer shortly thereafter. The tester should vary the release of the Timer for each trial from .5 to 2.0 seconds after giving the, "Ready" command. The examinee reacts by pressing the Timer against the wall with her/his ball of the

foot. The time is read from the line just above the big toe. Twenty trials are given. Trials during which the examinee obviously anticipated the release should not be counted and a retrial given.

Scoring.
The score is average of the 10 trials remaining after the 5 fastest trials and the 5 slowest trials have been discarded.

Norms.
Johnson & Nelson (1986, p. 257) mean time for college men.

REVIEW

PRISCILLA MACRAE, Ph.D.
Associate Professor
Sports Medicine
Pepperdine University
Malibu, CA 90263

The Nelson Foot Reaction Test is valid as indicated because the Timer will fall at a consistent rate based on gravitational pull. However, the validity of the test itself is questionable based upon the definition of reaction time. This test is supposed to be a measure of only reaction time, however, it really is a measure of response time (reaction and movement time).

The reliability of this test is questionable for any population other than college men, as its reliability has not been assessed with other populations. If the testers have not been trained in the correct use of the foreperiod, as well as proper positioning of the Timer relative to the placement of the examinee's foot, then there could be a lack of objectivity. It appears to be very important that the same tester conduct all the testing, particularly in pretesting and posttesting situations. The test does require active participation by the tester. This could affect the performance of the examinee.

This test is easy to administer. It requires a single tester who should be trained in the proper technique. The only requirement regarding the testing facility is that it should be in a quiet environment so the examinee can concentrate and not be distracted. The test requires a small amount of time and therefore a large number of trials are recommended. The test directions recommend 20 trials, with the slowest 5 trials and the fastest 5 trials discarded. This reviewer would recommend that 50 trials be completed, the first 5 to 10 trials to be discarded and all trials that are greater or less than two standard deviations from the mean discarded as outliers. The test is completely safe in terms of equipment and administration. It is important that the scoring be done by the tester for the purpose of accuracy since the Timer is scaled in thousandths of a second and very young children would have some difficulty in reading their score. There are no norms established for the test which is seen as a test weakness. This test is not suitable for research purposes because it is not precise enough.

SUMMARY

Major Strengths:

1. It is very easy to administer.

2. It does not require expensive equipment.

3. It gives a rough estimate of response time (reaction and movement time) of the foot that can be of value as a learning tool.

Major Weaknesses:

1. It is not an accurate measure of reaction time as it really measures both reaction time and movement time.

2. It is not a precise measure of reaction/movement time so it should not be used for research purposes.

3. The position of the examinee on the bench, with the foot in the proper position, is difficult to standardize.

4. The number of practice trials is too few. It is recommended that at least 50 trials be completed by the examinee.

The Nelson Foot Reaction Test is acceptable for teaching purposes and gives a rough estimate of response time. It is unacceptable for research purposes because it lacks precision and because of the fact that it is measuring total response time and not reaction time as defined in the literature. It would be important to give a sufficient number of trials (i.e., 50 or more) in order to obtain a stabilization of performance.

NELSON HAND REACTION TEST

References.

Nelson, F. B. (1965). The nelson reaction timer. Instruction Leaflet, Lafayette, LA.

Johnson, B. L., & Nelson, J. K. (1986). *Practical measurements for evaluation in physical education*. Edina, MN: Burgess Publishing, pp 255-256.

Additional Sources.

Barrow et al. (1989, p. 129); Hastad & Lacy (1989, pp. 273-274); Jensen & Hirst (1980, pp. 152-153); Verducci (1980, p. 253).

Purpose.

To measure the ability of an examinee to react to a visual stimulus with the hand.

Objectivity.

Not reported.

Reliability.

r = .89 using the test retest method.

Validity.

Face validity.

Age and Sex.

Suitable for females and males, age 8 - college.

Equipment.

A Nelson Reaction Timer and a table and chair or a student desk chair.

Space Requirements and Design.

A clear, level area approximately 3m (10') square in a quiet area with the table and chair or student desk chair placed in the center.

Directions.

The examinee sits with the her/his forearm resting on the table or desk top. The hand is positioned with the palm vertical and the fingers and thumb extended beyond the table's edge. The finger and thumb are held on the same horizontal plane about 2.54cm (1") apart ready to pinch the Nelson Reaction Timer. The tester holds the Timer between the examinee's finger and thumb with the base line on the Timer even with the top surface of the index finger and thumb. The tester then gives the command, "Ready," the examinee focuses on the concentration zone (i.e., the black shaded area on the Timer between the .120

and .130 lines), and pinches the Timer after it is released and he/she sees the concentration zone move. The tester should vary the time of the release for each trial from .5 to 2.0 seconds after giving the "Ready" command. The time for each trial is determined by reading the line just above the thumb. A total of 20 trials are given. Trials during which the examinee obviously anticipated the release should not be counted and a retrial given.

Scoring.

The score is the average of the remaining 10 trials after the 5 slowest trials and the 5 fastest trials are discarded.

Norms.

Corbin & Lindsey (1983, p. 123) sex and age not specified; Johnson & Nelson (1986, p. 256) mean times for college men, college women and small children.

REVIEW

WILLIAM R. SPIETH, Ph.D.
Professor of Physical Education
Georgia Southern College
Statesboro, GA 30460

The validity of the test is questionable based upon the definition of reaction time since movement is involved in order to stop the Timer. The test is reliable but its objectivity is questionable if the testers have not been trained in correct use of the foreperiod time lapse, the proper positioning of the Timer relative to the examinee's subjective finger-thumb position and the consistency of release of the Timer. The test does require the active participation of the tester.

The test is easy to administer. It requires but a single tester who should be trained. The only requirement regarding the testing facility is that it should be in a quiet environment so the examinee can concentrate and not be distracted in any way. A great number of trials can be administered as each one can be completed in about three seconds. It can be used by the designated age groups and it discriminates among these groups. The test is completely safe in terms of equipment and administration. Scoring should be done by the tester for the purpose of accuracy since the Timer is scaled in thousandths of a second and very young examinees would have some difficulty in reading their score. Some norms have been established for the test and numerous research studies regarding reaction time have indicated averages for the various age levels and sexes.

SUMMARY

Major Strengths:

1. It is very easy to administer.

2. It does not require expensive equipment.

3. It gives a rough estimate of reaction time that can be of value as a learning tool for the examinee.

Major Weaknesses:

1. It is not an accurate measure of reaction time.

2. It is in reality a measure of total response time and not reaction time.

3. These is no way to assure that examinees have their thumb and index finger one inch apart.

4. There is no stabilization of the tester's arm on release of the Timer.

5. The number of practice trials is too few.

The Nelson Hand Reaction Test is acceptable for teaching purposes and giving a rough estimate of reaction time. It is unacceptable for research purposes because it lacks a precise measurement and the fact that it really is measuring total response time. Research has shown that 15 practice trials should be permitted prior to the actual scoring of any reaction time test and then the mean score of trials 16 to 30 be used as the examinee's score. A stabilizing support should be made available for the tester to rest his/her forearm so the release of the Timer would be smooth and consistent in its drop.

REACTION/MOVEMENT TIME TESTS

FOUR-WAY ALTERNATE RESPONSE TEST

References.

Jensen, C. R. (No Date). Practical measurements of reaction time, response time and speed. Unpublished study, Brigham Young University.

Jensen, C. R., & Hirst, C. C. (1980). *Measurement in physical education and athletics.* New York: MacMillan, pp 154-155.

Additional Sources.
None.

Purpose.
To measure the ability of an examinee to react and move in a given direction.

Objectivity.
Not reported.

Reliability.
Not reported.

Validity.
Face validity.

Age and Sex.
Suitable for females and males.

Equipment.
A stopwatch, measuring tape, and marking tape.

Space Requirements and Design.
A clear, level area approximately 20m (60') square with a 9.14m (30') square marked in the center of the area. An X is marked in the center of the square (Figure 10-1).

Directions.
The examinee takes a standing ready stance over the X in the center of the square facing the tester who is approximately 3m (10') away. The tester starts the test by giving the command, "Ready," followed by the movement of one hand in one of four directions to indicate the direction the examinee should move. Simultaneous with the hand movement, the tester starts the stopwatch. The tester stops the watch when the examinee crosses the correct boundary line of the square. The time is recorded to the nearest tenth of a second. A total of 20 trials are given, 5 in each of the four directions. The trials in each direction

may be given in any order. To help in administering the test, the tester places 5 small cards with forward written or typed on them, 5 with backward on them, 5 with left on them, and 5 with right on them. The tester places these 20 cards in a hat and draws one out to determine the direction of movement for each trial. The tester should use an interval of .5 to 2.0 seconds between the command, "Ready," and the hand movement starting the test.

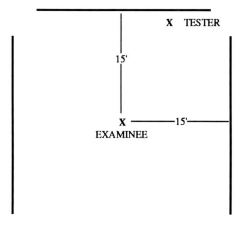

Figure 10-1. Four Way Alternate Response Test.

Scoring.
The score is the total time for all 20 trials.

Norms.
Not reported.

REVIEW

T. GILMOUR REEVE, Ph.D.
Professor
Health and Human Performance
Auburn University
Auburn, AL 36849-5323

The Four-Way Alternate Response Test is intended to measure the ability to react and move in a given direction. Thus, the test combines two distinct basic motor abilities: reaction time (the ability to initiate a response quickly) and speed of movement (the ability to move quickly following response initiation). Performance in movement situations requiring these basic abilities is highly dependent on the task demands. That is, choice reaction time is affected by the number of response choices, the compatibility between the stimulus to move and the corresponding response, and the complexity of the movement, whereas speed of movement is affected by the extent and accuracy requirements of the movement. Thus, the Four-Way Alternate Response Test may provide only limited information about performances in sport or movement situations which require task demands that differ from those required in the test.

The scientific aspects of the test are unknown. Although face validity is stated, the lack of relationship of this test to specific sport situations makes even face validity questionable. Construct validity must be established to define those situations for which the test may provide a valid measurement of performance. For example, does this test relate to athletic performance in sports such as football, racquetball, or tennis? Because the test procedures are simple and performance is measured with a stopwatch, the test most likely has satisfactory reliability and objectivity. However, reliability and objectivity coefficients must be established for the test prior to its use in critical measurement situations.

The facility, equipment, and administration requirements make the test practical to use in large group situations. The test could be easily administered, either outside or inside. Only one tester is required; however, the use of an assistant to record performance times would expedite the testing. Unfortunately, the test cannot be self administered. The equipment require-ments are minimal; a tape measure and marking tape to prepare the test site and a stopwatch and score sheet to administer the test. The test poses little risk to the examinee. Norms for the test are not available.

Several problems with the response test are evident in the instructions for administering the test. The test directions specify 20 trials (5 trials for each of four directions). However, no guidelines are provided regarding false starts or movements in the wrong direction. Because performance is calculated as the total time for the 20 trials, the guidelines must be clear regarding what constitutes an error trial and how to handle such trials. Moreover, the instructions do not specify how the examinee is to respond. For example, when the hand signal indicates that movement is to be to the line located behind the examinee, is the examinee to run backwards to the line or to turn and run forward to the line?

SUMMARY

Major Strengths:

1. Little equipment is required.

2. The test site is easy to prepare.

3. Only one tester is required to administer and score the test.

Major Weaknesses:

1. The lack of scientific development of the test.

2. The lack of generalizability of performances on the test to other sport or physical activities.

3. The lack of precise instructions regarding test administration.

Overall, the Four-Way Alternate Response Test is an unacceptable test. The test has little utility for research or sport specific situations in teaching and coaching.

NELSON CHOICE RESPONSE MOVEMENT TEST

References.
Nelson, J. K. (1967). Development of a practical performance test combining reaction time, speed of movement and choice of response. Unpublished study, Louisiana State University.

Johnson, B. L., & Nelson, J. K. (1986). *Practical measurements for evaluation in physical education*. Edina, MN: Burgess, pp 259-261.

Additional Sources.
None.

Purpose.
To measure the ability of an examinee to react and move quickly in the correct direction indicated by a choice stimulus.

Objectivity.
r = .83.

Reliability.
r = .87 for college men using the test-retest method.

Validity.
Face validity.

Age and Sex.
Suitable for boys and girls.

Equipment.
A stopwatch, tape measure, and marking tape.

Space Requirements and Design.
A clear, level area approximately 3m x 20m (10' x 60') with three parallel lines marked 6.40m (21') apart.

Directions.
The examinee straddles the center line in a basketball defensive stance facing the tester who is standing several meters (yards) forward. The tester holds the stopwatch overhead and gives the command, "Ready," pauses .5 to 2.0 seconds and then quickly moves it left or right simultaneously starting the watch. The examinee then runs as quickly as possible in the direction the watch was moved. The tester stops the watch when the examinee crosses the correct line 6.40m (21') away. The time is recorded to the nearest tenth of a second. Should the examinee initially move in the wrong direction, he/she must reverse directions and run across the correct finish line. A total of 10 trials, 5 to the left and 5

to the right, are given in random order. To help the tester in determining the intended direction of movement for a trial, 5 small note cards with left written on them and 5 with right written on them could be placed in a hat and randomly drawn out for each trial. A rest of 20 seconds should be allowed between trials.

Scoring.
The score is the average time of all 10 trials.

Norms.
Johnson & Nelson (1986, p. 253) men and women.

REVIEW

DALE G. PEASE, Ph.D.

Associate Professor and Chair
Health and Human Performance
University of Houston
Houston, TX 77204-5331

This test, although categorized as a reaction time test, is primarily a movement time or more accurately a general performance time measure of an examinee moving 21 feet. Reaction time is a very small component of the time measured, especially considering the testing conditions suggested by the test constructor. The technique of hand signalling direction and starting the watch will reduce reliability and especially the objectivity of the test administration. Since the test can be administered by one tester standing at the middle line, a good visual line to determine when the examinee passes the finish line is not available and adds to the variability in scoring. The choice direction component appears to be a simple way of attempting to control for the anticipation factor.

The test is easy to administer, requires limited equipment and can be administered indoors or outdoors. Norms are available, but for college age examinees only. The nature of the test, both performance and scoring, would seem to make it appropriate for most age and gender groups. Limiting the testing to 10 trials with rest periods would seem to reduce fatigue factors. Each examinee should require approximately five minutes for testing.

SUMMARY

This test is acceptable for providing a general performance measurement for short distance running when initial direction is unknown. Due to the test administration procedures, the test has limited use as a research tool. Its generalization to specific sports and other physical activities is unknown.

NELSON SPEED OF MOVEMENT TEST

References.
Nelson, F. B. (1965). The nelson reaction timer. Instruction Leaflet, Lafayette, LA.

Johnson, B. L., & Nelson, J. K. (1986). *Practical measurements for evaluation in physical education*. Edina, MN: Burgess Publishing, pp 257-258.

Additional Source.
Jensen & Hirst (1980, pp. 153-154).

Purpose.
To measure the ability of an examinee to react and move the hands.

Objectivity.
Not reported.

Reliability.
r = .75 for college men.

Validity.
Face validity.

Age and Sex.
Suitable for females and males, age 8 - college.

Equipment.
A Nelson Reaction Timer, a small table, a chair, marking tape, and a ruler.

Space Requirements and Design.
A clear, quiet area approximately 3m (10') square with the table in the center and the examinee seated in the chair at the table. Two tape lines, 30.48cm (12") apart from the outer edge of each line, are placed on the edge of the table. Another tape line, thinner and shorter than the other two, is placed on the table's edge exactly halfway between these two lines.

Directions.
The examinee places her/his hands on the table with the palms facing each other and the inside edges of the little fingers resting parallel to the outer edges of the tape lines. The tester holds the Nelson Reaction Timer midway between the hands so that the base line, marked on the Timer, is level with the top edge of the examinee's palms. The tester then gives the command, "Ready" and releases the Nelson Reaction Timer. The tester should vary the release of the Timer from .5 to 2.0 seconds after having given the command, "Ready." The examinee tries to stop the timer as quickly as possible by moving the hands together horizontally. The score for each trial is the time showing on the Timer just above the upper edge of the palms. A total of 20 trials are given. Trials during which the examinee obviously anticipated the release should not be counted and a retrial given.

Scoring.
The score is the average of the 10 trials remaining after the 5 fastest trials and the 5 slowest trials are eliminated.

Norms.
Johnson & Nelson (1986, p. 257) mean time for college men.

REVIEW
ROBERT E. STADULIS, Ed.D.

Associate Professor
Physical Education
Kent State University
Kent, OH 44242

The test appears to achieve the purpose of measuring the combined reaction and movement speed of the hands; however, caution must be exercised to avoid generalizing to hand movements of a different distance, complexity, or organization. Reliability is reported at an acceptable level (r = .75), but whether this refers to internal or external reliability is unclear. Objectivity may be a problem - the tester can markedly affect the procedure by providing anticipation cues, by being too consistent (or too variable) in timing the period between "Ready" and release, and/or by not judging consistently the starting height of the Timer in relation to the upper borders of the examinee's hands.

The test requires minimal space, equipment, and time, seems easy to administer, and is not dangerous. A large age range can be served; however, norms are not available. Using the test as a drill would not seem advisable. Although the scoring scale is objective, the objectivity of the scores may be questioned. Using the scores for research purposes seems ill advised without further assessment of the scientific aspects of the test. The scoring procedure seems overly complex for many of the age groups served; providing an odd number of trials and determining the median score is recommended (e.g., if fewer trials were used, perhaps 11, then drop the 5 fastest trials and 5 slowest trials).

SUMMARY

Major Strengths:

1. Very inexpensive.

2. Easy to administer.

Major Weaknesses:

1. Questionable objectivity.

2. Potential for overgeneralization.

3. No norms.

4. Complicated scoring procedure.

The test is adequate for teaching purposes, especially for examinees at the upper age level. Caution must be exercised relative to overgeneralizing the test results to other hand movements. Without further investigation, the test appears to be inadequate for research purposes.

TWO-WAY ALTERNATE RESPONSE TEST

Reference.
Jensen, C. R., & Hirst, C. C. (1980). *Measurement in physical education and athletics.* New York: MacMillan, p 155.

Additional Sources.
None.

Purpose.
To measure the ability of an examinee to react and move in a given direction.

Objectivity.
Not reported.

Reliability.
Not reported.

Validity.
Not reported.

Age and Sex.
Suitable for females and males.

Equipment.
A stopwatch, measuring tape, and marking tape.

Space Requirements and Design.
A clear, level area approximately 3m x 20m (10' x 60') with three parallel lines approximately 2m (6')long marked off 4.57m (15') apart.

Directions.
The examinee stands straddling the center line facing the tester who is several feet forward. The tester gives the command, "Ready, Go," and then moves one hand left or right, simultaneously starting the stopwatch. The examinee then runs as quickly as possible in the direction the hand was moved. The tester stops the watch when the examinee crosses the correct line. The time is recorded to the nearest tenth of a second. A total of 10 trials are given, 5 to each side. The tester should use an interval of .5 to 2.0 seconds between the command, "Ready," and the hand movement starting the test. In determining the test trial directions, 5 small note cards with left typed or written on them and 5 with right typed or written on them, should be placed in a hat and drawn out one at a time for each trial.

Scoring.
The score is the total time for all 10 trials.

Norms.
Not reported.

REVIEW

JOY L. HENDRICK, Ph.D.
Assistant Professor
Physical Education
State University College at Cortland
Cortland, NY 13045

The measurement of response time is not an easy task since it is comprised of an examinee's reaction time plus the individual's speed of movement. Each component is specific to the test conditions (e.g., the type of stimulus, type of movement, and extent of movement). The reader is referred to Johnson and Nelson (1986) for a good discussion of these factors.

In most athletic activities, speed is considered to be the movement of the entire body by means of leg power. The Two-Way Alternate Response Test is relevant at least on face validity since it involves moving the body as a whole from a standing position. Although no objectivity or reliability values were given, the test appears to have a reasonable level of each.

The only two measurement books found that mention this particular test are Neilson and Jensen (1972) and Jensen and Hirst (1980). However, this particular test is similar to the Nelson Choice-Response Movement Test (Nelson, 1967). In fact, these two tests are so similar that one test appears to be an earlier version of the other test. The major difference is that the Nelson test has published reliability and objectivity coefficients (.87 and .83, respectively) and norms for high school and college females and males.

The best practical aspect about this test is that it is economical in terms of time, equipment, and space. The test appears to be valid for all age groups and ability levels, however no norms are provided.

Problems could arise in the tester's ability to simultaneously move the arm to signal the direction and start the stopwatch. It appears that much practice is needed to coordinate these actions perfectly. This problem will have an influence on reliability and objectivity.

In addition, test directions do not include the administration of practice trials nor do the directions include the handling of mistrials (e.g., the examinee beginning the movement too early or too late). It is well established that reaction time improves with practice; therefore, enough practice should be given so that learning is not a confounding factor. The appropriate number of practice trials needs to be investigated. Perhaps 12 or 14 trials could be given and then the fastest and slowest trial(s) be discarded to arrive at a more stable score.

Another factor that influences reaction time is the length and regularity (fixed or variable) of the preparatory interval. The test directions take this effect into account by telling the tester to vary the preparatory interval between .5 and 2.0 seconds.

SUMMARY

Major Strength:

1. The test is economical in terms of time, equipment, and space.

Major Weaknesses:

1. The lack of reliability and objectivity coefficients.

2. The lack of published norms.

Based on the above reasons, this test is unacceptable. Since the Nelson Choice-Response Movement Test is so similar to this test and has established acceptable levels of reliability and objectivity as well as a table of norms, the use of the Nelson Choice-Response Movement Test is recommended.

REVIEW REFERENCES

Jensen, C. R., & Hirst, C. C. (1980). *Measurement in physical education and athletics.* New York: MacMillan.

Johnson, B. L., & Nelson, J. K. (1986). *Practical measurements for evaluation in physical education.* Edina, MN: Burgess.

Neilson, N. P., & Jensen, C. R. (1972). *Measurement and statistics in physical education.* Belmont, CA: Wadsworth.

Nelson, J. K. (1967). Development of a practical performance test combining reaction time, speed of movement and choice of response. Unpublished study, Louisiana State University.

Chapter 11

SPEED

RUNNING SPEED TESTS

DASH FOR A SPECIFIED DISTANCE TEST

Reference.
None.

Additional Sources.
Barrow et al. (1989, p. 118); Baumgartner & Jackson (1982, p. 215); Baumgartner & Jackson (1987, p. 281); Baumgartner & Jackson (1991, p. 264); Clarke & Clarke (1987, p. 160); Hastad & Lacy (1989, pp. 272-273);

Jensen & Hirst (1980, p. 156); Johnson & Nelson (1986, pp. 259, 366); Kirkendall et al. (1980, p. 243), 272; Kirkendall et al. (1987, pp. 153, 410); Safrit (1980, p. 242); Safrit (1986, pp. 442-443); Safrit (1990, pp. 243-244, 414-415); Verducci (1980, pp. 252-253, 285-286, 288).

Purpose.
To measure the ability of an examinee to run a specified distance in the least amount of time.

Objectivity.
Usually high depending primarily on the testers' ability to start and stop their watches at the same time.

Reliability.
Usually high (e.g., 50 yard dash: r = .86 Fleishman, 1964B, p. 59 and r = .95, Jackson & Baumgartner, 1969).

Validity.
Face validity.

Age and Sex.
Suitable for females and males, age 8 - adult.

Equipment.
Two stopwatches or one stopwatch with a split timer.

Space Requirements and Design.
A clear, level and straight course of the specified distance (usually 30-60 meters/yards) with an additional area of appropriate length so the examinee may safely stop.

Directions.
For safety reasons, all examinees taking the test should be in appropriate shoes and should warm up adequately.

The examinee takes a standing position just behind the starting line. Upon the signal, "Ready, Go," the examinee starts running as fast as possible straight ahead. The stopwatch is started on the signal, "Go" and stopped when the examinee's chest breaks the plane of the finish line. Two to six trials are given with a five minute rest between trials.

Scoring.
The score is the time of the best trial measured to the nearest tenth of a second.

Norms.
Alabama (1988, pp. 44-45) boys and girls for 50 yard dash; American Alliance (1975, pp. 30, 38, 47, 52, 57, 59-60) girls, boys, men and women for 50 yard dash; American Alliance (1990, p. 48) boys and girls for 50 yard dash;

Barrow et al. (1989, p. 123) boys and girls for 50 yard dash; Baumgartner & Jackson (1982, pp. 176, 216) high school and college women volleyball players for 20 yard dash and boys and girls for 50 yard dash;

Baumgartner & Jackson (1987, p. 286) boys and girls for 50 yard dash; Baumgartner & Jackson (1991, pp. 220-221, 261) high school and college women volleyball players for 20 yard dash, college football players for 40 yard dash, boys and girls for 50 yard dash; Canadian Association (1980, pp. 37-68) boys and girls for 50 meter dash; Chrysler-AAU (1990, p. 6) boys and girls for 50-100 yards; Harrison & Bradbeer (1982, pp. 24-25) boy and girl athletes for 40 yard dash; Hastad & Lacy (1989, p. 273) boys and girls for 50 yard dash;

Hawaii (1989, pp. 19-20) boys and girls for 35 yard dash; Jackson & Baumgartner (1969, p. 710) male college physical education major students for 20, 30, 40 and 50 yard dashes; Johnson & Nelson (1986, p. 260) boys and girls for 50 yard dash;

Kirkendall et al. (1980, p. 279-280, 287-288, 334) boys and girls for 40 yard dash, and boys and girls for 50 yard dash; Kirkendall et al. (1987, p. 159, 410-412) boys, girls, and special populations for 50 yard dash; Miller (1988, p. 232) boys and girls for 50 yard dash;

National Marine (no date, p. 15) boys and girls for 50 yard dash; New York (1958, pp. 51-60) boys and girls for 50 yard dash; New York (1966, pp. 45-62) boys and girls for 50 yard dash; President's Council (1987, pp. 2-6) USSR boys and girls for 60m dash and USSR boys and girls for 100m dash; President's Council (1988, p. 6) boys and girls for 50 yard dash;

Pyke (1986, p. 8) boys and girls for 50 yard dash; Safrit (1986, pp. 282-283) boys and girls for 50 yard dash; Safrit (1990, p. 415) boys and girls for 50 yard dash; Shannon (1989, p. 45) high school football players for 40 yard dash; Texas (no date, no page numbers) boys and girls for 50 yard dash.

NOTE: Some measurement experts recommend that running speed tests should be administered with the examinee using either a crouch or "flying" start. Since the crouch start, as used by elite track sprinters, involves a greater element of skill than the standing start, the tester must give proper instruction and allow ample practice to master its technique. The "flying" start can be used to eliminate the effects of starting technique and make the test a truer measure of running speed. If electronic equipment is not available, the "flying" start introduces another variable for potential error (i.e., when to start the stopwatch). In administering a running speed test where the "flying" start is used, the examinee generally starts running 10 to 20 yards/meters behind the starting line. The tester must then signal (e.g., by swinging an arm down) the timer located at the finish line to start the stopwatch when the examinee crosses the starting line.

REVIEW

RONALD K. HETZLER, Ph.D.
Assistant Professor
Health, Physical Education and Recreation
University of Hawaii at Manoa
Honolulu, HI 96822

This test is possibly the best measure of sprinting speed and should serve as the gold standard. The test is easy to administer and requires a minimal amount of training and equipment. A potential user should be able to follow the test instructions without difficulty. As stated in the description of the test, the Dash for Specified Distance has good objectivity, high reliability, and face validity. The safety considerations should be closely adhered to, with a special emphasis on warm up and stretching exercises prior to a maximal effort by the examinee.

Two to six separate trials were recommended, although two trials would probably be sufficient in most instances. However, additional trials may be necessary for very precise results. If space is available, the longer recommended distances would reduce the influence of reaction time at the start on the test results. A real strength of the test is that normative data do exist for a variety of populations. This should aid in interpretation of the results for both the tester and the examinee.

SUMMARY

In summary, the Dash For A Specified Distance is a highly recommended test to assess sprinting speed. Close attention should be given to the safety considerations. Normative data does exist and can be used to help interpret the results of the test.

DASH FOR A SPECIFIED TIME TEST

Reference.

None.

Additional Sources.

Hastad & Lacy (1989, pp. 274-275); Johnson & Nelson (1986, 4 sec. dash, pp. 258,367-368,379; 6 sec. dash, pp. 258-259).

Purpose.

To measure the ability of an examinee to run as great a distance as possible in a specified time.

Objectivity.

Usually high depending primarily on the testers' ability to start and stop their watches at the same time.

Reliability.

Usually high.

Validity.

Face validity.

Age and Sex.

Suitable for females and males, age 8 - college.

Equipment.

A stopwatch, whistle, and suitable material for marking the course.

Space Requirements and Design.

A clear, level and straight course marked off with lines every 1, 2, or 5 yards/meters which are parallel to the starting line plus an additional area of appropriate length so the examinee being tested may stop safely. A football field with its line markings will save time in preparing the test site.

Directions.

The examinee takes a standing position behind the starting line. Upon the signal, "Ready, Go," the examinee starts running as fast as possible straight ahead. At the end of the specified time (usually four seconds for eight year olds and eight seconds for those in their teens) the starter/timer blows a whistle and an observer notes the location of the examinee at the instant the whistle blew. The observer runs to the location and determines the distance run to the nearest yard. Two trials are given with a minimum rest of five minutes between trials.

For convenience in administering the test, the tester can have the group divide into pairs with one examinee taking the test and the other serving as an observer. For safety reasons, all examinees taking the test should be in appropriate shoes and warm up adequately.

Scoring.

The score is the sum distance run during the best trial measured to the nearest yard/meter.

Norms.

Corbin & Lindsey (1983, p. 126) men and women for 3 second dash; Johnson & Nelson (1986, pp. 258-259, 370-371, 380) girls, men and women for 4 second dash and boys and girls, for 6 second dash; Texas (no date, no page numbers) for 8 second dash.

NOTE: Some measurement experts recommend that running speed tests should be administered with the examinee using either a crouch or "flying" start. Since the crouch start, as used by track sprinters, involves a greater element of skill than the standing start, the tester must give proper instruction and allow ample practice to master its technique. The "flying" start can be used to eliminate the effects of starting technique - making the test a truer measure of running speed. If electronic equipment is not available, the "flying" start introduces another variable for potential error (i.e., when to start the stopwatch). In administering a running speed test where the "flying" start is used, the examinee generally begins running 10 to 20 yards/meters behind the starting line. The tester must then signal (e.g., by swinging an arm down) the timer located at the finish line to start the stopwatch when the examinee crosses the starting line.

REVIEW

DUANE MILLSLAGLE, Ed.D.

Associate Professor
Physical Education
Northern State University
Aberdeen, SD 57401

The Dash For Specified Time is a field test designed to measure the motor ability of speed. The administration of the test requires little equipment and can be conducted within a reasonable amount of time.

The stated purpose of the test is to determine the ability to run as great a distance as possible in a specified time. The purpose is misleading, not in the test's outcome (i.e., distance run), but in the evaluation of the underlying motor ability of speed. The professional in the field should recognize that one's speed is being evaluated and the distance run in a certain time is the measurement of speed.

The test is similar in intent to other tests of speed. The AAHPERD Youth Fitness Test measures speed by a 50 yard dash time whereas the Texas Physical Fitness Test measures the distance run over eight seconds. Varying the running from four to eight seconds, based on the age of the examinees, has merit. Generating speed over time requires a considerable amount of strength and power which young children may not have developed. But exercise physiology and track and field studies with college and elite sprinters have reported that one can maintain top speed for only short time. Since little or no research has been conducted to determine the period of seconds the child or young adult can run before muscular fatigue or anaerobic ability becomes a factor, the four second period for 8 to 12 year olds and eight seconds for those in their teens could be a developmental concern for the professional in the field.

The test requires each examinee to exert a great amount of effort over two trials. The reliability of the score could be affected by the recovery period between trials. A fully recovered examinee may attain a greater distance on each trial than an examinee who may not have recovered. This test does not specify guidelines pertaining to the recovery period of the examinees. Other factors that may affect the reliability and objectivity of the measurement are: (a) the examinee's starting position, (b) the observer's determination of distance covered when the whistle was blown, and (c) the starter's ability to time the signal to stop while the stopwatch is running. Due to the high probability that these factors will affect both the objectivity and reliability of the measure from one trial to another causes administrative concerns in conducting this test.

Standardizing the starting position for each examinee or allowing a running start, providing adequate rest between trials, having more than one observer in determining distance covered, and acquiring a timing device which can be initiated and which activates a sound after set periods of time can ensure more objectivity and reliability. The ease of convenience in the administration of this test with relatively little equipment and space restraints, other than a flat surface, are positive considerations in adopting this test. The appropriateness of this test for both age and sex, and intended purpose serve the professional who would like to evaluate the motor ability of speed in a field setting.

SPEED CURVE TEST

Reference.
Brooks, C. (1981). Use a speed curve to measure sprint speed. *Scholastic Coach,* 50(6):66, 68, 83-85.

Additional Sources.
None.

Purpose.
To measure an examinee's maximum running speed.

Objectivity.
Not reported.

Reliability.
Not reported.

Validity.
Not reported.

Age and Sex.
Not reported, but suitable for females and males, age 6 - adult.

Equipment.
A stopwatch, a tape measure, and two hurdles or plastic cones.

Space Requirements and Design.
A clear, level area approximately 2m x 80m (2 yards x 80 yards) with a measured distance of 60'(18.29m) marked off at the start and the finish with the two hurdles. Approximately 40m (40 yards) should be in front of the starting hurdle for gaining speed and 20m (20 yards) after the finish hurdle for stopping.

Directions.
The examinee stands anywhere in the 40 yard run up area facing the measured 60' distance. When ready, the examinee runs progressively faster toward the hurdles achieving maximum speed at the first hurdle. The examinee should maintain maximum speed until after he/she passes the second hurdle. The tester should stand in the middle of the 60' distance and at right angles to the running lane (Note: the perpendicular distance away from the running lane is not specified). The tester starts the stopwatch when the examinee reaches the first hurdle and stops it when the examinee reaches the second hurdle.

Scoring.
The score is the time required to run the 60' distance which is converted to feet per second. Brooks (1981, p. 84) provides a chart for making this conversion.

Norms.
Not reported.

REVIEW

JAMES KLINZING, Ph.D.
Associate Professor
Health, Physical Education and
Recreation
Cleveland State University
Cleveland, Ohio 44115

The purpose of this test is to measure pure sprint running speed in order to identify potential sprinters. The acceleration and deceleration phases of a sprint are eliminated in this test. This is accomplished by using an untimed 40 yard acceleration distance prior to entering the 60 foot timed distance, and since the overall distance is short, deceleration should not occur. The test should consistently identify examinees with the speed required to become potential sprinters. The possibility of inaccurate timing exists, but this can be minimized if two or three timers are used and each examinee is given two or three trials. The time for the best trial should be used to determine peak running velocity.

This test is an efficient means of identifying examinees with natural speed, which can then be further developed for sport activities. An outdoor track or other suitable running space is needed. Because the tester(s) needs to see both the starting and finishing marks, as identified by the hurdles, there must be adequate space so that the tester(s) can be positioned about 40 yards perpendicular away from the center of the timed running area. This will reduce the amount of parallax which will occur from closer distances. The equipment necessary for this test should be readily available and the personnel required to administer the test should be easily recruited and trained.

The time necessary to administer the test will depend upon the size of the group being measured. However, an efficient organization should allow the administration of two or three trials in a reasonable length of time. Although the directions do not clearly indicate the number of trials, more reliable results will be recorded if two or three trials are given with an adequate recovery period of at least five minutes between each trial.

This test can be used in any situation where it is desirable to measure maximum sprint speed. Therefore, it is suitable for both females and males ages six to adult. The necessity for accurate timing limits this test to measurements made by qualified test administrators. Repetitive sprints of this distance could provide a component of a speed training program. Partner monitoring of sprint times may be suitable in such a training situation. The demand for all out effort in this test requires thorough warm up prior to testing to insure maximum performance and for the prevention of injury.

This test could be used in a research situation if the timing is done by automatic timer rather than by hand. The investigators would then be more assured that any changes in time were true indicators of performance. Because no norms are provided, it is suggested that individuals planning to extensively use this test develop their own norms as adequate data becomes available.

SUMMARY

The Speed Curve Test is an excellent test when used to measure maximum running velocity because the acceleration and deceleration phases of sprint are eliminated.

Major Strengths:

1. Identifies examinees with potential for success in sports where speed is essential.

2. The test is very practical to administer, requiring readily available equipment, facilities, and reasonable amounts of time.

3. A velocity chart allows easy conversion of running time to velocity.

Major Weaknesses:

1. More than one trial needs to be administered to insure reliable results.

2. The distance for acceleration should be exact, such as 40 yards, and the examinees being tested should be required to attain maximum speed as soon as possible after starting the sprint to insure maximum speed throughout the 60 foot timed distance.

3. Because of the distance needed to the side of the timing zone, it is only suitable to outdoor testing, unless automatic timing is available.

If used properly, this is an excellent test both for research and teaching situations. It allows teachers, coaches, or investigators to measure maximum running speed accurately. When appropriate motivation, warm up, and timing procedures are used the data collected will be accurate and useful. However, it is not the intended purpose of the test to determine the ability to accelerate at the start of a sprint nor the ability to delay deceleration at the end of a longer sprint. Other testing must be used to measure these important phases of sprinting and appropriate training methods used for their development.

THE SPEED TEST

Reference.
New York State Education Department (1977). *The New York state physical fitness screening test.* Albany, NY: State Department of Education, pp. 12-15, 34-42.

Additional Sources.
None.

Purpose.
To measure an examinee's running speed.

Objectivity.
Not reported.

Reliability.
Test-retest reliability coefficients for boys ranged from .85 to .93 and for girls .75 to .93.

Validity.
Not reported.

Age and Sex.
Suitable for boys and girls, grades 4 - 12.

Equipment.
A stopwatch and two objects, such as plastic cones or Indian clubs, which can be used as turning markers.

Space Requirements and Design.
A clear, level area approximately 5m x 25m (15' x 75') with a distance of 13.72m (45') between the two cones which serve as turning markers. A starting/finishing line approximately 3m (10') long should be drawn through the center of one cone (1.5m to each side) and perpendicular to the line connecting the centers of the two cones. The 1.5m to the right of the cone is the starting line and the 1.5m to the left of the cone is the finishing line. At least 3m (9') of unobstructed space should be allowed beyond the start/finish line so that the examinee will have an adequate distance in which to stop after crossing the finish line. At least 3m (9') of unobstructed space should be left beyond both turning markers so that the examinee will have a safe distance to run around the markers.

Directions.
The examinee takes a standing position behind the starting line to the right of the first cone. At the command, "Ready, Go," the examinee runs forward, around the other cone, and then back and around the cone at the starting line. The examinee runs around each cone in a counterclockwise direction. For grades 4 to 6, a total of two laps should be run and for grades 7 to 12, a total of three laps should be run. If the examinee knocks down either turning cone while running the course, a retrial must be given after a sufficient rest period.

Scoring.
The score is the time, measured to the nearest half-second, it takes to run the required distance.

Norms.
New York (1977, pp. 34-42) boys and girls.

REVIEW

RUSSELL H. LORD, Ed.D.
Professor and Chair
Educational Foundations and
Counseling
Eastern Montana College
Billings, MT 59101-0298

The face validity of having people run around markers placed 45' apart for the purpose of measuring their running speed seems obvious. Less obvious are (1) the possible dimensions of the physical component that may be overlooked by use of a general label for a physical skill, and (2) the ways that administration of the test might distort results.

If one were one to judge the running speeds of a 60m sprinter and a 1500m runner 45' from a common start, how validly would you have measured their respective "running speed?" Would you have only measured different aspects of "running speed?" As research has firmly established, motor skills are more specific than general. Does it not also seem reasonable that fourth grade and twelfth grade males would differ? Similarly, would not different runners' times be affected to different degrees by having to make turns sharply enough to reduce time but not so sharply as to knock over the marker?

These questions raise concerns over the attachment of a generic label "running speed" on the basis of elapsed time in one specific running task.

Will not different boys and girls between the fourth and twelfth grades be affected quite differently by the presence of their peers as either spectators or timers during the performance of a "test" of running speed? Over 100 years of social facilitation research clearly informs us that the presence of others affects motor performance. What is less clear, is the specific facilitation effects of such presence on an individual's performance. Indeed, eleventh grade girls showed the only large drop in test-retest reliability (down to .75 from .89 in eighth grade); which could have been due to many factors, but at least hints at social facilitation effects.

Despite these caveats concerning the validity of general labels and social effects on performance, the Speed Test showed respectably high test-retest reliability when 2,033 boys and girls in grades 5, 8, and 11, were tested with approximately three weeks between test administrations. The objectivity of the Speed Test should be quite high because times are simply recorded from a stopwatch. Of course, inaccurate reading of the watch or sloppy administration of the test could reduce the test's inherent objectivity, but that would be a flaw in a specific administration, not the test itself.

Although variously referred to in the New York Manual as a screening test, a means for evaluating "the total product of the physical education program, or the total effectiveness of any individual teacher," an "aid in planning a program of instruction," and having "the specific function of [this test is the] identification of physically underdeveloped pupils," the Speed Test does not have the kinds of validity data needed to support such claimed uses. Its reliability seems quite acceptable, but validity evidence beyond the face validity referred to earlier is lacking.

The Speed Test is very practical; imposing no administration requirements that should exceed the skills of a practicing educator. About the only instance where the Speed Test might cause confusion is in its use of unusual achievement level norms distributed across 11 equal units. Instead of the use of other, more widely recognized normative scales, the Speed Test norms range "along a theoretical scale of physical fitness" consisting of 11 equal units; the amount of difference in physical fitness being the same from any one level to the next. These achievement levels correspond to a normal distribution, with percentile equivalents clearly matched to achievement levels. Scoring is accomplished very easily, with conversion of raw scores to achievement levels explained clearly, and norm tables that are followed easily.

The Speed Test involves no dangers other than those always associated with having individuals running around in proximity to one another. As a drill for promoting learning or conditioning, The Speed Test seems inappropriate. Again, relying upon the research on specificity of skills, it would seem that only the skilled examinees would learn from training on the Speed Test would be the specific task of running in circles around markers. The task is appropriate for examinees between fourth and twelfth grades, and assumes no prior development of specific skills. Consequently, it seems unlikely that it disadvantages examinees who lack certain background experiences in sport. However, the extent to which it sufficiently discriminates those who are "physically fit" from those who are "physically underdeveloped so that programs of remedial training" can be designed for them is unsupported in the manual, and such discriminability seems unlikely.

Though the normative data are over a decade old, norms are clearly presented for gender and grades 4 to 12. They are based upon sufficiently large groups, and would be extremely easy for any interested practitioner to follow in developing local norms for comparative purposes.

SUMMARY

Major Strengths:

1. Use of facilities and equipment already available in every physical education program.

2. Ease of administration, scoring, and normative comparisons.

3. High reported reliability.

4. High safety factor.

5. Objectivity of scoring.

6. Suitability across the intended age range.

Major Weaknesses:

1. Unknown generalizability of "running speed" as assessed in this specific task.

2. Unknown extent to which the presence of others affects different examinees, especially as they may differ across age and gender.

3. Creation and use of an unique standard scale for the achievement levels.

4. Dated norms.

The Speed Test seems to be an acceptable test; adequate for research and teaching, so long as care is taken to prevent too many inferences about examinees based solely on their test scores. With some well constructed research, up- dating of norms based upon scores obtained from well designed investigations, the Speed Test might well be refined into an excellent test.

Chapter 12

STRENGTH

DYNAMIC - HIGH REPETITION STRENGTH TESTS

YMCA BENCH PRESS TEST

Reference.
Golding, L. A. et al. (eds.) (1989). *Y's way to physical fitness: The complete guide to fitness testing and instruction.* Champaign, IL: Human Kinetics, pp 110-111, 113-124.

Additional Source.
Baumgartner & Jackson (1991, pp. 228, 230).

Purpose.
To measure the strength and endurance of an examinee's arm extensor muscles.

Objectivity.
Not reported.

Reliability.
Not reported.

Validity.
Not reported.

Age and Sex.
Females and males, age 18 - 65 + .

Equipment.
A 15.90kg (35 lb.) barbell for females, a 36.36kg (80 lb.) barbell for males, a metronome, and a weight training bench.

Space Requirements and Design.
A clear, level area approximately 3m (10') square with the bench in the center.

Directions.
The examinee assumes a supine position on the bench with the knees bent 90 degrees and the feet flat on the floor. The tester then places the barbell in the examinee's hands which are shoulder width apart. The examinee begins the test with the weight in the down position just above the chest and the elbows flexed. The examinee presses the weight upward until the elbows are fully extended and then lowers the weight to the original starting position. This sequence equals one repetition. The examinee tries to do as many repetitions as possible, executing each up movement and each down movement in rhythm with the metronome, which is set at 60 beats per minute. The test is terminated when the examinee is unable to fully extend the elbows during the up movement of a given repetition or is unable to keep the proper cadence.

Scoring.
The score is the number of properly completed repetitions.

Norms.
Barrow et al. (1989, pp. 139-140) men and women; Baumgartner & Jackson (1991, p. 230) men and women; Golding et al. (1989, pp. 113-124) men and women.

REVIEW

KATHLEEN E. MILLER, Ph.D.

Professor
Health and Physical Education
Associate Dean, School of Education
University of Montana
Missoula, MT 59812-1055

The YMCA Bench Press Test is one item in a battery of tests. The purpose of the test is to measure strength and endurance of the extensor muscles of the arms. A more accurate description would be that it is a measure of the strength and absolute endurance of the arm extensor muscles. It has been consistently reported in the literature that there is a high positive correlation (.75 to .97) between dynamic strength and absolute dynamic endurance but a very low correlation (.04 to -.19) between dynamic strength and relative dynamic endurance.

This test has demonstrated face validity although no validity has been reported. Measures of reliability and objectivity could easily be determined and should, because of the nature of the test, be quite high.

Administration of the test requires one tester, but he/she should have no affect on the examinee's score.

Equipment and space requirements could be a problem for mass testing. It might be difficult to obtain sufficient numbers of weights and benches. The test is relatively easy to administer. Half of the examinees could spot and count, then trade places to measure the other half. Time for the test is not a problem as a top score of 45 would only require about one and one-half minutes. One trial is all that examinees should be asked to perform since they are expected to continue to the point of fatigue. However, some kind of mild warm up might be in order. Repetition of the test over a period of time would result in conditioning. Norms indicate discrimination by gender and age and appear to have been updated recently.

Two safety problems seem to exist: (1) dropping weights and (2) lower back strain. As fatigue sets in, an examinee could easily drop the weights. This could be resolved by using an actively involved spotter. Because of varying bench heights and body sizes, it may not be possible for all examinees to have their feet flat on the floor with the knees bent at 90 degrees. Consequently, as the examinee starts to experience fatigue, poor lifting technique may begin to appear and the examinee may begin to arch the lower back to help complete the lift. This problem may be solved by having the examinees flex at the knees and hips and place their feet near their buttocks on the end of the bench.

Examinees could score themselves, but self testing with free weights and no spotter is not recommended. Prudent practice requires a spotter.

The bench press test has been used in many research studies to measure relationships between strength and endurance (both relative and absolute). One problem that may exist is that a score of zero is possible with an absolute endurance test. Use of a relative test where the weight is based on a percentage of 1-RM might be desirable in a population where zero is an unacceptable score and/or comparison between examinees is necessary. Absolute tests are appropriate for within examinee comparisons.

SUMMARY

Major Strengths:

1. Face validity is good.

2. Minimal equipment and administrative support are needed.

3. Ease of scoring.

4. Not too time consuming.

5. Can be used as part of a conditioning program.

6. Can be self administered and scored with slight modifications for safety.

7. Good norms.

Major Weaknesses:

1. Safety concern without spotters and for potential back strain problems.

2. Does not differentiate as to when absolute or relative tests are appropriate.

The YMCA Bench Press Test is an acceptable test and is adequate for research and/or teaching with the following cautions/qualifications. Testers need to know exactly at which point an examinee is to be stopped because of not keeping up with the cadence. Does the test stop the first time the examinee is a little off, or does the examinee get "warned" and then continue until the next time the cadence is missed? Many step tests and sit up tests executed to a cadence allow for a "catch up to the cadence" procedure. The within or between examinee comparison question for research is an important distinction that should be addressed so the appropriate absolute or relative measure can be used.

Regardless of how the test results are to be used, the safety factors should not be overlooked. Judicious practice would require the use of a spotter at all times and strong consideration of placing the examinee's feet on the bench rather than on the floor to help alleviate back problems as well as the use of the back and hips to help lift the weight once fatigue becomes a factor.

YMCA LEG EXTENSION STRENGTH TEST

Reference.
Westcoff, W. L. (1987). *Building strength at the YMCA*. Champaign, IL: Human Kinetics, pp 86-87.

Additional Sources.
None.

Purpose.
To measure the strength of an examinee's knee extensor muscles.

Objectivity.
Not reported.

Reliability.
Not reported.

Validity.
Not reported.

Age and Sex.
Not reported, but norms are designed for adult females and males.

Equipment.
A Nautilus leg extension machine, a body weight scale, and a stopwatch.

Space Requirements and Design.
A clear, level area approximately 3m (10') square with the leg extension machine in the center.

Directions.
The examinee's body weight is determined following standard procedures. The selector pin is then placed in the weight stack so that the resistance is approximately 30 percent of the examinee's body weight. The examinee sits on the bench of the machine so that the knee joints are aligned with the machine's axis of rotation and the ankles are behind the roller pad. The examinee then fastens the seat belt and places the hands on the hand grips. Once properly positioned on the machine, the examinee takes 2 seconds to fully extend the knees, holds the extended position for 1 second, and takes 4 seconds to lower the weight stack to a level just above the remaining weights not in use. This sequence marks the completion of one repetition. If the examinee is able to complete 10 such repetitions with the 30 percent resistance, the selector pin is moved in the weight stack to provide a resistance of 40 to 50 percent of the examinee's body weight. After a two minute rest, the examinee tries to complete 10 more repetitions in the same manner described above. If the examinee is able to complete the 10 repetitions with the 40 to 50 percent resistance, the selector pin is once again moved in the weight stack to provide a resistance of 60 to 70 percent of the examinee's body weight. After the examinee is given a two minute rest, he/she tries to complete 10 more repetitions in the manner described above. If the examinee is successful at that percentage, more resistance is added in the same manner until the examinee cannot complete 10 repetitions.

Scoring.
The score is the greatest resistance lifted 10 repetitions by the examinee, divided by her/his body weight.

Norms.
Westcoff (1987, p. 87) men and women.

REVIEW

JAMES M. MANNING, Ph.D.
Associate Professor
Movement Science and Leisure Studies
The William Paterson College of New Jersey
Wayne, NJ 07470

The YMCA Leg Extension Strength Test seems to be a test with several shortcomings. Muscular strength is defined as the maximum force that can be generated by a muscle or muscle group. The measurement of muscular strength has historically been assessed by: (1) one repetition maximum or 1-RM, (2) cable tensiometry, (3) dynamometry, or (4) computerized assessment of strength. These tests have been used extensively and have had their objectivity, reliability, and validity criteria established. Most strength tests aim to obtain the maximum force which can be exerted in one trial thus allowing the measurement of that muscle group's maximum strength.

The specific directions for this test, using variable resistance equipment in order to obtain a maximum strength measure, seems to involve too many repetitions such that fatigue may become a factor. Starting the test at 30 percent of an examinee's body weight seems quite low. Understandably every examinee is different, so specific directions may not be applicable but Westcoff/YMCA should consider a direction such as: select a weight close to but below the examinee's maximum, then add small increments until maximum capacity is achieved. It is generally agreed that the maximum should be obtained in three or four trials in order to eliminate the influence fatigue may play, especially if numerous trials or repetitions are used.

The scoring should be the greatest resistance lifted in one trial not the amount lifted in 10 repetitions, divided by the examinee's body weight.

Specific breathing techniques for performing this type of exercise need to be explained. The specific directions should include, "examinee should exhale during exertion."

This test, for the above reasons, does not consist of suitable precision to be used for research purposes.

Norms are available for females and males.

SUMMARY

Major Strengths:

1. Directions for use of the specific equipment are precise.

2. Norms for females and males are given.

Major Weaknesses:

1. Test does not measure maximal strength as commonly defined in the literature, that is, the test is not valid.

2. Reliability measures are not given.

3. Objectivity measures are not given.

4. This test could be influenced by fatigue in its attempt to obtain a maximum strength measure.

5. Correct breathing procedures are not given.

6. Specific equipment is necessary.

This test does not measure maximal muscular strength as commonly defined in the literature. Without objectivity, validity, and reliability measures adequately established, the use of such a test for research and/or teaching is not recommended.

DYNAMIC - LOW REPETITION STRENGTH TESTS

BENCH PRESS TEST

Reference.
Johnson, B. L., & Nelson, J. K. (1986). *Practical measurements for evaluation in physical education.* Edina, MN: Burgess, pp 111-113, 119-121.

Additional Sources.
Barrow et al. (1989, p. 141); Baumgartner & Jackson (1982, pp. 196, 248); Baumgartner & Jackson (1987, p. 188); Baumgartner & Jackson (1991, p. 227); Clarke & Clarke (1987, p. 174); Hastad & Lacy (1989, pp. 207-208); Safrit (1986, p. 315).

Purpose.
To measure the force producing capability of an examinee's arm and shoulder muscles during a pushing movement.

Objectivity.
r = .97 by Bennett and Long (1972) cited in Johnson and Nelson (1986, p. 111).

Reliability.
r = .93 for test-retest.

Validity.
Face validity.

Age and Sex.
Females and males, age 12 - college.

Equipment.
A 1.5m - 1.8m (5' - 6') long weight lifting bar, an adequate number of weight plates, a bench approximately 1.2m (4') long, and a body weight scale.

Space Requirements and Design.
A clear, level area approximately 3m (10') square with the bench in the center and the weights at one end of the bench.

Directions.
The examinee's body weight is determined following standard procedure. The desired amount of weight is first placed on the bar. The examinee should be familiar with the bench press and the approximate maximum amount of weight that he/she can lift. If the examinee is not familiar with the approximate maximum amount of weight that can be lifted, then the administering of more than two trials may be needed to determine the best score. The examinee takes a supine position on the bench. The bar is placed in the examinee's hands and across the chest by two spotters. The hands are placed approximately shoulder width apart. On command, the examinee pushes the bar away from the chest in a vertical motion until the arms are fully extended with the elbows straight. Upon completion, the spotters remove the bar and place it on the floor. The amount of weight then may be reduced or increased and a second trial allowed. Generally two trials are given, but if both trials are unsuccessful, the weight load may be further reduced and after a brief rest, the examinee retested. Throughout the execution of the bench press, the examinee's head, shoulders, and buttocks must remain in contact with the bench.

Scoring.
The score is derived by dividing the maximum weight the examinee lifted by the examinee's body weight.

Norms.
Baumgartner & Jackson (1982, p. 200) men and women; Baumgarnter & Jackson (1987, p. 181) college football players; Baumgartner & Jackson (1991, pp. 221, 229) college football players, men and women; Greenberg & Pargman (1989, p. 80) men and women; Hoeger (1986, pp. 35, 39) men and women; Johnson & Nelson (1986, p. 113) men and women; Miller (1988, p. 172) men and women; Pollock & Wilmore (1990, pp. 349, 672-683) men and women; Pollock, Wilmore & Fox (1978, p. 106) men and women on a weight machine; Shannon (1989, p. 45) high school football players.

REVIEW

THOMAS E. BALL, Ph.D.

Assistant Professor
Physical Education
Northern Illinois University
DeKalb, IL 60115

The Bench Press Test for maximal lifting capacity is a test commonly used to assess muscular strength. The difficulty in determining the validity of the Bench Press Test as a measure of muscular strength lies with the reluctance of the scientific community to come to a common, acceptable definition of muscular strength. This debate is reviewed by Atha (1981) and he concludes by proposing that strength be defined "as the ability to develop force against an unyielding resistance in a single contraction of unrestricted duration." Given this definition of strength, the Bench Press Test is not a valid measure of muscular strength. If we adopt the more common definition that strength is the ability of a muscle group to develop force in a single maximum effort, then we can accept the Bench Press Test as having face validity as a measure of muscular strength.

The reliability of the Bench Press Test is acceptably high, and if the instructions are precisely followed and the tester well trained, reliability coefficients of r. = 95 can be achieved. In addition, the objectivity of the Bench Press Test is also acceptably high, again if all testers are trained and follow the instructions precisely. A problem with the Bench Press Test, as with many other tests, is that the tester can significantly alter test results if not sufficiently trained, or if instructions are not followed precisely.

The Bench Press Test does appear to be a practical test with space and equipment costs being moderate. In addition, the bench can be any bench of sufficient size and strength, and does not need to be an expensive bench press bench. The test is relatively easy to administer. It requires only one trained tester and possibly one or two spotters. One major drawback to the Bench Press Test is that it requires approximately 10 to 15 minutes to test one examinee. With only one bench and one tester, it could take several periods to test a class.

The test may be used with a wide variety of people and with a large age range. There is concern about prepubescent children doing maximal bench press tests and about using the test with the aged. In addition, there is the possibility that an examinee could drop a weight or strain a muscle. Personal experience suggests that this seldom happens if the examinee is trained in the appropriate technique and warmed up prior to the test.

Another advantage of the test is that it is easily scored, the score simply being the total weight lifted. Examinees can score themselves without having to wait for the tester to explain the procedure to them. Many people recommend using what is referred to as relative strength. To arrive at relative strength, the absolute strength score is divided by body weight. This results in a unitless ratio. The interpretation of this ratio is difficult at best. The procedure may unfairly disadvantage people with larger muscle masses (Ball, 1989).

While the test has been used for research purposes, the debate in the scientific community over the definition of strength, and the precision of the test (the accuracy is +/- 5 pounds) limits its usefulness in a research setting.

Norms are available for the Bench Press Test for a variety of groups. (Baumgartner & Jackson, 1987; Heyward, 1984; Pollock et al., 1984).

SUMMARY

In summary, the Bench Press Test does measure the ability of the chest and arm musculature to develop force in a single maximal contraction. The test can be easily administered and scored and only requires a moderate amount of equipment. The Bench Press Test should not be used with prepubescent children or aged adults, and may take several hours to administer to a group. The Bench Press Test is a very good test for teaching and/or for fitness evaluations. It gives a more accurate measure of the functional capacity of muscles than a calisthenic test (e.g., push ups). The acceptability of the Bench Press Test for research is more limited due to its precision. One may add five pounds but no less than five pounds may be added at one time, so one examinee may actually be able to lift 179 pounds and another examinee 176 pounds but they both receive scores of 175 pounds.

REVIEW REFERENCES

Atha, J. (1981). Strengthening muscle. In Miller, D. J. (ed.). *Exercise and Sport Science Reviews,* Vol. 9. Salt Lake City: The Franklin Institute Press.

Ball, T. E. (1989). Unpublished data.

Baumgartner, T. A., & Jackson, A. S. (1987). *Measurement for evaluation.* Dubuque: Wm. C. Brown.

Heyward, V. H. (1984). *Designs for fitness.* Minneapolis: Burgess.

Pollock, M. C., Wilmore, J. H., & Fox, S. M. (1984). *Exercise in health and disease.* Philadelphia: W. B. Saunders.

BENCH SQUAT TEST

Reference.
Johnson, B. L., & Nelson, J. K. (1986). *Practical measurements for evaluation in physical education.* Edina, MN: Burgess, pp 108-109.

Additional Sources.
Johnson & Nelson (1986, p. 118-120); Safrit (1986, pp. 309-311); Safrit (1990, pp. 478, 480).

Purpose.
To measure an examinee's leg and back strength in lowering to, and standing from, a seated position.

Objectivity.
r = .99 was derived by Recio (1972) cited in Johnson and Nelson (1986, p. 108).

Reliability.
r = .95 for test-retest.

Validity.
Face validity.

Age and Sex.
Females and males, age 12 - college.

Equipment.
A 1.5m - 1.8m (5' - 6') long weight lifting bar, an adequate number of weight plates, a thick towel for padding the bar, a bench which can be adjusted to knee cap level, and a body weight scale.

Space Requirements and Design.
A clear, level area approximately 3m (10') square with the bench, bar, and the examinee in the center.

Directions.
The examinee's body weight is determined following standard procedure. The desired amount of weight is then loaded on the bar. The examinee stands close to the bench, which is knee cap level, with her/his feet a comfortable distance apart. Two spotters place the bar in the examinee's hands and on the examinee's shoulders behind the neck. On command, the examinee lowers to a seated position on the bench while keeping her/his back erect. The examinee then returns to a standing position without using any type of rocking motion. The two spotters remove the bar and the amount of

weight may then either be reduced or increased for a second trial. If the examinee is not familiar with the lift, it may take more than two trials to derive a maximum effort. The amount of weight may be reduced if the first trial is unsuccessful. If the second trial is unsuccessful, the weight may be further reduced and after a brief rest, the examinee is retested.

Scoring.
The score is derived by dividing the maximum weight the examinee lifted, on the best of two trials, by the examinee's body weight.

Norms.
Johnson & Nelson (1986, p. 109) men and women; Shannon (1989, p. 45) high school football players.

REVIEW

JAMES E. GRAVES, Ph.D.
Assistant Research Scientist
College of Medicine
University of Florida
Gainesville, FL 32610

The Bench Squat Test is a one repetition maximum (1-RM) test that measures the strength of the knee and hip extensors (primarily the quadriceps and gluteus muscles). The observed 1-RM load is divided by body weight to produce a relative measure of muscular strength. Although it is stated in the description of the test that the purpose is "to measure an examinee's leg and back strength . . .," it is questionable if the test can provide a valid measure of back strength. The back muscles are important stabilizers for this exercise but they are not prime movers. To accurately quantify the strength of the lumbar extensors, pelvic stabilization is required.

The test may be applied to females and males ranging in age from 12 years to well beyond college age, although norms exist only for college men and women. Reliability and objectivity are sufficiently established and are generally not a limitation associated with 1-RM testing. Like all 1-RM tests, the Bench Squat Test is limited to identifying strength at the weakest position in the range of motion (often referred to as the "critical joint angle" or "sticking point"). The test provides little or no information about strength through the full range of motion of the particular muscle groups involved.

The knee and hip extensors are large muscle groups that play an important role in many sport related activities. Thus, there is a high degree of practical application for the Bench Squat Test. The test is suitable as a drill to promote conditioning and lifting technique. However, proper instruction is required to achieve these goals.

Because the muscles involved in the Bench Squat Test are relatively large, powerful muscles, heavy weight loads are usually required to obtain the 1-RM. Thus, safety is a major concern. Two spotters are required to handle the weight and monitor the test. A third spotter, to stand behind the examinee and guide the movement, should be encouraged. The examinee must be instructed to carefully control the descent to avoid extreme compression forces on the spine. The use of a squat rack instead of a bench is strongly recommended to minimize the risk of injury. Pins can be placed on the rack to indicate the correct height for lowering the weight and facilitate test standardization.

The test requires only standard weight lifting equipment, a scale to determine body weight, an adjustable bench (or preferably a squat rack), and a minimal amount of floor space. The equipment required is relatively inexpensive and can be used to perform many strength tests. The test is easy to administer but inexperienced testers may not be efficient at selecting appropriate amounts of weight. Experienced testers can obtain the 1-RM with a minimal number of trials which can minimize fatigue that is often associated with multiple trial strength tests.

There is a considerable amount of technique involved in the proper execution of the squat exercise. Therefore, skilled examinees may have an advantage and score higher than novice examinees regardless of their true level of strength.

It may be advantageous to have examinees practice the proper execution of the bench squat with a light resistance prior to initiation of the test to minimize the influence of variations in technique on the strength measurement.

When properly administered, the test is suitable as a criterion measure for research purposes. This is especially true when a strength test requiring a component of skill is desired. The bench squat exercise itself may provide an effective training modality for strength training research. When lifting technique is an undesirable variable, a leg press test on any of a number of commercially available weight training machines may provide a suitable alternative to the bench squat exercise to measure hip and leg strength.

SUMMARY

Major Strengths:

1. The test is easy to administer.

2. Objectivity and reliability are high.

3. Major muscle groups are tested. Thus, a high degree of practical application exists.

4. The equipment required is inexpensive and can be used for other strength tests.

5. Space requirements are minimal.

Major Weaknesses:

1. Two or preferably three spotters are required.

2. One repetition maximum testing is limited to the weakest position in the range of motion.

3. There is a component of skill that may influence the results.

4. Heavy weight loads may be required.

The Bench Squat Test is an acceptable test for measuring the 1-RM strength of the hip and knee extensors. Because the test will often involve lifting heavy loads, safety is a primary concern. The use of a squat rack rather than a bench is recommended. The test is adequate for research purposes and as a training exercise when administered properly and adequate attention is given to lifting technique.

DIP STRENGTH TEST

Reference.
Johnson, B. L., & Nelson, J. K. (1986). *Practical measurements for evaluation in physical education.* Edina, MN: Burgess, pp 105-108.

Additional Source.
Miller (1988, p. 181).

Purpose.
To measure an examinee's arm and shoulder strength in vertical descending and push up movements.

Objectivity.
r = .99 derived by Prestidge (1972) cited in Johnson and Nelson (1986, p. 105).

Reliability.
r = .98 for test-retest.

Validity.
Face validity.

Age and Sex.
Males, age 12 - college.

Equipment.
A body weight scale, weight plates, straps, chair, and parallel bars positioned high enough so the examinee's feet will not touch the floor when he assumes a lowered bent arm position. The bars should be approximately shoulder width apart.

Space Requirements and Design.
A clear, level area approximately 3m (10') square with parallel bars mounted to a wall or with a set of gymnastic parallel bars positioned in the center. The chair is positioned in front of the bars.

Directions.
The examinee's body weight is determined following standard procedure. The examinee straps the preferred amount of weight to his waist and then steps up on the chair. The examinee then assumes a straight arm support position on the parallel bars and the chair is removed. On command, the examinee lowers his body until the tester indicates the elbows are at a right angle. With a vertical push, the examinee returns to a straight arm support position and the chair is placed under the examinee's feet. The

examinee then steps off the chair. The examinee may either reduce or increase the amount of weight used for a second trial. If the examinee is not familiar with his approximate maximum, the administering of more than two trials may be needed to determine the best score. During the vertical push, the examinee cannot swing or kick.

Scoring.
The score is derived by dividing the examinee's maximum weight lifted, during the best of two trials, by his body weight. An examinee who is unable to perform the movement with no extra weight is given a score of zero.

Norms.
Johnson & Nelson (1986, p. 107) men.

NOTE: The motivation and measurement of examinees unable to perform one dip using their own body weight may be achieved by the following method. A one inch interval scale is attached along and perpendicular to the parallel bars in line with the movement of the shoulders. The examinee's score is determined by measuring the distance obtained in the upward push motion in relation to the straight arm support position. For example, an examinee who comes within two inches of obtaining the straight arm support position would receive a higher score than an examinee coming within four inches of the straight arm position.

REVIEW

THOMAS J. KILROY, M.Ed.

Assistant Professor
Physical Education
Paul Smiths College
Paul Smiths, NY 12970

All of the scientific aspects of this test seem to be appropriate with the possible exception of age and sex. This will be expanded in subsequent paragraphs.

The practical aspects of the test are generally in order but a few questions remain. Facility and space requirements should pose no problem as should the equipment necessary. This reviewer would prefer to use a squat belt with a chain attached for the test. This piece of equipment is available commercially and may be referred to as a dip belts. The use of the word "straps" could be confusing and are not fully explained. Administering the test and the time needed to do so should be no problem if only two trials are the rule. If, however, the tester is trying to establish a one repetition maximum (1-RM), it is doubtful if most examinees can be measured accurately with only two trials. It is also doubtful if two trials are sufficient or reliable in terms of a 1-RM which defines strength.

This test is very suitable for learning and conditioning as it is synonymous with the principle of overload. The more it is practiced, the more strength is affected.

This reviewer has strong reservations about the suitability of the test, especially for preteens and late adolescents. The reviewer's experience with middle/junior high school students is that this muscle group is very undeveloped and is the weakest area of the body at this age. The test will not discriminate among its intended users.

The test does have some dangerous aspects. What would happen if the examinee were unable to support the weight and fall beneath the bars causing trauma to the shoulder complex? Examinees need to be instructed on how to release or fall between the bars.

The scoring of the test is objective and the results are easily interpreted for self evaluation. The norms may present a problem. The test needs more up to date norms and, norms for younger age groups. This test is unsuitable for research purposes.

SUMMARY

Major Strengths:

1. Its validity.

2. Ease of administration.

3. Simplicity of equipment required.

4. Its drill and conditioning value.

Major Weaknesses:

1. Its suitability for early teens and/or prepubescent boys.

2. Safety aspects.

3. Lack of up to date and suitable norms.

4. Its research value.

This test is an acceptable test for the purpose purported. The test needs further application to examinees under the age of 18. With the seeming lack of norms for that population and the age of the norms, the test is in need of further research.

ONE REPETITION MAXIMUM (1-RM) LEG STRENGTH TESTS

Reference.
Baumgartner, T. A., & Jackson, A. S. (1987). *Measurement for evaluation in physical education*. Dubuque: Wm. C. Brown, pp 193, 196.

Additional Sources.
Baumgartner & Jackson (1982, pp. 200-201); Baumgartner & Jackson (1991, pp. 233-235); Safrit (1986, pp. 303-308); Safrit (1990, pp. 473-477); Verducci (1980, pp. 245-246).

Purpose.
To measure the maximum force producing capability of an examinee's hip and knee extensor muscles.

Objectivity.
Not reported.

Reliability.
Not reported.

Validity.
Construct validity was established.

Age and Sex.
Not reported, but suitable for children through adult.

Equipment.
A goniometer and a Universal gym or similar weight training machine.

Space Requirements and Design.
A clear, level area approximately 5m (15') square with the Universal gym in the center.

Directions.
Baumgartner and Jackson recommend two different tests (leg press and leg extension) to measure leg strength. The examinees should practice the tests prior to test day so they will know approximately what they can lift 1-RM. A weight that the examinee can lift easily the first trial is recommended.

Leg Press

The examinee sits in the leg press station's chair and adjusts it so her/his knees are at a 120 degree angle. The tester checks the angle with the goniometer. On command, the examinee grasps the handles and exerts maximum force with her/his hip and knee extensor muscles in an effort to fully straighten the legs. The examinee then returns her/his legs to the starting position. Weight is added each trial until the maximum value is determined.

Leg Extension

(Also known as Knee Extension) - The examinee sits on the bench of the leg extension machine and leans slightly backward with one hand gripping each side of the bench. The examinee's knees are bent 90 degrees so that her/his lower legs hang vertically behind the padded lever arm of the machine. On command, the examinee exerts maximum force with her/his knee extensor muscles in an effort to fully straighten the legs. The examinee then returns her/his legs to the starting position and adds weight each trial until the maximum value is determined.

Scoring.
The score for each test is the maximum amount of weight used in the completion of one of the trials. The examinee may have as many trials as needed to determine the maximum effort.

Norms.
Baumgartner & Jackson (1982, p. 200) men and women for leg press; Baumgartner & Jackson (1987, pp. 181, 196) college football players, men and women, for leg press and leg extension; Baumgartner & Jackson (1991, pp. 221, 235) college football players, men and women, for leg press and leg extension;

Greenberg & Pargman (1989, p. 80) men and women for leg press; Hoeger (1986, p. 39) men and women for leg extension and leg press; Miller (1988, p. 172) men and women for leg press; Pollock, et al. (1978, p. 106) men and women for leg press;

Pollock & Wilmore (1990, p. 350) men and women; Safrit (1986, pp. 305, 307) men and women for leg extension and leg press; Safrit (1990, pp. 475, 477) men and women for leg extension and leg press.

REVIEW

JAMES B. GALE, Ph.D.

Professor
Physical Education and Health
Sciences
Sonoma State University
Rohnert Park, CA 94928

The strength tests described are typical of dynamic (isotonic) maximal strength tests. Examinees are asked to lift increasing weights until a maximum weight is determined by failure to lift the next weight in the series. The validity of these tests is affected by the volitional effort applied by the examinee and by fatigue. Learning curves have been demonstrated for strength testing and it is important that examinees be familiar with the test equipment and that they have attempted maximal lifts prior to the actual testing.

The tests are valid, within the constraints noted above. However, because there may be a learning curve, the tests may not be reliable unless previous practice sessions have been utilized. Because motivation is a factor affecting 1-RM testing, it is important to give the same instructions and encouragement to all examinees. Either the same tester should administer all of the tests or administration should be practiced by all testers for uniformity. In addition, it is important to provide a warm up period and to establish a constant recovery interval between each of the trials. Examinees may not be willing to exert maximally if they fear injury from lack of warm up; there will be a great deal of variability in recovery intervals if this is left to the discretion of the examinees.

The tests take only the space needed for the stationary equipment. Many facilities have some type of resistive training equipment which utilizes weight stacks that can be adjusted quickly. However, the results cannot be accurately compared from one machine to another. Mechanical leverage differences and even maintenance and lubrication of the equipment will affect results. This is an important factor to consider when performing pretesting and posttesting with equipment which has been used for training during the interim period.

The tests are simple to administer in that only one tester is required, and the time to complete a test is short. On the other hand, if the test is to be reliable, previous training must be performed to reduce the effects of the learning curve (see above). A single 1-RM test may not yield true maximal strength, and, if accuracy is important, pretesting should be used in order to begin the actual test at a weight near maximum in order to reduce the number of trials and the subsequent fatigue. One-RM efforts have been suggested as a part of strength training programs and if used regularly this could improve the validity of the posttest (though the validity of the strength training study, itself, may be compromised.)

The tests can be used with any age group for whom the equipment is intended. Leg length may preclude the use of the knee extension test for some shorter examinees. Certain precautions should be taken to protect the examinee from injury. Both of these tests may be contraindicated for examinees with a previous knee joint injury, instability, or a history of patellar dislocation. There is always the risk of serious musculotendinous injury when a maximal effort is performed and the investigator should determine if the need to know is worth the risk, however minimal. Slippage of the leg below the footplate can also result in serious injury.

Scoring is objective if the tester requires a consistent range of movement. Resolution is limited by the difference in weights between the plates in the stack. Smaller weights which can be added to the stack are recommended. While the absolute values determined may not be transferable to other laboratories, this type of testing has been accepted in published reports of the effects of strength training methods.

Because of the differences in equipment, norms would be of little value. If the equipment is well maintained it would be possible to establish norms for examinees tested at a particular site with the same machine.

SUMMARY

These tests are acceptable and similar to tests which are used for both research and to evaluate the results of strength training programs. They are simple to administer and pose little risk to healthy examinees. They require equipment which is available in many institutions and are suited to a broad range of ages and body sizes. However, because these, and all other strength tests, may be affected by learning and motivation, care must be given to the interpretation of the results. Because the type of equipment and its state of repair may affect the values, comparison of results between sites must be performed cautiously.

ONE REPETITION MAXIMUM (1-RM) UPPER BODY STRENGTH TESTS

Reference.
Baumgartner, T. A., & Jackson, A. S. (1987). *Measurement for evaluation in physical education.* Dubuque: Wm. C. Brown, pp 186-193.

Additional Sources.
Baumgartner & Jackson (1982, pp. 196-197, 248); Baumgartner & Jackson (1991, pp. 227-229); Bosco & Gustafson (1983, p. 86); Hastad & Lacy (1989, pp. 204-207); Safrit (1986, pp. 303-308, 312-318); Safrit (1990, pp. 473-477); Verducci (1980, pp. 245-246).

Purpose.
To measure the maximum force producing capability of an examinee's upper body muscles.

Objectivity.
Not reported.

Reliability.
Not reported.

Validity.
Construct validity was established.

Age and Sex.
Not reported, but suitable for children through adult.

Equipment.
An Universal gym or similar weight training machine.

Space Requirements and Design.
A clear, level area with the Universal gym positioned in the center.

Directions.
Baumgartner and Jackson recommend three different tests (Bench Press, Curls, and Latissimus Dorsi Pull, more commonly known as the Lat. Pull) to measure upper body strength. The examinees should practice the tests prior to test day so that they will know approximately what they can lift 1-RM. The examinees should use a weight that they can easily lift during the first trial of each test and continually increase the amount of weight each trial until they reach their maximum values.

Bench Press
The examinee assumes a supine position on the bench at the bench press station. The examinee can use any grip greater than shoulder width.

Throughout the test the examinee must keep her/his back flat on the bench and her/his feet on the floor. A successful lift is credited when the examinee pushes the weight upward until the elbows are fully extended.

Curls
The examinee stands with the shoulders and buttocks against a wall and the feet 30cm to 38cm (12" - 15") from the wall. A sheet of paper is placed behind the buttocks. The examinee must keep the paper pinned against the wall and should it fall during the lift, that particular trial is not counted. The low pulley station is so positioned that when the examinee holds the bar of the weight machine with the arms straight, the weight to be lifted is held slightly above the extra weights. A successful lift is credited when the examinee completely flexes the elbows and the bar touches the chin.

Lat. Pull
The examinee grips the bar of the lat. station and kneels below it. The arms should be straight. A successful lift is credited when the examinee pulls the bar down behind the head to a level even with the top of the shoulders.

Scoring.
The score for each test is the maximum amount of weight used in the completion of one of the trails. The examinee may have as many trials as needed to determine her/his maximum effort.

Norms.
Baumgartner & Jackson (1982, pp. 197, 199) men for bench, curl and lat. pull; Baumgartner & Jackson (1987, pp. 189-190, 193) men and women for bench press, curl, and lat. pull; Baumgartner & Jackson (1991, p. 299) men and women for bench, curl, and lat. pull;

Hoeger (1986, pp. 35, 39) men and women for curl and lat. pull; Miller (1988, p. 172) men and women on weight machine; Pollock et al. (1978, p. 106) men and women for the bench press and curl; Safrit (1986, pp. 305, 307) men and women for curl and lat. pull; Safrit (1990, pp. 475, 477) men and women for bench, curl, and lat. pull.

REVIEW

BEN R. LONDEREE, Ed.D.

Associate Professor
Physical Education
University of Missouri
Columbia, MO 65211

The tests were described originally by Jackson and Smith in 1974 at the National Convention of AAHPERD. They were published first in the 1982 edition of the current source. In 1982 the primary procedure was to use a constant weight and measure the number of repetitions to failure (absolute endurance); the 1-RM approach was listed as an alternative. The current source describes both forms of the tests but emphasizes the 1-RM format.

The 1-RM versions are valid by definition (i.e., isotonic strength typically is defined as the 1-RM value). The objectivities and reliabilities of the tests were not reported by the test constructors; however, Johnson and Nelson (1986) reported a reliability of .93 and an objectivity of .97 for the bench press.

The description of the arm curl test was not clear in the 1987 version. The 1982 version showed a photograph with the examinee using the Universal low pulley station. As such, the position of the machine relative to a wall will influence the angle of the resistance; the picture showed the chain at about a 30 degree angle to the floor. Examinee height will modify this angle some.

Universal equipment was recommended by the test constructors. Since users should develop their own norms, other equipment probably could be substituted as long as the procedures are standardized and the equipment is similar to that described here. Since strength is influenced by examinee size, norms should be provided for different body weights.

To insure that examinees adhere to proper procedures, a tester must be at each station. One tester probably could observe more than one station by alternating; in other words, observe one station while another examinee is getting ready at a second station. Other individuals could assist and spot, but a skilled tester should judge for proper execution.

Time of administration is a problem with 1-RM tests. However, if the examinees have practiced on previous days, they should know their proper weights and be able to reduce the number of trials.

Tests involving maximal effort involve some risk, especially if examinees do not warm up properly. In addition, spotting by other individuals is imperative to avoid accidents; this is important particularly when using free weights.

SUMMARY

Major Strengths:

1. Valid tests of upper body strength when administered properly.

2. Reliable and objective when administered with appropriate standardization of procedures.

Major Weaknesses:

1. Tests are time consuming with inexperienced examinees.

2. Tests require expensive equipment as described.

In summary, these tests are excellent for research and teaching. They appear to be valid, reliable, and objective when administered properly. Users will need to develop local norms. The tests are time consuming if the examinees are inexperienced. The description of the arm curl test is vague regarding equipment positioning. Equipment substitutions probably are acceptable as long as standard procedures and local norms are used. Appropriate warm up and spotting should be used.

REVIEW REFERENCE

Johnson, B. L., & Nelson, J. K. (1986). *Practical measurements for evaluation in physical education,* Edina, MN: Burgess.

PULL-UP WITH WEIGHTS TEST

Reference.
Johnson, B. L., & Nelson, J. K. (1986). *Practical measurements for evaluation in physical education.* Edina, MN: Burgess, pp 105-106.

Additional Sources.
Miller (1988, pp. 175-177); Safrit (1986, pp. 311-312); Safrit (1990, p. 481).

Purpose.
To measure an examinee's arm and shoulder strength in the pull up movement.

Objectivity.
r = .99 was derived by Taylor (1972) cited in Johnson and Nelson (1986, p. 105).

Reliability.
r = .93 for test-retest.

Validity.
Face validity.

Age and Sex.
Males, age 12 - college.

Equipment.
A horizontal bar or chinning bar which is high enough to prevent the tallest examinee's feet from touching the floor when hanging in a straight arm position, an adequate number of weight plates, a chair, and a strap used to fasten the weight plates around the examinee's waist, and a body weight scale.

Space Requirements and Design.
A clear, level area approximately 2m (6') square with the horizontal bar in the center.

Directions.
The examinee's body weight is determined following standard procedure. The examinee straps the preferred amount of weight around his waist and then steps up on to the chair. The examinee takes a firm grip on the bar with his palms forward (i.e., forearms pronated) and about shoulder width apart. The chair is removed and the examinee assumes a straight arm hanging position with his feet above the floor. On command, the examinee exerts a maximum pull in an upward motion until his chin is above the bar. The chair is then replaced under the examinee who lowers his feet until contact is made. The examinee is assisted off the chair. The examinee may reduce or increase the amount of weight to be used for a second trial. During the upward movement, the examinee's legs must remain straight and the body cannot be permitted to swing.

Scoring.
The score is derived by taking the maximum weight the examinee lifted on the best of two trials and dividing it by the examinee's body weight. An examinee who is unable to perform the movement with no extra weight is given a score of zero.

Norms.
Johnson & Nelson (1986, p. 106) men.

NOTE: The motivation and measurement of examinees who are unable to pull up their own body weight may be achieved by the following method. A cloth tape is hung from the center of the bar so that the examinee's chin slides along the tape as he pulls upward. The score is determined by how close the chin is raised in relation to the bar. A score of a minus three means the examinee was able to raise his chin to within three inches of the bar.

REVIEW

BARRY BEEDLE, Ed.D.
Associate Professor
Health, Physical Education and
Leisure
Elon College
Elon College, NC 27244-2177

The test is valid, to some degree, but because the test constructors used face validity, validity is assumed and not actually demonstrated. If a quantitative assessment had been used, validity would be higher if the test were better at discriminating among examinees. The test-retest reliability is good, but the test constructors did not mention who served as examinees. Moreover, objectivity was not determined by the test constructors, but reported by Taylor. They should have obtained an objectivity coefficient. The test has the advantage of not requiring the active participation of another individual.

Space and facility requirements are not a problem as long as there are an adequate number of pull up bars and weight plates. The test is easy to administer, but the tester can only administer the test to one examinee at a time. The number of trials is adequate, and taking the best score seems to be the practical thing to do. Because of the time it takes to add plates, this is probably not an adequate test to use as a drill.

The test is suitable for the intended age levels but it does not discriminate as well as it should, mainly because it is the type of test that is not practiced much, if not at all, and, therefore, is fairly difficult to perform. There are other tests which discriminate more effectively for arm and shoulder strength (e.g., Baumgartner's Modified Pull-Up Test and the Modified Pull-Up Test from the National Children and Youth Fitness Study II). There are no dangerous aspects to the test. The scoring appears to be objective; however, an explanation should be given as to why a score of zero is given to those who can perform the movement but without any extra weight. For those who cannot perform one pull up, the modification is helpful, but how does a score on the modified version correspond to a score on the "regular" test? Since a calculation is necessary to determine the final test score, there is an increased chance that incorrect scores could be recorded if examinees determine their own

scores. Because the score is in continuous units, it is harder to understand the meaning of the score.

This test would be suitable for research purposes if a quantitative measure and large enough value of validity had been reported. Norms are available for college men, but the norms are outdated (1976) as reported in Johnson and Nelson's (1986) textbook.

SUMMARY

Major Strengths:

1. The test demonstrated good reliability and the test constructors reported good objectivity.

2. The test is relatively easy to administer and does not require expensive equipment.

Major Weakness:

1. The test does not discriminate well enough to gather an adequate amount of information about the examinees. Most tests of this type, designed to assess upper arm and shoulder strength, do not discriminate well enough because of the number of examinees who cannot perform one pull up. It is an exercise that is not performed very often by most individuals.

This is an acceptable test which is adequate for teaching but not for research. The test would not demonstrate satisfactory discrimination, has not been shown to have quantitative validity, is somewhat time consuming to administer, and has not been demonstrated satisfactorily to be important to health or in sports skill performance.

SIT-UP WITH WEIGHTS TEST

Reference.
Johnson, B. L., & Nelson, J. K. (1986). *Practical measurements for evaluation in physical education.* Edina, MN: Burgess, pp 108-110.

Additional Sources.
Miller (1988, p. 173); Safrit (1986, p. 312).

Purpose.
To measure the force producing capability of an examinee's abdominal muscles.

Objectivity.
r = .98 was derived by Garcia (1972) cited in Johnson and Nelson (1986, p. 108).

Reliability.
r = .91 for test-retest.

Validity.
Face validity.

Age and Sex.
Females and males, age 12 - college.

Equipment.
A mat, a body weight scale, a 1.52m - 1.82m (5' - 6') long weight lifting bar, dumbbell bar, a ruler, marking tape, and an adequate variety of weight plates.

Space Requirements and Design.
A clear, level area approximately 2m (6)' square with the mat in the center.

Directions.
The examinee's body weight is determined following standard procedures. The examinee may perform the sit up using either a weight plate, a dumbbell, or a barbell held behind the neck. Weight plates with a circumference no larger than a standard five pound plate can be used on the barbell or dumbbell. The examinee takes the preferred amount of weight and places it on the mat in a position from which it can easily be positioned against the back of the neck when he/she reclines on the mat. The examinee flexes her/his knees in order to hold a ruler under them. The examinee then slides the feet outward until the ruler drops from under the knees. The position of the feet when the ruler drops, determines the placement of the heels in relation to the buttocks. A strip of tape is placed at the back of the heels and in front of the buttocks to show where each must remain during the sit up. On command, the examinee grips the weight, holds it behind the neck and raises the trunk of the body until her/his back is vertical. A partner should then remove the weight completing the first trial. The examinee may then reduce or increase the amount of weight to be used for a second trial.

Scoring.
The score is derived by taking the maximum weight the examinee lifted during the best of two trials and dividing it by her/his body weight. An examinee who is unable to perform the movement with no extra weight is given a score of zero.

Norms.
Johnson & Nelson (1986, p. 110) men and women.

REVIEW

N. KAY COVINGTON, Ph.D.

Assistant Professor
Health, Recreation and Physical
Education
Southern Illinois University at
Edwardsville
Edwardsville, IL 62026-1126

The Sit-Up Test with Weights was developed as a measure of muscular strength of the abdominal muscles. The test is an indicator of abdominal strength, but is a measure of the trunk flexors. Even though the lower legs are not stabilized during the sit up, it is very difficult for the examinee to execute the sit up without involving the trunk flexors. Therefore, the test seems only to have satisfactory face validity. Reliability has been obtained and scores are consistent across multiple trials with the same examinees. The test is easy to score and objectivity is excellent. The endpoint of the test is when the examinee reaches vertical. Testers need to be clear as to what constitutes vertical, so that the endpoint for each examinee and trial is consistent.

The space requirements are appropriate and testing facilities will usually have access to a mat. The standard weight equipment may be problematic, since execution of each trial is dependent on the correct poundage.

Placing a weight plate, dumbbell, or a barbell behind the neck poses safety concerns. As a sit up without weight is performed, the examinee should be curling or rolling the body up to the vertical position. Placing a weight plate, dumbbell, or barbell behind the neck raises the examinee's center of gravity so that curling or rolling become more difficult. Lower back injuries tend to occur when the examinee does not curl or roll. Also, if the examinee does not curl or roll, the abdominals are not utilized as effectively and the lower back becomes a dominant assistant. In essence, the sit up test no longer measures primarily abdominal strength, but measures lower back strength. Because of the concern related to safety with this test, a major change is recommended in the protocol associated with the usage and placement of the weight plate, dumbbell, or barbell. Examinees may find that using a barbell behind the neck is difficult to balance. Therefore, curling or rolling to a vertical position may be awkward and clumsy. One recommendation is the elimination of the barbell suggested weight equipment. The weight plate or dumbbell is appropriate equipment for this test. The second recommendation concerns the placement of the weight plate or dumbbell. The weight plate or dumbbell should be placed on the chest with the arms crossed and the plate held with both hands. This reduces the stress placed on the lower back and decreases the chance of injury by enabling the examinee to curl or roll more effectively and decrease the involvement of the lower back muscles.

The test is suitable for the age levels designated, but the scoring assumes that an examinee can perform a sit up with weight. Possibly, an examinee who is unable to perform a sit up with weight would be able to do a sit up without weight. The tester could use the norms for the sit up without weight for those examinees who cannot perform with weight. The norms in Johnson and Nelson (1986) were developed from college age examinees, yet the test is recommended for females and males, aged 12 to college. The norms do not address the 12 to 18 year old population.

SUMMARY

Major Strengths:

1. The test is reliable, objective, and has face validity for abdominal strength and trunk flexion.

2. Even without norms for the 12 to 18 year old population, the test has value as a pretest and posttest for measuring strength.

3. The test is easy to administer.

Major Weaknesses:

1. With the established protocol, injury of the lower back is a major concern.

2. Normative data are available for only the college aged population.

3. Use of the barbell may be ineffective as weight for the sit up.

4. Examinees may have difficulty executing a correct sit up with the weight plate and/or dumbbell behind the neck.

5. The test assumes that an examinee can efficiently perform a sit up.

The Sit-Up with Weight is recommended for field testing of abdominal strength and trunk flexion, with the suggested change in protocol. The test is more effective with trained examinees (e.g., athletes) who can usually perform a sit up. The test is not as effective with novice or untrained examinees. It is not recommended for use with examinees aged 12 to 18 years since normative data is unavailable for this group. For the 12 to 18 year old population, the test is effective as a pretest and posttest instrument. The test is acceptable for research purposes with the suggested change in protocol and the tester being aware of the safety factor associated with the sit up.

STANDING VERTICAL ARM PRESS TEST

Reference.
Johnson, B. L., & Nelson, J. K. (1986). *Practical measurements for evaluation in physical education*. Edina, MN: Burgess, pp 111, 113-114.

Additional Source.
Bosco & Gustafson (1983, pp. 86, 89).

Purpose.
To measure an examinee's arm extension strength in a vertical overhead press movement.

Objectivity.
r = .99 was derived by Prestidge (1972) cited in Johnson and Nelson (1986, p. 111).

Reliability.
r = .98 for test-retest.

Validity.
Face validity.

Age and Sex.
Males, age 12 - college.

Equipment.
A body weight scale, a 1.5m to 1.8m (5' - 6') long weight lifting bar, and an adequate number of weight plates.

Space Requirements and Design.
A clear, level area approximately 3m (10') square with the weight lifting bar and weight plates in the center.

Directions.
The examinee's body weight is determined following standard procedure. The preferred amount of weight is loaded on the bar and the bar is then placed by two spotters in the hands of the examinee at chest level. The examinee's hands (palms forward) and feet are spread approximately shoulder width apart. On command, the examinee extends the arms in a vertical overhead motion until the elbows are straight. After the elbows are straightened, the examinee holds the bar for a count of three, to exhibit control. The bar is then returned to the floor. While performing the press, the examinee is not permitted to bend his knees or hips or arch his back. The spotters should be ready to catch the barbell in case the examinee looses balance and/or control of the bar. A total of two trials are generally given. If the examinee is not familiar with the lift, it may take more than two trials to derive maximum effort. The amount of weight may be reduced if the first trial is unsuccessful. If the second trial is also unsuccessful, the weight may be further reduced and after a brief rest the examinee retested.

Scoring.
The score is derived by dividing the maximum weight the examinee lifted by his body weight.

Norms.
Johnson & Nelson (1986, p. 114) men; Miller (1988, p. 172) men and women on weight machines; Greenberg & Pargman (1989, p. 80) men and women.

REVIEW

DONALD R. CASADY, Ph.D.

Professor of Exercise Science
The University of Iowa
Iowa City, IA 52242

The Standing Vertical Arm Press Test (sometimes called the Military Press) is assumed, on logical grounds, to be a valid test of muscular strength. As with other muscular strength tests, this test yields a sample of overall strength that is based on the force exerted by only a few muscles; consequently, it does not necessarily reflect the strength level of other non involved muscle groups. In addition, this is an isotonic strength test in which the barbell is moved through a range of motion. As such, it is not an accurate measure of either static (no movement) or isokinetic (force measured at all points throughout the pressing movement) muscular strength.

Both the reliability and objectivity of the military press test have been consistently in the .90's, when reported.

If those being tested are experienced in this lift, the stability of their test scores is improved because of a more constant motivational level plus an increased knowledge of what constitutes a maximum poundage with which they can succeed.

One potential problem with the objectivity of those judging the lift lies in the fact that the examinees can "cheat" when performing this lift. It is difficult to draw the line as to when "hunching" (an illegal movement of shrugging the shoulders or moving the hips or ankles) has been used to begin the pressing movement. Even more difficult to judge is deciding if a legal or acceptable lift was made whenever the lifter begins the press with an arched back body position or if the back is increasingly arched during the pressing movement. In addition, the tester must judge if the hands remained level with each other throughout the lift. Because of the above problems, the standing arm press was, several years ago, eliminated as one of the three "olympic lifts" from all olympic weight lifting competition.

A barbell and various size weight plates are often available with which to administer the Standing Vertical Arm Press Test. However, the need to repeatedly change the poundage plates and refasten the safety collars requires a significant amount of testing time. Many schools and institutions, however, are more likely to have weight training machines which are usually constructed for performing vertical arm presses while seated; such weight training stations are unsuitable for a standing position.

The vertical arm press is easy to administer, but one spotter should stand on each side of the examinee, ready to give assistance and protection when necessary. This fact, coupled with the need to place the barbell in a starting resting position on the chest plus the necessity for lowering the barbell to the floor afterwards, requires trained helpers and extra time.

In most weight lifting competition three trials are standard. While the use of only two trials for the Standing Vertical Arm Press Test saves some time, it does so at the expense of lessening the accuracy of a measure of maximum strength. In fact, these types of tests are unlikely to consistently obtain a maximum exertion from those being tested.

Another factor weighing against this test is that if the examinee loses control of the barbell while it is in an overhead position, it is both awkward and difficult for spotters to give assistance with safety. This, together with the fact that trained spotters with adequate strength are seldom available, makes this test unacceptable for use in evaluating instructional outcomes. The need for spotters can be critical in the few instances when a lifter "gets stuck" during the pressing movement and strains for a few seconds when the barbell is at face level and loses consciousness because of restricted arterial blood flow to the brain while the breath is held. This phenomenon, sometimes called the Valsalva effect, further indicates that this test of strength is unacceptable for general use.

Tests such as the Standing Vertical Arm Press readily lend themselves to self evaluation. Its discriminatory capacity, however, is limited because: (1) it is intended for use only with males which is an untrue expectation for today's society, (2) practice and training are necessary for it to yield the most accurate measures, and (3) only a few local norms for males are available for this test; certainly, the use of past national and olympic records for various body weight classes would be meaningless.

SUMMARY

The Standing Vertical Arm Press has a number of weaknesses that overcome any possible reasons for using it as a measure of muscular strength. Most measurement and evaluation textbooks dating from 1970 on do not list this test. Because of its need for trained spotters and examinees and because of the difficulty of having all examinees perform the press in a uniform body position, this test is unacceptable for use in either teaching or research. Other tests of muscular strength such as the bench press and the maximum hand grip strength tests are superior tests.

STATIC STRENGTH TESTS

ARM PULL (HORIZONTAL) TEST

Reference.
Fleishman, E. A. (1964B). *The structure and measurement of physical fitness.* Englewood Cliffs: Prentice Hall, pp 46, 59.

Additional Sources.
None.

Purpose.
To measure the force producing capability of an examinees's arm and shoulder muscles during a pulling movement.

Objectivity.
Not reported.

Reliability.
r = .83 for test-retest.

Validity.
Construct validity was established.

Age and Sex.
Not reported, but appears suitable for females and males, age 6 - adult.

Equipment.
A dynamometer with the capability of measuring forces up to 205kg (450 lb), a pillar or a sturdy vertical pole approximately 2m (6') in height which is firmly secured, and a strap.

Space Requirements and Design.
A clear, level area approximately 2m (6') square is needed next to the pillar. One end of the strap is run through one of the handles of the dynamometer and around the pillar. Both ends are fastened thus forming a loop around the pillar with the dynamometer attached.

Directions.
The examinee stands in an upright position with the dynamometer at shoulder level. The examinee grips the dynamometer in one hand and places the other hand against the pillar in order to brace the body. The strap is adjusted to the length that will enable the examinee's arm, which is braced against the pillar, to be straight. On command, the examinee exerts a maximum horizontal pull while keeping the forearm and legs straight. A total of three trials are given with a minimum rest of 30 seconds between trials.

Scoring.
The score is the maximum force obtained on the best of three trials.

Norms.
Beunen et al. (1988, pp. 32, 81, 93) boys; Fleishman (1964B, p. 59) mean and standard deviation for men; Ostyn et al. (1980, pp. 102-103, 127-140) boys; Simons et al. (1990, pp. 99, 129, 138-141) girls.

REVIEW

RICHARD MUNROE, Ed.D.

Associate Professor
Exercise and Sport Sciences
University of Arizona
Tucson, AZ 85721

No validity coefficient was given for this test. If the factor loading (.71) from Fleishman's factor analysis is taken as the validity coefficient, that is very moderate. Intercorelations with other "strength" tests produced no coefficient above .55 indicating the tests apparently measured different qualities. A reliability coefficient of .83 is not especially high, and since this was stated as a test-retest value, it may not be appropriate. Objectivity was not addressed, but reading a dynamometer should provide high consistency. Although the test involves only the examinee being measured, the self bracing aspect could cause considerable variance in repeated scores; perhaps this was a limiting factor in the obtained reliability measure.

Space and equipment problems seem minimal, however, the cost of a dynamometer for such a specific application may be unwarranted. Test administration is relatively simple, but may lead to low reliability since there are few if any controls on positioning, bracing, etc. The test is essentially self administered. Strength testing by its nature requires little time and/or very few trials, and this item seems to be appropriate for most examinees (as long as the dynamometer is sensitive enough to record a full range of potential scores). The safety factor is open to question, particularly with respect to the possibility of the bracing hand slipping from the post. The test is scored directly and should be objective and meaningful. This test has questionable validity, moderate reliability, and generally is not sufficiently precise for research work.

SUMMARY

Major Strength:

1. The strength of this test lies mainly in its practicability; it utilizes a simplified approach suitable for field testing, not research.

Major Weakness:

1. It requires specialized equipment to measure one muscle group, and does not isolate that group particularly well.

The Arm Pull is an unacceptable test, particularly when better tests are available. Fleishman's study selects the hand grip test above the Arm Pull, and certainly the Oregon cable tension strength tests are superior even though they may be outdated themselves.

CLARKE CABLE TENSION STRENGTH TESTS

References.

Clarke, H. H., & Clarke, D. H. (1978). *Developmental and adapted physical education.* Englewood Cliffs: Prentice Hall, pp 101-126.

Clarke, H. H., & Munroe, R. A. (1970). *Test manual: Oregon cable tension strength test batteries for boys and girls from fourth grade through college.* Eugene, OR: Microform Publications, University of Oregon.

Additional Sources.

Bosco & Gustafson (1983, pp. 82-86); Jensen & Hirst (1980, pp. 85-86); Kirkendall et al. (1980, pp. 228-229); Kirkendall et al. (1987, p. 106); Safrit (1986, p. 301); Safrit (1990, p. 472); Verducci (1980, pp. 242-244).

Purpose.

To measure an examinee's strength of 38 individual muscle groups which act over the major joints of the body.

Objectivity.

r = .90 and above when given by experienced testers (Clarke & Clarke, 1978, p. 101).

Reliability.

Not reported.

Validity.

Not reported.

Age and Sex.

Females and males, age 9 - adult.

Equipment.

A cable tensiometer, the appropriate diameter cable, a specially designed testing table, the proper pulling assembly, a chair with arm rests, and a goniometer (see Clarke & Clarke, 1978, pp. 101-107).

Space Requirements and Design.

A clear, level area approximately 5m (15') square next to a wall with the proper hooks screwed into the wall. The special testing table is aligned perpendicular to the wall in front of the wall hooks. The chair can be positioned in the area as needed.

Directions.

For each of the 38 tests, the exact body position of the examinee is specified so as to produce the maximum force application of the muscle group being measured. The position of the examinee's other body parts are also specified as well as the blocking and bracing duties of the tester and/or assistants. The goniometer is used to ensure the proper joint angle for each test. In positioning the pulling assembly, the tester should make sure that it is aligned perpendicular to the body part the examinee is attempting to move. The tester should also be sure the cable is taut immediately before asking the examinee to exert a maximum force in the specified position. The examinee should exert maximum force in a steady, progressive manner over a period of 5 to 8 seconds duration.

NOTE: For a written description of each of the 38 individual muscle group tests, the reader is referred to Clarke and Clarke (1978, pp. 107-124). An illustration of most of the tests is also included in the reference.

Scoring.

The score is determined by converting the cable tension reading of the tensiometer into pounds of force on a calibration chart supplied with each tensiometer.

Norms.

Clarke & Munroe (1970, pp. 32-65) provide validated test batteries and norms for upper elementary school, junior high school and senior high school boys and girls, and for college men and women.

NOTE: When purchasing a tensiometer, it is necessary to specify the maximum capacity desired as instruments of greatest capacity do not test well for the lower strength amounts. Clarke and Munroe (1970) recommend tensiometers that provide for more than one maximum capacity unless testing only elementary age children. For junior high, senior high, and college age populations, two or three instruments are needed. Recommended ranges for the three tensiometers are 10 to 200 lbs., 100 to 400 lbs., and 100 to 800 lbs. Tensiometers may be obtained from the Pacific Scientific Company, HTL Caribe Incorporated, P.O. Box 559, Luquillo, PR 00673.

REVIEW

CHARLES J. ANSORGE, Ph.D.

Professor of Physical Education
University of Nebraska-Lincoln
Lincoln, NE 68588-0229

If muscular strength is defined as the maximum force that a muscle group can exert over a brief time, then this force as measured by a calibrated tensiometer using an appropriate testing protocol would represent a valid measure of static strength.

No reliability data have been reported by Clarke and Clarke (1978) although an objectivity coefficient of .90 was reported when the strength tests were administered by experienced testers. If different testers were able to obtain high intercorrelations, this would suggest that the reliability of the tests is also quite high.

For each of the strength tests, one tester and an assistant to brace or stabilize the examinee is recommended. Various sources (e.g., Clarke & Munroe, 1970; Clarke & Clarke, 1978) present information regarding how each of the strength tests is to be administered.

The space requirements are not great, but the equipment needed for administering the tests extends beyond the tensiometer(s) required. A variety of pulling assemblies are needed which are used in conjunction with the tests (Clarke & Clarke, 1978, pp. 102-107). In addition, a testing table is recommended. Finally, a goniometer is needed to determine the appropriate joint angles for the various tests. The price for all this equipment is not excessively expensive, but would be priced too high for some settings.

The training required to administer or assist in static strength testing is not extensive. However, the time required to administer all 38 tests to one examinee is extensive. Clarke and Munroe (1970) have recommended strength test batteries for use with females and males at four

levels: upper elementary, junior high, senior high, and college. From the 38 Clarke Cable Tension Strength Tests, three item batteries were selected for each sex at each level. The time for administering such a battery would not be inordinate.

No information is provided regarding the number of trials recommended for each of the tests. Various measurement and evaluation experts have suggested a variety of procedures for testing strength such as the best of several trials or the mean of a specified number of trials. Agreement among experts has not been reached about which procedure is best.

All of the strength tests were designed to be used with females and males, age nine through adult. If the correct tensiometer, pulling assembly, and cable are employed, a satisfactory range of scores is produced for the various tests.

There is minimal danger involved in strength testing. Suitable warm up should be employed before testing to minimize muscle strains or pulls, and care should be taken to maintain the integrity of pulling assemblies, cables, chains, connectors, and hooks to minimize any sudden breakage of the testing apparatus.

Scoring for the tests is objective. Tensiometers have a maximum pointer to facilitate reading an examinee's score. Self testing for any of the tests is practically impossible.

Researchers interested in measuring static strength at a particular joint angle will find the cable strength tests to be suitably precise for these purposes.

Norms are not available for individual tests. However, Seidler (1967), Becker (1967), and Lowenberger (1967) have prepared norms for the test batteries described earlier in this review. Nearly 3,000 subjects were involved in determining the norms. No evidence could be found of more recent norms.

SUMMARY

Major Strengths:

1. Ease in administration of tests.

2. Suitable for research purposes to determine static strength at a single joint angle.

Major Weaknesses:

1. Time consuming to administer since examinees must be tested individually.

2. Norms are not available for individual tests. Norms for test batteries involving some of the individual tests are over 20 years old.

3. Reliability data never were determined for the individual tests. Since objectivity coefficients reported are in the .90's, this should not be regarded as a serious weakness.

4. Strength of a muscle group is isolated at a particular angle, thus limiting information regarding strength at other angles. This is an inherent weakness of static strength tests and a reason why isokinetic tests have become so popular.

5. If three tensiometer units are purchased to accommodate various capacities and pulling assemblies, cables, tables, etc. are either purchased or built to specifications, the total expense may be prohibitive in many settings.

The Clarke Cable Tension Strength Tests are acceptable for research and, to a lesser extent, teaching, if there is an interest in measuring static strength. The weaknesses noted above should be studied before using these tests. Measuring isokinetic strength is usually considered to be superior to static strength, but the cost of isokinetic measuring devices is much greater. If cost is a factor, thought should be given to the measurement of static strength utilizing one or more of the Clarke Cable Tension Strength Tests.

REVIEW REFERENCES

Becker, B. J. (1967). *Developmental and adapted physical education.* Englewood Cliffs: Prentice Hall.

Clarke, H. H., & Clarke, D. H. (1978). *Developmental and adapted physical education.* Englewood Cliffs: Prentice Hall.

Clarke, H. H., & Munroe, R. A. (1970). *Test manual: Oregon cable tension strength test batteries for boys and girls from fourth grade through college.* Eugene, OR: Microform Publications, University of Oregon.

Lowenberger, A. G. (1967). Construction of a muscular strength test for college men. Unpublished doctoral dissertation, University of Oregon.

Neely, J. J. (1967). Construction of norms for cable-tension strength tests for upper elementary, junior high, and senior high school girls. Uunpublished doctoral dissertation, University of Oregon.

Seidler, M. G. (1967). Construction of norms for cable-tension strength tests for upper elementary, junior high, and senior high school boys. Unpublished doctoral dissertation, University of Oregon.

HAND GRIP STRENGTH TEST

Reference.
Fleishman, E. A. (1964B). *The structure and measurement of physical fitness.* Englewood Cliffs: Prentice Hall, pp 59, 113, 125, 166.

Additional Sources.
Baumgartner & Jackson (1987, pp. 190-192); Baumgartner & Jackson (1991, pp. 230-233); Bosco & Gustafson (1983, p. 79); Hastad & Lacy (1989, pp. 201-203);

Jensen & Hirst (1980, pp. 84-85); Johnson & Nelson (1986, pp. 123-124); Safrit (1986, p. 301); Safrit (1990, pp. 471-472); Verducci (1980, p. 242).

Purpose.
To measure the ability of an examinee to exert maximum force with the flexor muscles of the hand.

Objectivity.
Not reported.

Reliability.
r = .91 for test-retest.

Validity.
Face validity.

Age and Sex.
Suitable for females and males, age 8 - adult.

Equipment.
A hand dynamometer (a manuometer may be used) and magnesium carbonate to keep the hands dry.

Space Requirements and Design.
A clear, level area approximately 2m (6') square with the examinee in the center.

Directions.
The examinee stands erect with the dynamometer in the preferred hand. The dynamometer is positioned in the examinee's hand so that its base is solid in the palm. The upper gripping bar of the dynamometer is adjusted to fit in the examinee's fingers between the second and third knuckles. The examinee's arm is held at the side of her/his body with the thumb forward. The tester should make sure the examinee does not brace or rest any part of her/his

arm against the body. Upon the tester's command, the examinee squeezes the dynamometer with as much force as possible for 2 to 5 seconds. The tester notes where the pointer is positioned and records the force exerted. The pointer is then returned to zero. A total of three trials are given, with a rest of 20 to 30 seconds between trials.

Scoring.
The score is the greatest force, in kilograms or pounds, the examinee exerted during the best of three trials.

Norms.
Alexander et al. (1985, p. 9) Canadian women; Baumgartner & Jackson (1987, p. 193) men, women, and miners; Baumgartner & Jackson (1991, p. 233) men, women and, miners; Bosco & Gustafson (1983, p. 82) references for norms; Canadian Minister (1979, p. 17) men and women;

Corbin & Lindsey (1983, p. 52) boys, girls, men, and women; Corbin & Lindsey (1985, p. 55) men and women; Evans (1973, p. 386) rugby players; Fleishman (1964A, p. 53) boys and girls; Fleishman (1964B, p. 113) boys and girls; Fitness Canada (1986, p. 36) boys, girls, men, and women;

Harrison & Bradbeer (1982, pp. 24-25) boy and girl athletes; Johnson & Nelson (1986, pp. 124-125) boys, girls, men, and women using two hands; Stephens et al. (1986, p. 15) men and women; Stokes et al. (1986, p. 171) men and women; VanGelder & Marks (1987, p. 185) men and women; Montoye & Lamphier (1977, p. 113) men and women.

REVIEW

KATHLEEN TRITSCHLER, Ed.D.
Assistant Professor
Sport Studies
Guilford College
Greensboro, NC 27410

The Hand Grip Strength Test is a classic in the field of motor measurement. It has been used for the last quarter century in the assessment of grip strength for a wide variety of populations. Norms are available for boys, girls, and adult men and women (see references in the test description). Why would one want to measure grip strength? Although strength is considered to be a component of health related physical fitness, grip strength per se is not related to any particular lifestyle related disease or condition. Furthermore, it is known that grip strength has only a low to moderate correlation with the strength or muscular endurance of other upper or lower body muscle groups (Bell et al., 1985). The primary reason to measure grip strength seems to be its relationship to quality performance of many different sports skills. Weak grip strength may be especially problematic in striking skills in which a sports implement is held in one or both hands (Hatze, 1976; Missavage et al., 1984). Such skills are found in golf, all racket sports, and in baseball/softball batting. Grip strength can also be essential in selected gymnastic events such as the men's high bar. Thus, the measurement of grip strength is clearly an important concern of many motor performance teachers and coaches.

What's unclear, however, is the exact nature of the relationship between specific grip strength scores and sports skills performances. Just how much grip strength is needed for a quality tennis forehand drive? Will an increase in grip strength result in a concomitant increase in skill? If a woman is at the 85th percentile rank relative to other middle age women, does she have sufficient grip strength to succeed in learning to play golf? None of these questions can be answered using the age and gender related norms that are presently available for the Hand Grip Strength Test. Perhaps what needs to be developed are criterion referenced score values that represent the minimal strength required for successful performance of selected sports skills. Think how useful this could be to a teacher of a group of beginning tennis students! He/she could measure students' grip strength, then prescribe remedial strength development exercises for those whose scores fell below the criterion referenced standard. What a boon to teaching!

This grip test is relatively free of both psychometric and practical problems. Face validity is claimed, and the stated purpose of the test is consistent with common definitions of muscular strength. High test-retest reliability

$(r = .91)$ is typical of strength tests; it should be noted, though, that test constructors should report both the time period and population employed in reliability studies. The instrumentation (i.e., a grip dynamometer or manuometer) allows for excellent objectivity, and also contributes to high reliability if the dynamometer is calibrated prior to testing. No doubt test directions should include a reminder of the importance of calibration. Similarly, there should be a reminder to adjust the gripping bar appropriately for each examinee. If this is not done, there is the potential of score bias especially for examinees with smaller hands.

Practically speaking, the test is simple and easy to administer. The only training needed by the tester is in how to calibrate and adjust the dynamometer. The description of arm position might be clarified by explaining that the arm should be "at the side of the body, with elbow extended, and palm facing the side of the leg." Scoring is based on the best score recorded in three trials; three trials are surely adequate for the assessment of muscular strength. However, as a practical concern, it would clearly be advantageous in mass testing situations if the test could be administered validly and reliably in two, rather than three, trials. The third trial, if not truly needed from a psychometric viewpoint, adds 8 to 12 minutes of administration time for a group of 24 examinees.

Though the Hand Grip Strength Test is appropriate for the vast majority of children and adults, perhaps the greatest concern is that no precautions are offered for use of this test with certain at risk populations. All individuals, but especially elderly individuals, should be encouraged to exhale while squeezing the dynamometer to avoid an increase in thoracic pressure (i.e., a Valsalva manuever). And, it is no doubt an inappropriate test for anyone with diagnosed heart conditions or those with severe arthritis in the joints of the hands/fingers.

SUMMARY

Major Strengths:

1. Good psychometric qualities.

2. Appropriateness and norms for both genders.

3. Appropriateness and norms for children and adults.

4. Excellent practicality in terms of administrative time, equipment, and tester training.

Major Weaknesses:

1. Failure to caution against the holding of breath.

2. Failure to caution against use with coronary patients and arthritic populations.

In summary, the Hand Grip Strength Test is an excellent test, appropriate for use by both practitioners and researchers.

REVIEW REFERENCES

Bell, R.D., Hoshizaki, B., & Collis, M. L. (1985). The post 50 '3-S' physical performance test. *Canadian Gerontological Collection IV*. Winnipeg, Canada: Kellett Copy Center, Ltd.

Hatze, H. (1976). Forces and duration of impact and grip tightness during the tennis stroke. *Medicine and Science in Sports,* 8:88-95.

Missavage, R. J., Baker, J. A., & Putnam, C. A. (1984). Theoretical modeling of grip firmness during ball-racket impact. *Research Quarterly for Exercise and Sport,* 55:254-260.

PRESS TEST

Reference.
Johnson, B. L., & Nelson, J. K. (1986). *Practical measurements for evaluation in physical education*. Edina, MN: Burgess, pp 116-117.

Additional Sources.
None.

Purpose.
To measure an examinee's arm extension strength in a vertical overhead press motion.

Objectivity.
r = .99 was derived by Huntsman (1969) cited in Johnson and Nelson (1986, p. 116).

Reliability.
r = .96 for test-retest method.

Validity.
Face validity.

Age and Sex.
Females, age 12 - college.

Equipment.
A body weight scale, a S hook, a 75kg (160 lb) spring scale, one 1.52m (5') long piece of chain, one 61cm (2') long wooden bar with a screw hook inserted in the center, a wooden platform approximately 76cm x 46cm x 10cm (30" x 18" x 4") with a heavy duty eye hook attached in the center, and a 45cm (18") long piece of chain with the eye hook inserted through one of the links.

Space Requirements and Design.
A clear, level area approximately 2m (6') square with the test apparatus and the examinee in the center. The wooden platform with the 45cm (18") piece of chain is placed on the floor. The spring scale is attached to the chain followed by an S hook, the 1.52m (5') section of chain, and the wooden bar.

Directions.
The examinee's body weight is determined following standard procedure. The examinee then stands with her feet flat on the wooden platform. The wooden bar is held in front of the examinee's forehead. The examinee grasps the bar with her hands about shoulder width apart and the palms facing forward (i.e., the radioulnar joints are supinated). On command, the examinee exerts maximum force in a vertical motion in an attempt to straighten the arms. The examinee's legs and trunk must remain straight and erect while the feet are kept flat on the platform. A total of two trials are given. The examinee may rest a few seconds between trials.

Scoring.
The score is derived by taking the maximum force exerted by the examinee during the best of two trials and dividing it by her body weight.

Norms.
Johnson & Nelson (1986, p. 117) women.

REVIEW

SCOTT GOING, Ph.D.
Assistant Research Scientist
Exercise and Sport Sciences
University of Arizona
Tucson, AZ 85721

The scientific aspects of the test are acceptable; that is, the test is a valid measure of arm extension strength which has been demonstrated to be both reliable (r = .96) and objective (r = .99) (Huntsman, 1969). It is important that the users of the test differentiate between tests of maximal force production during a specific task or movement which involves several muscles or muscle groups as opposed to a test of the maximal force capacity of a single muscle or muscle group. The Press Test is a useful test of the maximal force produced by a set of agonists (e.g., triceps brachii, deltoid, and supraspinatus) recruited during a well defined movement and is not a test of the strength of a single muscle group per se.

The Press Test is also a practical test, potentially useful in both research and field situations. The equipment is simple and relatively inexpensive, and only a small amount of space is required. The test can be administered by one tester and unless the tester is unable to elicit a maximal effort, the test results should be consistent between different testers. Although suggested specifically for females, ages 12 to adulthood, the Press Test is suitable for use with healthy females and males of almost any age capable of understanding the instructions and giving a maximal effort, although the norms are available only for adult females. Because it is a test of maximal isometric force production, it is not recommended for use with individuals of compromised cardiovascular function and it has only limited value as a conditioning drill.

Although the Press Test is relatively simple to administer, to achieve the high degree of reliability and objectivity that has been reported and to obtain a valid measure of strength, carefully standardized procedures must be followed. Standardization of examinee position on the equipment is especially important if meaningful comparisons are to be made between repeated tests and between examinees. It is absolutely critical that the examinee be positioned as described so that additional muscle groups will not contribute to the measured force. The examinee must not be allowed to bend backward when force is exerted or an inappropriately high score unrepresentative of the examinee's true strength will be recorded.

The instructions given to the examinees, the number of trials, and the rest interval between trials must also be standardized. The examinees should be instructed to hold the bar so that the chain is fully stretched before beginning the trial. Examinees should not be allowed to jerk the chain which can lead to over estimates of strength when a spring scale is used. For this reason, it is usually best to instruct the examinees to exert a slow, steady push on the bar until the maximal force is achieved. In studies comparing rapid rates of force production with slower contraction speeds, very similar maximal forces were exerted. Although recovery from short duration maximal isometric efforts occurs relatively quickly, rest intervals should be standardized so that the conditions of each trial are similar. Thirty to 60 seconds rest between trials is recommended. The recommended number of trials is too few. With isometric tests, unless the examinees have been given previous practice, quite often there is a warm up or learning effect, and when only two trials are administered it is likely that strength will be under estimated. Three to five trials are usually sufficient to insure the examinees have achieved their maximal

strength capacity which is demonstrated by close agreement (percent difference) between two consecutive trials. When more than five trials are administered, it is likely that muscle fatigue will confound the results, unless longer rest intervals are given.

A final point needs to be made that is not addressed in the test's description. For the results to be valid when a spring scale is used, it is essential that the scale be calibrated regularly so that adjustments can be made for the change that occurs with time in the characteristics of the spring. This can be accomplished by gently hanging a series of standard weights from the scale and recording the associated readout for each weight. In this way, a chart or calibration line (i.e., a regression line) can be developed which is used to correct scale readings to the actual force exerted on the spring.

SUMMARY

Major Strengths:

1. Valid test of arm extension strength when a calibrated spring scale is used.

2. Highly reliable and objective with appropriate standardization of procedures.

3. Equipment is inexpensive and the test requires little space to administer.

Major Weaknesses:

1. Adequate attention is not given to the need for standardization of procedures including examinee position, instructions to the examinees, and rest intervals between trials.

2. Physical characteristics of the spring will change over time making calibration essential for results to be valid.

3. Available norms were developed from only a small sample of females at one institution and are not suitable for children.

The Press Test is especially well suited as a field test of isometric strength and may be used in a research setting. Adequate standardization of procedures is essential to obtain the high levels of reliability and objectivity that have been reported. The test is only valid if the spring scale is calibrated regularly against standard weights. With appropriate instruction, the Press Test could be used for self evaluation. The test is not recommended as a conditioning drill. Because of the acute effects on cardiovascular dynamics, the test is not recommended for individuals with cardiovascular disease. Norms are available for adults only. They were developed from a small sample at one institution and may not generalize to the population.

PUSH AND PULL STRENGTH TESTS

Reference.

Scott, M. G., & French, E. (1959). *Measurement and evaluation in physical education*. Dubuque: Wm. C. Brown, pp 291-292.

Additional Source.

Jensen & Hirst (1980, p. 85).

Purpose.

To measure the ability of an examinee to exert maximum force with the arms and shoulders toward the midline of the body for the push test and away from the midline of the body for the pull test.

Objectivity.

Not reported.

Reliability.

r = .91 for college women (push or pull not stated); r = .89 for pull; and r = .76 for push by Wilson (1944) cited in Scott & French (1959, p. 292).

Validity.

r = .49 by Wilson (1944) cited in Scott and French (1959, p. 292) when correlated with Rogers Short Strength Index.

Age and Sex.

College females.

Equipment.

A manuometer with a push-pull attachment.

Space Requirements and Design.

A clear, level area approximately 2m (6') square with the examinee in the center.

Directions.

Pull Test:

The examinee stands erect with her arms positioned parallel to the ground with her elbows bent. The examinee holds the manuometer in front of her chest with one hand on each handle. The instrument cannot be braced against the chest. Upon command, the examinee pulls outward with maximum force. The tester records the force obtained and resets the manuometer to zero. A total of two trials are allowed.

Push Test:

The directions and the position for the push test are the same as in the pull test, except the examinee pushes inward on the manuometer with maximum force.

Scoring.

The score is the greatest force obtained by the examinee on the best of two trials for each of the two tests.

Norms.

Scott & French (1959, p. 293) women.

REVIEW

EDGAR W. SHIELDS, JR., Ph.D.
Associate Professor
Physical Education, Exercise and
Sport Science
University of North Carolina
Chapel Hill, NC 27599-8605

These tests are two of six tests for arm and shoulder girdle strength presented in Chapter 8 of the reference text. Scott and French (1959) state that "Validity coefficients have been established in various studies and have always run fairly high," although they fail to cite those studies or report coefficients. The very nature of these tests would suggest that they are valid; however, as noted in the reference, Wilson's (1944) study of arm and shoulder girdle strength of college women resulted in a coefficient of only .49 when the scores from these tests were correlated with Rogers Short Strength Index. Further examination of the validity issue provides some explanation of this equivocalness. Scores on the Rogers Short Strength Index are computed by a formula which requires the number of pull ups and push ups (modified, right angle pull ups using rings suspended from a bar and knee push ups for girls), which are measures of dynamic or isotonic strength as opposed to the static or isometric strength measured by a dynamometer. Also, although not totally clear, it appears that validity was established for university freshmen and sophomore women. The reliability of the tests for college women, as reported by Scott and French (1959) is certainly satisfactory, although there is no differentiation given for the push item or pull item. Wilson's reported reliability coefficients for both push and pull items are lower. Both reliabilities appear to have been established by test-retest. Objectivity is not addressed, but the nature of the tests are such that objectivity should be high. Active participation by another individual is not required for either test.

Facility and space requirements are minimal and should present no problems. The purchase of a hand dynamometer with a push-pull attachment, while not costly compared to some other types of testing equipment, could present a problem for those who do not have access to such equipment. Assuming the availability of a dynamometer, the tests should be easy to administer and require minimum time. Only one tester is needed to record the scores and reset the dynamometer. If large groups were to be tested, additional dynamometers and testers would be desirable. The number of trials, two for each test, is acceptable for strength measurements.

Although both tests (i.e., push and pull) could be used to develop and/or maintain isometric strength in the specific muscle groups involved, the tests are not sufficient for conditioning and are not applicable in any practical sense to learning. No general or specific problems would be anticipated if these tests were to be administered to high school age or above females and males. There appears to be no dangerous aspect to the tests, although muscle strain and/or rupture is certainly possible. The nature of the tests is such that the ability of them to discriminate among their users may be assumed, although this issue is not addressed. The scoring is objective and the tests could be self administered and scored. The

tests could meet the precision requirements for research. Norms are available for college women. Any potential user of these tests should note that the norms were developed from the administration of the tests to 892 women at the University of Iowa, probably during the 1950's (no date was given in the reference). Of particular note, the table of norms consists of T-Scores for what appears to be the sum of the best scores from each of the two tests (there is no explanation which directs one to do this). It is also assumed that the scores are recorded to the nearest pound of force (this is not specified).

SUMMARY

Major Strength:

1. The simplicity and ease of administration.

Major Weaknesses:

1. Requires specialized equipment which may not be readily available.

2. There is no report of the ability of the tests to discriminate.

3. Validity findings are somewhat equivocal.

4. Available norms are significantly out of date and are applicable to a very narrow age range and to only one gender.

The Scott-French Push and Pull Strength Tests could be acceptable tests, adequate for research and/or teaching; however, due to the specific nature of the tests any potential user should examine them very closely to determine if they are valid for their purpose. It is this reviewer's recommendation that validity and reliability, specific to the group to be tested, be determined anew prior to any use of these tests. New norms, specific to the group to which they would be applied, would also need to be developed.

TRUNK PULL TEST

Reference.
Fleishman, E. A. (1964B). *The structure and measurement of physical fitness*. Englewood Cliffs: Prentice Hall, pp 47, 59, 65.

Additional Sources.
None.

Purpose.
To measure the maximum force producing capability of an examinee's abdominal muscles.

Objectivity.
Not reported.

Reliability.
r = .67 test-retest method.

Validity.
Factor loading .59.

Age and Sex.
Not reported, but suitable for females and males, age 8 - adult.

Equipment.
A dynamometer capable of measuring up to 200 kg (450 lb), a pillar or a sturdy vertical pole approximately 2m (6') in height which is firmly attached to the floor, two straps, and a bench.

Space Requirements and Design.
A clear, level area approximately 3m (10') square with the bench positioned next to the pillar or pole.

Directions.
The examinee sits erect on the bench with her/his back against the pillar. The examinee's arms are held next to the sides of her/his body with the elbows bent approximately 90 degrees. The end of one of the straps is inserted through one of the handles of the dynamometer and around the pillar thus forming a loop around the pillar with the dynamometer attached. The other strap is looped around the examinee's chest, as high as possible, and fastened to the other handle of the dynamometer. In order to reduce the potential use of the legs, a partner sits on the examinee's knees during the test. On command, the ex-aminee leans forward exerting as much force as possible. A total of three trials are given with a 30 second rest between trials.

Scoring.
The score is the maximum force obtained by the examinee on the best of three trials.

Norms.
Fleishman (1964B, p. 59) mean and a standard deviation for men.

REVIEW

JIM L. STILLWELL, P.E.D.

Chair, Human Performance Studies
The University of Alabama
Tuscaloosa, AL 35487

The Trunk Pull Test is an excellent measure of the force producing capabilities of the ab-dominal muscles because the protocol makes it easy to isolate the muscles. The test has both face validity and an acceptable level of reliability. Although there is not a value given for the objec-tivity of the test, it appears to have consistency. Since the force is applied by one and only one individual, the results are not affected by anyone else. This holds true even though a partner is used to sit on the examinee's knees to prevent the use of the leg muscles.

From a practical standpoint, the test is ap-propriate because it requires no particular space or facility other than normally available. The need for a specific piece of equipment is a con-cern. This test requires a device unique to most laboratories. If the equipment is available, the test can be administered easily. In fact it can be self administered for personal evaluation. It re-quires no special training for the tester, nor any great amount of time. The three trials allowed are sufficient. However, a 30 second rest be-tween trials is not sufficient for full recovery, especially in young examinees. The test is suitable for the age range described and should discriminate among its users. With regard to danger there is no need for concern, yet the test should not be administered to anyone with back pain. The test is not appropriate for conditioning nor as a tool to promote learning. Its best use is in a research setting, more so than as a tool in a fitness or a wellness setting. Norms are lacking and the mean and the standard deviation presented for men are outdated.

SUMMARY

Major Strengths:

1. It is easy to administer.
2. It isolates the abdominal muscles.

3. It is adequate as a research instrument.

Major Weaknesses:

1. It requires a piece of equipment unique to a laboratory setting.

2. It cannot be administered in mass.

3. Recovery time between trials is too short.

4. The straps may provide discomfort for females in the upper chest area.

TWO-HAND PUSH TEST

Reference.
Johnson, B. L., & Nelson, J. K. (1986). *Practical measurements for evaluation in physical education,* Edina, MN: Burgess, pp 114-116.

Additional Sources.
None.

Purpose.
To measure an examinee's arm and shoulder strength in a downward push movement.

Objectivity.
r = .99 was derived by Huntsman (1969) cited in Johnson and Nelson (1986, p. 114).

Reliability.
r = .97 for test-retest.

Validity.
Face validity.

Age and Sex.
Females, age 12 - college. Using a 300-pound scale, males can be tested satisfactorily.

Equipment.
A body weight scale, a 75kg (160 lb) spring scale, one 45cm (18") long piece of chain, one 1.52cm (5') long piece of chain, one chain link, one heavy duty eye hook, one S hook, and one 61cm (2') wooden bar with a screw hook inserted in the center.

Space Requirements and Design.
A clear, level area approximately 2m (6') square with the test apparatus in the center. One heavy duty eye hook is fastened securely overhead to the ceiling or a beam. A chain link is connected to the eye hook followed by the 45cm (18") long piece of chain with the heavy duty S hook attached to the bottom. The spring scale is connected to the S hook and has the 1.52cm (5') long piece of chain hooked to it. The wooden bar with a screw hook inserted in the center is connected to the piece of chain at the desired height.

Directions.
The examinee's body weight is determined following standard procedure. The examinee assumes a standing position next to the chain. The wooden bar is attached to the chain so that it hangs at the height of the examinee's waist. The examinee grips the bar with her/his hands, palms down, and about shoulder width apart. The examinee's head must remain erect and in the front of and in line with the chain. The examinee's body must also remain erect at all times with no bending of the knees and hips or twisting of the trunk. The examinee's feet must remain flat on the floor at all times. A partner may have to hold the examinee's hips in order to keep the examinee's feet on the floor. On command, the examinee exerts maximum force in a steady vertical downward motion in an attempt to straighten the arms. A total of two trials are given with a rest between trials.

Scoring.
The score is derived by taking the maximum force exerted by the examinee during the best of two trials and dividing it by the her/his body weight.

Norms.
Johnson & Nelson (1986, p. 116) men and women.

REVIEW

BETHANY SHIFFLETT, Ph.D.

Associate Professor
Human Performance
San Jose State University
San Jose, CA 95192-0054

The stated purpose of the Two Hand Push Test is to measure arm and shoulder strength. A problem with tests that require the use of multiple muscle groups is that following assessment, how do you advise someone who scores low? Is there a weakness in the shoulders or arms? The measure is difficult to interpret.

Inadequate information on objectivity was presented. The r = .99 apparently is a correlation coefficient. This is not the most appropriate statistic to employ to assess objectivity (or test-retest reliability). An intraclass R or coefficient alpha is more appropriate. Additionally it is unclear what was actually done to assess objectivity. Finally, with respect to objectivity and reliability, what were the characteristics of the sample from which these values were derived? These values, even if accurate, can be generalized only to similar groups.

Regarding validity, measures from the Two-Hand Push Test should have been correlated with a criterion measure for the group this test is intended. A simple statement of "face validity" is insufficient.

The description suggests that the test is reliable and valid for females, age 12 to college, and males (no ages specified) when a 300 pound scale is used, yet there is no evidence that reliability and validity were examined for each of these widely different groups.

The sample for the norms is too small to be used for comparative purposes. Additionally, it would be inappropriate to compare 12 year old girls' scores to these norms, yet the test is recommended for females aged 12 to college.

SUMMARY

Major Strengths:

1. Ease of administration.

2. Minimal space required.

Major Weaknesses:

1. Can test only one examinee at a time.

2. Partner necessary to keep examinee on the ground.

3. Lack of data regarding validity, reliability, and objectivity.

4. Inadequate normative data.

Appendix A

Measurement and Evaluation Books
in Exercise Science, Physical Education and Sport Science
Published Since 1980

Barrow, H. M., McGee, R., & Tritschler, K. A. (1989). *Practical measurement in physical education and sport*. Philadelphia: Lea & Febiger.

Baumgartner, T. A. & Jackson, A. S. (1987, 1991). *Measurement for evaluation in physical education and exercise science*. Dubuque, IA: Wm. C. Brown.

Bosco, J. S., & Gustafson, W. F. (1983). *Measurement and evaluation in physical education, fitness and sports*. Englewood Cliffs, NJ: Prentice Hall.

Clarke, H. H., & Clarke, D. H. (1987). *Application of measurement to health and physical education*. Englewood Cliffs, NJ: Prentice Hall.

Hastad, D. N., & Lacy, A. C. (1989). *Measurement and evaluation in contemporary physical education*. Scottsdale, AZ: Gorsuch Scarisbrick, Publishers.

Jensen, C. R., & Hirst, C. C. (1980). *Measurement in physical education and athletics*. New York: Macmillan.

Johnson, B. L., & Nelson, J. K. (1986). *Practical measurements for evaluation in physical education*. Edina, MN: Burgess.

Kirkendall, D. R., Gruber, J. J., & Johnson, R. E. (1980, 1987). *Measurement and evaluation for physical educators*. Champaign: Human Kinetics.

Miller, D. K. (1988). *Measurement by the physical educator: Why and how*. Indianapolis: Benchmark Press.

Mood, D. P. (1980). *Numbers in motion: A balanced approach to measurement and evaluation in physical education*. Palo Alto: Mayfield.

Safrit, M. J. (1981). *Evaluation in physical education*. Englewood Cliffs, NJ: Prentice Hall.

Safrit, M. J. (1986, 1990). *Introduction to measurement in physical education and exercise science*. St. Louis: C. V. Mosby.

Safrit, M. J.,& Wood, T. M. (1989). *Measurement concepts in physical education and exercise science*. Champaign, IL: Human Kinetics.

Verducci, F. M. (1980). *Measurement concepts in physical education*. St. Louis: C. V. Mosby.

Appendix B

References

NOTE: This reference list does not contain the additional references used by the reviewers.

(Alabama) Governor's Commission on Physical Fitness (1988). *Alabama youth fitness test manual.* Montgomery, AL: Chevron, U.S.A. Inc.

Alexander, M. J., Ready, A. E., & Fougere-Mailey, G. (1985). The fitness levels of females in various age groups. *Canadian AHPER Journal,* 51:8-12, March-April.

American Academy of Orthopaedic Surgeons (1963). *Measuring and recording of joint motion.* Detroit.

American Academy of Orthopaedic Surgeons (1965). *Joint motion: Methods of measuring and recording.* Chicago.

AAHPER (1965). *Youth fitness test manual.* Washington, DC: American Association for Health, Physical Education and Recreation.

AAHPER (1975). *Youth fitness test manual.* Washington, DC: American Alliance for Health, Physical Education and Recreation.

AAHPERD (1980). *AAHPERD health related physical fitness test manual.* Reston, VA: American Alliance for Health, Physical Education, Recreation and Dance.

AAHPERD (1984). *AAHPERD technical manual: Health related physical fitness.* Reston, VA: American Alliance for Health, Physical Education, Recreation and Dance.

AAHPERD (1985). *Testing for impaired, disabled and handicapped individuals.* Reston, VA: American Alliance for Health, Physical Education, Recreation and Dance.

AAHPERD (1988). *Physical best.* Reston, VA: American Alliance for Health, Physical Education, Recreation and Dance.

AAHPERD (1990). *Physical best instructor's guide.* Reston, VA: American Alliance for Health, Physical Education, Recreation and Dance.

AAHPERD, & Pate, R. R. (1985). *Norms for college students: Health related physical fitness test.* Reston, VA: American Alliance for Health, Physical Education, Recreation and Dance.

American College of Sports Medicine (1975, 1980, 1986). *Guidelines for graded exercise testing and exercise prescription.* Philadelphia: Lea & Febiger.

Arizona Association for Health, Physical Education, Recreation and Dance (1983). *Arizona journal of health, physical education, recreation and dance.* Special issue: Arizona Health Related Fitness Norms, 25(3):3-28.

Arnot, R., & Gaines, C. (1987). *Sports talent: Discover your natural athletic talents and excel in the sport of your choice.* New York: Penguin Books.

Astrand, P. O., & Ryhming, I. (1954). A nomogram for calculation of aerobic capacity (physical fitness) from pulse rate during sub-maximal work. *Journal of Applied Physiology.* 7:218-221.

Astrand, P. O., & Rodahl, K. (1986). *Textbook of work physiology.* New York: McGraw-Hill.

Ayalon, A., Inbar, O., & Bar-Or, O. (1974). Relationships among measurements of explosive strength and anaerobic power. *Biomechanics IV,* 1:572-577.

Bailey, D. A., Shephard, R. J., & Mirwald, R. L. (1976). Validation of a self administered home test of cardio-respiratory fitness. *Canadian Journal of Applied Sport Sciences,* 1:67-78.

Balogun, J. A., Abereoje, O. K., Olaogun, M. O., & Obajuluwa, V. A. (1989). Inter - and intratester reliabiltiy of measuring neck motions with tape measure and myrin gravity reference goniometer. *The Journal of Orthopaedic and Sports Physical Therapy,* 10(7):248-253.

Bar-Or, O. (1978). A new anaerobic capacity test: Characteristics and applications. Presented at the 21st World Congress in Sports Medicine, Brasilia.

Bar-Or, O. (1987). The wingate anaerobic capacity test: An update on methodology, reliability and validity. *Sports Medicine,* 4(6):381-394.

Barrow, H. M. (1953). A test of motor ability for college men. Unpublished doctoral dissertation, Indiana University).

Barrow, H. M., & McGee, R. (Tritschler, K. A. added in 1989) (1964, 1971, 1979, 1989). *A practical approach to measurement in physical education.* Philadelphia: Lea & Febiger.

Bass, R. I. (1939). An analysis of the components of tests of semicircular canal function and of static and dynamic balance. *Research Quarterly,* 10(2):33-52.

Battinelli, T. (1984). From motor ability to motor learning: The generality/specificity connection. *The Physical Educator,* 41(3):108-113.

Baumgartner, T. A. (1978). Modified pull-up test. *Research Quarterly,* 49(1):80-84.

Baumgartner, T. A., East, W. B., Frye, P. A., Hensley, L. D., Knox, D. F., & Norton, C. J. (1984). Equipment improvements and additional norms for the modified pull-up test. *Research Quarterly for Exercise and Sport*, 55(1):64-68.

Baumgartner, T. A., & Jackson, A. S. (1975, 1982, 1987, 1991). *Measurement for evaluation in physical education.* Dubuque, IA: Wm. C. Brown.

Baumgartner, T. A., & Jackson, A. S. (1975). *Measurement for evaluation in physical education: Review and resource manual.* Boston: Houghton Mifflin.

Bender, J., & Shea, E. J. (1964). *Physical fitness: Tests and exercises.* New York: Ronald Press.

Beunen, G. P., Malina, R. M., Van't Hof, M. A., Simons, J., Ostyn, M., Renson, R., & Van Gerven, D. (1988). *Adolescent growth and motor performance: A longitudinal study of Belgian boys.* Champaign, IL: Human Kinetics Books.

Bosco, C., Luhtanen, P., & Komi, P.V. (1983). A simple method for measurement of mechanical power in jumping. *European Journal of Applied Physiology*, 50:273-282.

Bosco, J. S., & Gustafson, W. F. (1983). *Measurement and evaluation in physical education, fitness and sports.* Englewood Cliffs, NJ: Prentice Hall.

Bovard, J. F., Cozens, F. W., & Hagman, E. P. (1930, 1949). *Tests and measurements in physical education.* Philadelphia: W. B. Saunders.

Brooks, C. (1981). Use a speed curve to measure sprint speed. *Scholastic Coach,* 50(6):66, 68, 83-85.

Brouha, L. (1943). The step test: A simple method of measuring physical fitness for muscular work in young men. *Research Quarterly,* 14(1):31-36.

Brouha, L., & Gallagher, J. R. (1943). A functional fitness test for high school girls. *Journal of Health and Physical Education,* 14(10):517, 550.

Brouha, L., & Ball, M. V. (1952). *Canadian red cross society's school meal study.* Toronto: University of Toronto Press. In Clarke, H. H. (1976). *Application of measurement to health and physical education.* Englewood Cliffs, NJ: Prentice Hall.

Brown, T., O'Neill, J., & Proud, N. (No Date). *First state fitness test: A measurement of functional health.* Delaware: Blue Cross & Blue Shield.

Bruininks, R. H. (1978). *Bruininks-Oseretsky test of motor proficiency.* Circle Pines, MN: American Guidance Service.

Burke, E. J. (1980). Physiological considerations and suggestions for the training of elite basketball players. *Toward an Understanding of Human Performance.* Burke, E. J. (ed.). Ithaca: Mouvement Publications, pp. 293-311.

Burpee, R. H. (1931). Differentiation in physical education. *Journal of Physical Education,* 28:130-136, March.

Burpee, R. H. (1940). *Seven quickly administered tests of physical capacity.* Bureau of Publications, Columbia University.

Callan, D. E. (1968). A submaximal cardiovascular fitness test for fourth, fifth and sixth grade boys. Unpublished doctoral dissertation, Ohio State University.

Campbell, W. R., & Tucker, N. M. (1967). *An introduction to tests and measurement in physical education.* London: G. Bell & Sons.

CAHPER (1980). *CAHPER fitness performance II test manual.* Canada: Canadian Association for Health, Physical Education and Recreation.

Canadian Minister of State (1979). *Standardized test of fitness: Assessment report.*

Canadian Standardized Test of Fitness (1986). (CSTF) (3 rd ed,). Ottawa, Ontario: Fitness and Amateur Sport Canada, pp. 10-11, 17, 28-29, 34-35.

Carlson, H. C. (1945). Fatigue curve test. *Research Quarterly,* 16(3):169-175.

Carver, R. P., & Winsmann, F. R. (1970). Study of measurement and experimental design problems associated with the step test. *Journal of Sports Medicine and Physical Fitness,* 10(2):104-113.

Chelladurai, P. et al. (1977). The reactive agility test. *Perceptual and Motor Skills,* 44:1319-1324, June (Part 2).

Chrysler Fund-AAU Physical Fitness Program (1990). *1989-90 test manual.* Bloomington, IN: Author.

Clarke, H. H. (Clarke, D. H. added in 1987), (1945, 1950, 1959, 1967, 1976, 1987). *Application of measurement to health and physical education.* Englewood Cliffs, NJ: Prentice Hall.

Clarke, H. H. & Clarke, D. H. (1978). *Developmental and adapted physical education.* Englewood Cliffs, NJ: Prentice Hall.

Clarke, H. H. (1971, 1987). *Physical and motor tests in the medford boys' growth study.* Englewood Cliffs, NJ: Prentice Hall.

Clarke, H. H. & Munroe, R. A. (1970, 1975). *Oregon cable tension strength test batteries for boys and girls from fourth grade through college.* Eugene, OR: Microform Publications.

Coleman, R. J., Wilke, S., Viscio, L., O'Hanley, S., Porcari, J., Kline, G., Keller, B., Hsieh, S., Freedson, P. S., & Rippe, J. (1987). Validation of 1 mile walk test for estimating VO^2 in 20-29 year olds. *Medicine and Science in Sports and Exercise,* 19(2):Sup 29.

Collins, D. R., & Hodges, P. B. (1978). *A comprehensive guide to sports skill tests and measurement.* Springfield, IL: C. C. Thomas.

Committee of Experts on Sports Research (1988). *Eurofit: Handbook for the eurofit tests of physical fitness.* Rome.

Cooper, K. H. (1982). *The aerobics program for total well-being.* New York: M. Evans & Co.

Corbin, C. B. (1977). A ball handling test for elementary school children. *Physical Educator,* 34(1):48-50.

Corbin, C. B. & Lindsey, R. (1985). *Concepts of physical fitness with laboratories.* Dubuque, IA: Wm. C. Brown.

Corbin, C. B. & Lindsey, R. (1983). *Fitness for life* (Teacher's ed.). Glenview, IL: Scott, Foresman & Co.

Cotten, D. J. (1971). A modified step test for group cardiovascular testing. *Research Quarterly,* 42(1):91-95.

Council of Europe (1988). *Eurofit: European test of physical fitness.* Rome.

Cozens, F. W., Cubberley, H. J., & Neilson, N. P. (1937). *Achievement scales in physical education activities for secondary school girls and college women.* New York: A. S. Barnes.

Cureton, T. K. (1951). *Physical fitness of champion athletes.* Urbana: University of Illinois Press.

Dawson, B., Ackland, T. & Roberts, C. (1984). New fitness test for team and individual sports. *Sports Coach,* 8(2):42-44.

deVries, H. A. (1971). *Laboratory experiments in physiology of exercise.* Dubuque, IA: Wm. C. Brown.

Eckert, H. M. (1974). *Practical measurement of physical performance.* Philadelphia: Lea & Febiger.

Edgren, H. D. (1932). An experiment in the testing of ability and progress in basketball. *Research Quarterly,* 3(1):159-171.

Evans, E. G. (1973). Basic fitness testing of rugby football players. *British Journal of Sports Medicine,* 7:384-387.

Fairbanks, J. G. (1978). Submaximal walking test: Prediction of max VO2 and physical fitness in adult males. Unpublished doctoral dissertation, Brigham Young University.

Faulkner, R. A., Sprigings, E. J., McQuarrie, A., & Bell, R. D. (1989). A partial curl up protocol for adults based on analysis of two procedures. *Canadian Journal of Sport Sciences,* 14(3):135-141.

Field, R. (1989). Simple field tests for track and field athletes. *Modern Athlete and Coach,* 21(4):37-38.

Fitness Canada (1986). *Canadian standardized test of fitness (CSTF) operations manual.* Ottawa, Canada: Government of Canada Fitness and Amateur Sport.

Fitness Institute (1981). *The fitness institute bulletin.* 4: (Pages are not numbered), May.

Fleishman, E. A. (1964 A). *Examiner's manual for the basic fitness tests.* Englewood Cliffs, NJ: Prentice Hall.

Fleishman, E. A. (1964 B). *The structure and measurement of physical fitness.* Englewood Cliffs, NJ: Prentice Hall.

Forbes, J. M. (1950). Characteristics of flexibility in boys. Unpublished doctoral dissertation, University of Oregon.

Fox, E. L., & Mathews, D. K. (1981). *The physiological basis of physical education and athletics.* Philadelphia: W. B. Saunders.

Francis, K. & Cuipepper, M. (1988). Validation of a three minute height adjusted step test. *The Journal of Sports Medicine and Physical Fitness,* 28(3):229-233.

Franks, B. D. (1989). *YMCA youth fitness test manual.* Champaign, IL: Human Kinetics Books.

Franks, B. D. & Deutsch, H. (1973). *Evaluating performance in physical education.* New York: Academic Press.

Gallaher, J. R. & Brouha, L. (1943). A simple method of testing the physical fitness of boys. *Research Quarterly,* 14(1):23-30.

Gates, D. D., & Sheffield, R. P. (1940). Tests of change of direction as measurements of different kinds of motor ability in boys of the seventh, eighth, and ninth grades. *Research Quarterly,* 11(3):136-147.

Gauthier, R., Massicotte, D., Hermiston, R., & Macnab, R. (1983). The physical work capacity of canadian children, aged 7 to 17 in 1983. A comparison with 1968. *Canadian AHPER Journal,* 50(2):4-9.

Gauthier, R. R., Massicotte, D., & Weihren, S. J. (1988). Canadian norms of predicted maximal oxygen uptake of children aged 6-17. *Journal of Human Movement Studies,* 15:129-140.

Getchell, B. (1983). *Physical fitness: A way of life.* New York: John Wiley & Sons.

Gillian, G. M., & Marks, M. (1983). 300 yard shuttle run. *National Strength and Conditioning Association Journal,* 5(5):46.

Glencross, D. J. (1960). The measurement of muscular power; a test of leg power and a modification for general use. Microcarded doctoral dissertation, University of Western Australia).

Golding, L., Meyers, C. R., & Sinning, W. E. (eds.) (1989). *Y's way to physical fitness: The complete guide to fitness testing and instruction.* Champaign, IL: Human Kinetics Books.

Governor's Commission on Physical Fitness. (no date). *Texas physical fitness-motor ability test.* Austin, TX.

Greenberg, J. S., & Pargman, D. (1989). *Physical fitness: A wellness approach.* Englewood Cliffs, NJ: Prentice Hall.

Greipp, J. F. (1982). The assessment of shoulder flexibility. *Pennsylvania Journal of Health, Physical Education, and Recreation,* 52:19-20, Fall.

Groppell, J. L. (1989). How fit are you? Take this fitness test. *Tennis,* 24(12):97-100.

Hagerman, F. C., Starr, L. M., & Murray, T. F. (1989). Effects of a long term fitness program on professional baseball players. *The Physician and Sportsmedicine,* 17(4):101-104, 107-108, 115-119.

Harrison, P. W., & Bradbeer, P. A. (1982). Physiological fitness norms for gifted young British athletes. *Athletics Coach,* 16(1):21-25.

Harrison, P. W., & Bradbeer, P. A. (1982). Battery tests for the assessment of physiological fitness norms. *Athletics Coach*, 16(2):6-12.

Harvey, V. P. & Scott, G. D. (1970). The validity and reliability of a one-minute step test for college women. *Journal of Sportsmedicine and Physical Fitness*, 10(3):185-192.

Haskins, M. J. (1971). *Evaluation in physical education*. Dubuque, IA: Wm. C. Brown.

Hastad, D. N., & Lacy, A. C. (1989). *Measurement and evaluation in contemporary physical education*. Scottsdale, AZ: Gorsuch Scarisbrick Publishers.

(Hawaii) Aizawa, H. M. (1989). Memo to district superintendents, principals, and physical education department heads. Honolulu, HI: Department of Education.

Haydon, D. F. (1986). Physical education and fitness levels in Texas youth: A report and recommendations from the governor's commission on physical fitness. *Texas HPERD Association Journal*, 54(2):16, 55-57.

Hensley, L. D., & East, W. B. (1989). Testing and grading in the psychomotor domain. In Safrit, M.S., & Wood, T.M. (eds.). *Measurement Concepts in Physical Education and Exercise Science*. Champaign, IL: Human Kinetics Books.

Hockey, R. V. (1981). *Physical fitness: The pathway to healthful living*. St. Louis, MO: Mosby.

Hodgkins, J., & Skubic, V. (1963). Cardiovascular efficiency scores for college women in the United States. *Research Quarterly*, 34(4):454-461.

Hoeger, W. W. (1986, 1989). *Lifetime physical fitness and wellness: A personalized program*. Englewood, CO: Morton Publishing.

Hongan, J. S. ,& Hongan, J. S. (1982). Measurement bias in representing accuracy of movement on linear-positioning tasks. *Perceptual and Motor Skills*, 55(3):971-981.

Hsieh, C., & Yeung, B. W. (1986). Active neck motion measurements with a tape measure. *The Journal of Orthopaedic and Sports Physical Therapy*, 8(2):88-92.

Jackson, A., Bruya, L., Baun, W., Richardson, P., Weinberg, R., & Caton, I. (1982). Baumgartner's modified pull-up test for male and female elementary school-aged children. *Research Quarterly for Exercise and Sport*, 53(2):163-164.

Jackson, A. S., & Baumgartner, T. A. (1969). Measurement schedules of sprint running. *Research Quarterly*, 40(4):708-711.

Jackson, A. S., & Ross, R. M. (1986). *Understanding exercise for health and fitness*. Houston, TX: Mac J-R Publishing.

Jensen, C. R., & Hirst, C. C. (1980). *Measurement in physical education and athletics*. New York: Macmillan.

Jensen, C. R. (no date). Practical measurements of reaction time, response time and speed. Unpublished study, Brigham Young University.

Jette, M. (1979). A comparison between predicted VO2 max from the Astrand procedure and the Canadian home fitness test. *Canadian Journal of Applied Sport Science*, 4(3):214-218.

Johnson, B. L. (1966). A kinesthetic obstacle test. Unpublished study, Louisiana State University.

Johnson, B. L. (1966). A progressive inverted balance test. Unpublished study, Northeast Louisiana University.

Johnson, B. L. (1966). The shuffleboard control of force test. Unpublished study, Lousiana State University.

Johnson, B. L. (1971). Modification of shuffleboard and bean bag kinesthesis. Unpublished study, Lousiana State University.

Johnson, B. L. (1977). *Practical flexibility measurement with the flexomeasure*. Portland, TX: Brown & Littleman Co.

Johnson, B. L. (1978). Flexibility assessment. In Blair, S. N. (ed.). *SDAAHPER Proceedings*, pp. 63-69.

Johnson, B. L., & Fitch, J. (1968). Dynamic test of positional balance. Unpublished study, East Texas State University.

Johnson, B. L., & Leach, J. (1968). A modification of the bass test of dynamic balance. Unpublished study, East Texas State University.

Johnson, B. L., & Nelson, J. K. (1969, 1974, 1979, 1986). *Practical measurements for evaluation in physical education*. Edina, MN: Burgess.

Johnson, L. W. (1934). Objective tests for high school boys. Unpublished master's thesis, State University of Iowa.

Johnson, R., & Lavay, B. (1988). *Kansas adapted/special physical education test manual: Health-related fitness and psychomotor testing*. Topeka, KS: Kansas State Department of Education.

Kalamen, J. L. (1968). Measurement of maximum muscular power in man. Unpublished doctoral dissertation, Ohio State University. In Fox E. L., & Mathews, D. K. (1981). *The physiological basis for physical education and athletics*. Philadelphia, PA: W. B. Saunders.

Kammermann, S., Doyle, K., Valois, R. F., & Cox, S. G. (1983). *Wellness R.S.V.P.* Menlo Park, CA: Benjamin/Cummings.

Karpovich, P. V. (1965). *Physiology of muscular activity*. Philadelphia: W. B. Saunders.

Kasch, F. W. (1961). A comparison of the exercise tolerance of post-rheumatic and normal boys. *Journal of the Association for Physical and Mental Rehabilitation*, 15:35-40.

Kirby, R. F. (1971). A simple measure of agility. *Coach and Athlete*, 33(11):30-31.

Kirkendall, D. R., Gruber, J., & Johnson, R. E. (1980, 1987). *Measurement and evaluation for physical educators*. Champaign, IL: Human Kinetics Books.

Kline, G. M., Porcari, J. P., Hintermeister, R., Freedson, P. S., Ward, A., McCarron, R. F., Ross, J., & Rippe, J. M. (1987). Estimation of VO^2max from a one-mile track walk, gender, age and body weight. *Medicine and Science in Sports and Exercise*, 19(3):253-259.

Kraus, H., & Hirshland, R. P. (1954). Minimum muscular fitness tests in school children. *Research Quarterly*, 25(2):178-188.

Kurucz, R. L., Fox, E. L., & Mathews, D. K. (1969). Construction of a submaximal cardiovascular step test. *Research Quarterly*, 40(1):115-122.

Kurucz, R. L. (1967). Construction of the Ohio State University cardiovascular fitness test. Unpublished doctoral dissertation, Ohio State University.

Lamb, D. R. (1984). *Physiology of exercise: Responses and applications*. New York: Macmillan

Larson, L. A. (ed.) (1974). *Fitness, health, and work capacity: International standards for assessment*. New York: Macmillan.

Larson, L. A., & Yocom, R. D. (1951). *Measurement and evaluation in physical, health, and recreation education*. St. Louis, MO: C. V. Mosby.

Latchaw, M., & Brown, C. (1962). *The evaluation process in health education, physical education and recreation*. Englewood Cliffs, NJ: Prentice Hall.

Leger, L., & Boucher, R. (1980). An indirect continuous running multistage field test: The Universite de Montreal track test. *Canadian Journal of Applied Sport Sciences*, 5(1):77-84.

Leger, L., & Gadoury, C. (1989). Validity of the 20m shuttle run test with 1 minute stages to predict VO2max in adults. *Canadian Journal of Sports Sciences*, 14(1):21-26.

Leger, L., & Lambert, J. (1982). A maximal multistage 20m shuttle run test to predict VO2max. *European Journal of Applied Physiology*, 49:1-12.

Leger, L., Lambert, J., Goulet, A. Rowan C., & Dinelle, Y. (1984). Capacite aerobic des Quebecois de 6 a 17 ans - test navette de 20 metres avec paliers de 1 minute. *Canadian Journal of Applied Sport Sciences*, 9(2):64-68.

Leger, L., Mercier, D., Gadoury, C., & Lambert, J. (1988). The multistage 20 metre shuttle run test for aerobic fitness. *Journal of Sport Sciences*, 6:93-101.

Leighton, J. R. (1955). An instrument and technique for the measurement of range of joint motion. *Archives of Physical Medicine and Rehabilitation*, 36:571-578, September.

Lindsey, R., Jones, B. J., & Whitley, A. V. (1989). *Fitness for the health of it*. Dubuque, IA: Wm. C. Brown.

Lohman, T. G. (ed.) (1988). *Anthropometric standardization reference manual*. Champaign, IL: Human Kinetics Books.

Manahan, J. E., & Gutin, B. (1971). The one-minute step test as a measure of 600-yard run performance. *Research Quarterly*, 42(2):173-177.

Margaria, R., Aghemo, P. & Rovelli, E. (1966). Measurement of muscular power (anaerobic) in man. *Journal of Applied Physiology*, 21:1662-1664, September.

Maryland Commission on Physical Fitness (1986). *Project superfit test manual*. Baltimore, MD: Author.

Mathews, D. K. (1958, 1963, 1968, 1973, 1978). *Measurement in physical education*. Philadelphia: W. B. Saunders.

Maud, P. J., & Shultz, B. B. (1989). Norms for the Wingate anaerobic test with comparison to another similar test. *Research Quarterly for Exercise and Sport*, 60(2):144-151.

Maughan, R. J., Harmon, M., Leiper, J. B., Sale, D., & Delman, A. (1986). Endurance capacity of untrained males and females in isometric and dynamic muscular contractions. *European Journal of Applied Physiology*, 55:395-400.

McArdle, W. D., Pechar, G. S., Katch, F. I., & Magel, J. R. (1973). Percentile norms for a valid step test on college women. *Research Quarterly*, 44(4):498-500.

McArdle, W. D., Katch, F. I., Pechar, G., Jacobson, L., & Ruck, S. (1972). Reliability and interrelationships between maximal oxygen intake, physical work capacity, and step test scores in college women. *Medicine and Science in Sports*, 4(4):182-186.

McArdle, W. D., Katch, F. I. & Katch, V. L. (1986). *Exercise physiology: Energy, nutrition, and human performance*. Philadelphia: Lea & Febiger.

McCaughan, L. R. (1975). A physical ability test battery for New Zealand schools. *Canadian AHPER Journal*, 42(2):8-17, November-December. Reprinted from the *New Zealand Journal of HPER*, V. 7, November, 1974.

McCollum, R. H., & McCorkle, R. B. (1971). *Measurement and evaluation: A laboratory manual*. Boston: Allyn & Bacon.

McCloy, C. H., & Young, N. D. (1939, 1942, 1954). *Tests and measurements in health and physical education*. New York: Appleton Century Crofts.

McCristal, K. J., & Adams, W. C. (eds.) (1965). *Foundations of physical activity*. Champaign, IL: Stipes.

Mercier, D., Leger, L. A., & Lambert, J. (1983). Relative efficiency and predicted VO2 max in children. *Medicine and Science in Sports and Exercise*, 15(2):143.

Metheny, E., Bookwalter, C., Burch, G., Carpenter, A., Espenschade, A., Glassow, R., Hodgson, P., Purbeck, M., & Rodgers, E. (1945). Physical performance levels for high school girls. *Journal of Health and Physical Education*, 16(6):308-311, 354-357.

Metton, A. I. (1947). Army air forces aviation psychology program research reports. *Apparatus Tests*, Report No. 4.

Meyers, C. R. (1974). *Measurement in physical education*. New York: Ronald Press.

Meyers, C. R., & Blesh, T. E. (1962). *Measurement in physical education*. New York: Ronald Press.

Miller, D. K. (1988). *Measurement by the physical educator: Why and how*. Indianapolis, IN: Benchmark Press.

Montoye, H. J. (1978). *An introduction to measurement in physical education*. Boston: Allyn and Bacon.

Montoye, H. J. (ed.) (1970). *An introduction to measurement in physical education*, Volumes 1-5. Indianapolis, IN: Phi Epsilon Kappa.

Montoye, H. J., & Lamphier, D. E. (1977) Grip and arm strength in males and females, age 10 to 69. *Research Quarterly*, 48(1):108-120.

Mood, D. P. (1980). *Numbers in motion: A balanced approach to measurement and evaluation in physical education*. Palo Alto, CA: Mayfield.

Moore, M. L. (1978). Clinical assessment of joint motion. In Basmajian, J. V. (ed.) (1978). *Therapeutic Exercise*. Baltimore, MD: Williams & Wilkins.

Myers, B. (1986). Testing for field and multi-events athletes. *Athletic Journal,* 66:1-12, May.

Nagle, F. J., Seals, D. R., & Hanson, P. (1988). Time to fatigue during isometric exercise using different muscle masses. *International Journal of Sports Medicine,* 9(5):313-315.

National Marine Corps League (No date). *Physical fitness program: Designed for youth age 8 through high school.* Arlington, VA: Author.

Neilson, N. P., & Jensen, C. R. (1972). *Measurement and statistics in physical education.* Belmont: Wadsworth.

Nelson, F. B. (1965). The nelson reaction timer. Instruction leaflet, Lafayette, LA.

Nelson, J. K. (1968). The Nelson balance test. Unpublished study, Louisiana State University.

Nelson, J. K. (1976). Fitness testing as an educational process. *Physical Education, Sports and Sciences.* Broekhoff, J. (ed,). Eugene, OR: Microform Publications.

Nelson, J. K., & Johnson, B. L. (1979). *Measurement of physical performance: Resource guide with laboratory experiments.* Minneapolis, MN: Burgess.

New York State Education Department (1958, 1966, 1977, 1984). *The New York state physical fitness screening test.* Albany, NY.

O'Dwyer, S. (1987). AGCO: The construction of an agility coordination test. Paper presented at First World Congress of Science and Football, Liverpool.

O'Connor, M. E., & Cureton, T. K. (1945). Motor fitness tests for high school girls. *Research Quarterly,* 16(4):302-314.

O'Hanley, S., Ward, A., Zwiren, L., McCarron, R., Ross, J., & Rippe, J. M. (1987). Validation of a one mile walk test in 70-79 olds. *Medicine and Science in Sports and Exercise,* 19(2):Sup 28.

Ostyn, M., Simons, J., Beunen, G., Renson, R., & Van Gerven, D. (1980). *Somatic and motor development of Belgian secondary schoolboys: Norms and standards.* Belgium: Leuven University Press.

Paliczka, V. J., Nichols, A. K., & Boreham, C. A. G. (1987). A multistage shuttle run as a predictor of running performance and maximal oxygen uptake in adults. *British Journal of Sports Medicine,* 21(4):163-165.

Pate, R. R., Ross, J. G., Baumgartner, T. A., & Sparks, R. E. (1987). The modified pull up test. *Journal of Physical Education, Recreation and Dance,* 58(9):71, 73.

Phillips, D. A., & Hornak, J. E. (1979). *Measurement and evaluation in physical education.* New York: John Wiley.

Pollock, M. L., & Wilmore, J. H. (1990). *Exercise in health and disease.* Philadelphia: W. B. Saunders.

Pollock, M. L., Wilmore, J. H., & Fox, S. (1978). *Health and fitness through physical activity.* New York: John Wiley.

Porcari, J. P., Ebbeling, C. B., Ward, A., Freedson, P. S., & Rippe, J. M. (1989). Walking for exercise testing and training. *Sports Medicine,* 8(4):189-200.

Powell, R. L. (1984). Dynamic balance testing. *National Strength and Conditioning Association Journal,* 6(4):42D.

Prentice, W. E., & Bucher, C. A. (1988). *Fitness for college and life.* St. Louis, MO: Times Mirror/Mosby.

President's Council on Physical Fitness and Sports (1987). *USSR youth physical performance test.* Washington, DC: U.S. Government Printing Office.

President's Council on Physical Fitness & Sports (1988). *Normative data from the 1985 school population fitness survey.* Washington, D C: U.S. Government Printing Office.

President's Council on Physical Fitness and Sports (1989). *President's challenge physical fitness program: Test manual.* Washington, DC: U.S. Government Printing Office.

Pyke, J. (1986). Australian health and fitness survey 1985: The fitness, health and physical performance of school children. *The ACHPER National Journal,* 111:7-12, March.

Ramsbottom, R., Brewer, J., & Williams, C. (1988). A progressive shuttle run test to estimate maximal oxygen uptake. *British Journal of Sports Medicine,* 22(4):141-144.

Rechnitzer, R. A., Cunningham, D. A., & Howard, J. H. (1989). The self-selected walking pace test and beta blockade. *Canadian Journal of Sport Sciences,* 14(3):178-181.

Redding, D. (1989). Head strength and conditioning coach, Kansas City Chiefs. Personal correspondence, December 6.

Renson, R., Beunen, G., Van Gerven, D., Simons, J., & Ostyn, M. (1980). Description of motor ability tests and anthropometric measurements. In Ostyn, M., Simons, J., Beunen, G., Renson, R., & Van Gerven, D. (eds.) (1980). *Somatic and motor development of Belgian secondary schoolboys: Norms and standards.* Leuven: Leuven University Press.

Rhode Island Department of Education (1989). *Rhode Island State assessment program: 1988-1989 basic skills, health and physical fitness testing results.* Rhode Island.

Rockport (1989). *The Rockport guide to fitness walking.* Marlboro, MA.

Rogers, F. R. (1926). *Physical capacity tests in the administration of physical education.* New York: Columbia Teachers College.

Ross, J. G., Dotson, C. O., Gilbert, G. G., & Katz, S. J. (1985). New standards for fitness measurement (NCYFS). *Journal of Physical Education, Recreation and Dance,* 56(1):62-66.

Ross, J. G., Pate, R. R., Delpy, L. A., Gold, R., & Svilar, M. (1987). New health-related fitness norms. *Journal of Physical Education, Recreation and Dance,* 58(9):66-70.

Rowan, C., Leger, L., & Lavoie, J. (1986). Aerobic multi-stage field tests. *Coaching Review,* 9:43-46, 50, November/December.

Safrit, M. J. (1973, 1981), *Evaluation in physical education.* Englewood Cliffs, NJ: Prentice Hall.

Safrit, M. J. (1986, 1990). *Introduction to measurement in physical education and exercise science.* St. Louis, MO: C. V. Mosby.

Safrit, M. J., Hooper, M., Ehiert, A., Costa, M. G., & Patterson, P. (1988). The validity generalization of distance run tests. *Canadian Journal of Sport Sciences,* 13(4):188-196.

Safrit, M. J., & Wood, T. M. (1989). *Measurement concepts in physical education and exercise science.* Champaign, IL: Human Kinetics Books.

Sargent, D. A. (1921). The physical test of a man. *American Physical Education Review,* 26:188.

Scott, M. G. (1939). The assessment of motor ability of college women through objective tests. *Research Quarterly,* 10(3):63-83.

Scott, M. G. (1943). Motor ability tests for college women. *Research Quarterly,* 14(4):402-405.

Scott, M. G., & French, E. (1959). *Measurement and evaluation in physical education.* Dubuque, IA: Wm. C. Brown.

Seashore, H. G. (1947). The development of a beam-walking test and its use in measuring development of balance in children. *Research Quarterly.* 18(4):246-259.

Seils, L. G. (1951). The relationship between measures of physical growth and gross motor performance of primary-grade school children. *Research Quarterly,* 22(2):244-260.

Semenick, D. (1984). Anerobic testing - practical applications. *National Strength and Conditioning Association Journal,* 6(5):45, 72-73.

Shannon, C. E. (1989). Off season testing: evaluation and motivation. *Texas Coach,* 33(8):44-45.

Sharkey, B. J. (no copyright date). *Coaches guide to sport physiology.* Champaign, IL: Human Kinetics Books.

Sharkey, B. J. (1984). *Physiology of fitness.* Champaign, IL: Human Kinetics Books.

Sheehan, T. J. (1971). *An introduction to the evaluation of measurement data in physical education.* Reading, MA: Addison Wesley.

Shephard, R. J., & Lovallee, H. (eds.) (1978). *Physical fitness assessment.* Springfield, IL: C. C. Thomas.

Shephard, R. J., Cox, M., Corey, P., & Smyth, R. (1979). Some factors affecting accuracy of Canadian home fitness test scores. *Canadian Journal of Applied Sport Sciences,* 4(3):205-209.

Siconofi, S. F. et al. (1985). A simple valid step test for estimating maximal oxygen uptake in epidemiological studies. *American Journal of Epidemiology*, 121(3):382-390.

Sills, F. D., & Everett, P. W. (1953). The relationship of extreme somatotypes to performance in motor and strength tests. *Research Quarterly*, 24(2):223-228.

Simons, J., Beunen, G. P., Renson, R., Claessens, A. L., Vanreusel, B., & Lefevre, J. A. (1990). *Growth and fitness of flemish girls: The leuven growth study.* Champaign, IL: Human Kinetics Books.

Sjostrand, T. (1947). Changes in the respiratory organs of workmen at an ore smelting works. *Acta Medica Scandinavia,* 196 Suppl:687-699.

Skubic, V., & Hodgkins, J. (1963). Cardiovascular efficiency test for girls and women. *Research Quarterly,* 34(2):191-198.

Skubic, V., & Hodgkins, J. (1964). Cardiovascular efficiency test scores for junior and senior high school girls in the United States. *Research Quarterly,* 35(2):184-192.

Smithells, P. A., & Cameron, P. E. (1962). *Principles of evaluation in physical education.* New York: Harper.

South Carolina Association for Health, Physical Education, Recreation and Dance (1983). *South Carolina physical fitness test manual.* South Carolina: Author.

State Education Department (1958). *The New York State physical fitness test: For boys and girls grades 4-12.* Albany, NY: Author.

State Education Department (1977). *The New York State physical fitness screening test: For boys and girls grades 4-12.* Albany, NY: Author.

State Education Department of Public Instruction (1977). *North Carolina motor fitness battery.* Raleigh, NC: Author. In Barrow, H. M., & McGee, R. (1979). *A practical approach to measurement in physical education.* Philadelphia: Lea & Febiger.

Stephens, T., Craig, C. L., & Ferris, B. F. (1986). Physical fitness levels and participation patterns of the Canadian population. *The ACHPER National Journal,* 111:13-15, March.

Stokes, R., Moore, A. C., & Moore, C. (1986). *Fitness: The new wave.* Winston-Salem: Hunter.

Stone, W. J. (1987). *Adult fitness programs.* Glenview, IL: Scott, Foresman & Co.

(Texas) Governor's Commission on Physical Fitness (no date). *The Texas physical fitness - motor ability test: Physical fitness awards - instructions, norms - tables.* Austin, TX: Author.

Tharp, G. D., Newhouse, R. K., Uffelman, L., Thorland, W. G., & Johnson, G. O. (1985). Comparison of sprint and run times with performance on the Wingate anaerobic test. *Research Quarterly for Exercise and Sport,* 56(1):73-76.

Thomson, J. M. (1981). Prediction of anaerobic capacity: A performance test employing an optimal exercise stress. *Canadian Journal of Applied Sport Sciences,* 6(1):16-20.

Tomita, P. H. (1989). Take the flex test, *Shape,* 8(11):88-89.

Van Gelder, N., & Marks, S. (1987). *Aerobic dance exercise instructor manual.* San Diego, CA: International Dance Exercise Association (IDEA) Foundation.

Van Mechelen, W., Hlobil, H., & Kemper, H. C. (1986). Validation of two running tests as estimates of maximal aerobic power in children. *European Journal of Applied Physiology,* 55:503-506.

Verducci, F. M. (1980). *Measurement concepts in physical education.* St. Louis, MO: C. V. Mosby.

Vermont Governor's Council on Physical Fitness (1982). *School fitness test manual.* Montpelier, VT.

Virginia Department of Education (1988). *Physical fitness testing guidelines.* Richmond, VA: Author.

Viitasalo, J. T. (1988). Evaluation of explosive strength for young and adult athletes. *Research Quarterly for Exercise and Sport,* 59(1):9-13.

Wahlund, H. (1948). Determination of the physical working capacity. *Acta Medica Scandinavia,* Suppl:215.

Ward, A., Wilkie, S., O'Hanley, S., Trask, C., Kallmes, D., Kleinerman, J., Crawford, B., Freedson, P., & Rippe, J. (1987). Estimation of VO_2max in overweight females. *Medicine and Science in Sports and Exercise,* 19(2):Sup 29.

Weiss, R. A., & Phillips, M. (1954). *Administration of tests in physical education*. St. Louis, MO: C. V. Mosby.

Wells, K. F., & Dillon, E. K. (1952). The sit and reach - a test of back and leg flexibility. *Research Quarterly,* 23(1):115-118.

Westcoff, W. L. (1987). *Building strength at the YMCA*. Champaign, IL: Human Kinetics Books.

Wilkerson, G. B. (1983). Time expectations for a well-conditioned athlete in the 1 1/2 mile. *National Strength and Conditioning Association Journal,* 5(5):44-45.

Wilkie, S., O'Hanley, S., Ward, A., Zwiren, L., Freedson, P., Crawford, B., Kleinerman, J., & Rippe, J. (1987). Estimation of VO^2 max from a 1-mile walk test using recovery heart rate. *Medicine and Science in Sports and Exercise,* 19(2):Sup 28.

Willgoose, C. E. (1961). *Evaluation in health education and physical education*. New York: McGraw Hill.

Windsor, R. A., Baranowski, T., Clark, N., & Cutter, G. (1984). *Evaluation of health promotion and education programs*. Palo Alto, CA: Mayfield.

Witten, C. (1973). Construction of a submaximal cardiovascular step test for college females. *Research Quarterly,* 44(1):46-50.

Young, O. G. (1945). A study of kinesthesis in relation to selected movements. *Research Quarterly,* 16(4):277-287.

Yuhasz, M. S. (1967). The western motor ability test. In Campbell, W. R.. & Tucker, N. M. (1967). *An introduction to tests and measurement in physical education*. London: G. Bell & Sons.

Zuti, W. B., & Corbin, C. B. (1977). Physical fitness norms for college freshmen. *Research Quarterly,* 48(2):499-503.

Index